Suicide Prevention
The Global Context

Suicide Prevention
The Global Context

Edited by

Robert J. Kosky
University of Adelaide
Adelaide, South Australia, Australia

Hadi S. Eshkevari
Women's and Children's Hospital
and University of Adelaide
Adelaide, South Australia, Australia

Robert D. Goldney
University of Adelaide
Adelaide, South Australia, Australia

and

Riaz Hassan
Flinders University of South Australia
Bedford Park, South Australia, Australia

Plenum Press • New York and London

Library of Congress Cataloging-in-Publication Data

Suicide prevention : the global context / edited by Robert J. Kosky
... [et al.].
      p.   cm.
"Proceedings of the XIXth Congress of the International
Association for Suicide Prevention, held March 23-27, 1997, in
Adelaide, South Australia, Australia"--T.p. verso.
  Includes bibliographical references and index.
  ISBN 0-306-45815-2
  1. Suicide--Congresses. 2. Suicide--Prevention--Congresses.
3. Suicidal behavior--Congresses.   I. Kosky, Robert.
II. International Association for Suicide Prevention. Congress
(19th : 1997 : Adelaide, S. Aust.)
HV6545.S8423 1998
362.28'7--dc21   98-9502
                                                                    CIP

Proceedings of the XIXth Congress of the International Association for Suicide Prevention,
held March 23 – 27, 1997, in Adelaide, South Australia, Australia

ISBN 0-306-45815-2

© 1998 Plenum Press, New York
A Division of Plenum Publishing Corporation
233 Spring Street, New York, N.Y. 10013

http://www.plenum.com

10 9 8 7 6 5 4 3 2 1

Printed in the United States of America

FOREWORD

Munara, ngai wanggandi Marni na pudni
Lairma yertaamma. Wortangga, Mami na
pudni Banba-banbalyanna. Tirramangkotti
turiduri ngarkuma birra. Ngai Birko-mankolankola
Tandanyanku. Naityo Yungadalya, Yakkandulya.

First, let me welcome you all to Kaurna country. Next, I welcome you all to the Suicide Prevention Conference as an ambassador of the Adelaide people.

For thousands of years, Kaurna people have held conferences in this country with the Nukunu, the Ngadjuri, and the Narrunga. Whole groups of Aboriginal people came together and had Banba-banbalya, which was a conference, discussed their differences and new ideas. This country has always had education and the Kaurna people were the educators. I'm proud to say they led the way in conferencing and education. All of the universities in this state have Kaurna names for their Aboriginal Education Units. The University of South Australia has the Kaurna Higher Education Centre as its main campus and the *Yunguni* ("to communicate") building at the new campus, *Yunggondi,* which means "to give information," is at the Flinders University. The Adelaide University has *Woldo Yerlo,* which means "sea eagle" and is the totem of my aunt.

Aunty Glad was the matriarch of the Kaurna people in this city and also helped found Tauondi, which became the Aboriginal College. She helped introduce Aboriginal people to formalized education. Her grandson, Paul Hughes, got an honorary doctorate from the Flinders University, a Master of Arts from Harvard, a Graduate diploma from the University of South Australia, and a teaching diploma from the Western Teachers College. He ran the Aboriginal Education Unit in the South Australian Education Department, and two years ago went to Geneva to accept the Comenius Medal (UNESCO) on behalf of the Aboriginal Education Unit.

The educational involvement of the Aboriginal people continues in Adelaide today. The First National Programme for Aboriginal Education in the tertiary sector was held in this city at the Institute of Technology. Aboriginal people have always, and will continue, to be involved in education here. *Ngaityo utungandalya, yakkandallya.* Thank you my brothers, my sisters.

Mr. Lewis O'Brien, Elder of the Kaurna People of the Adelaide Plains
Opening Ceremony of the XIX Congress of the International
Association of Suicide Prevention
Bonython Hall, University of Adelaide, 22 May, 1997

PREFACE

At the XIX Congress of the International Association of Suicide Prevention over 150 papers by authors from 38 different countries were delivered. These papers included scholarly discourses, theoretical explorations, reports of research, and descriptions of developments on suicide prevention programs around the world. They confirmed the world wide concern about suicide as a public health and social problem, and illustrated the efforts being made by governments, charitable organizations, voluntary groups, clinicians, researchers, care-givers and groups of survivors and the families of those who have suicided. Members of the organizing committee of the Congress were amazed at the numbers and variety of people with interests in this subject.

It is not possible to contain within the printed pages of this book the excitement and stimulation that the Congress provided. People who had worked in the field for 50 years met with and talked to people who, against great odds and taboos were carrying a message for the first time to their governments about suicide as a public health problem. Some clinicians came to Adelaide from countries where the person who suicides and their family are punished as criminals, or where there are heavy religious sanctions on the act of suicide. For those delegates who came from modern, Western, and increasingly secular countries, these attitudes seem strange, but they should be reminded that only recently was suicide decriminalised in Britain, and that one of the founders of this organization, Erwin Stengel, played a leading part in that achievement. The coming together of so many people from so many different backgrounds and cultural diversities was an astonishing experience for many delegates.

We have selected some papers for publication that we hope will give a flavour of this diversity as well as informaton on the work that is currently being done around the world. The main speakers are represented, but we have also published papers from others we felt would provide the reader with insight into activities in parts of the world where literature on suicide is scarce. Consequently the papers are not only included for their scientific merit, but also because some represent brave experiments and courageous activities in suicide prevention. We believe that the publication of these interesting papers will remind the reader that attitudes toward suicide and attempted suicide differ from community to community, and that we cannot take contemporary Western attitudes in the area for granted when we are thinking about the problem of suicide in other parts of the world.

We have also included abstracts of all papers that were presented at the conference. We have done this because we believe these abstracts will give the reader access to what is being done in many places in the world and to the people who are working there. We hope that this will provide a network of communication among the researchers and clinicians in the suicide area throughout the world.

We have included tributes to two individuals who have made an outstanding contributions to suicide research and prevention: Norman Farberow & Erwin Stengel. The XIX Congress in Adelaide was held on the one-hundredth anniversary of the publication of Emile Durkheim's Le Suicide, and to celebrate this event, the Scientific Committee established a Durkheim Oration, which is contained in this book.

For the first time since the IASP was founded in 1961, this Congress, provided a truly global perspective for suicide prevention. This book reflects this increasingly wide-ranging look at suicide and suicide prevention.

The Editors would like to thank Mrs. Gail Weaver and Mrs. Mary Prisk for their help and secretarial assistance with the preparation of this book.

The Editors

CONTENTS

Attempted Suicide

Prevention

OPENING CEREMONY OF THE 19TH CONFERENCE OF THE INTERNATIONAL ASSOCIATION FOR SUICIDE PREVENTION MARCH 22nd–27th 1997

Opening Address from the South Australian Minister of Health

The Honorable Doctor Michael Armitage, and MP

In the presence of the Chancellor of the University of Adelaide and the
    Ambassador of the Kaurna People
Bonython Hall
University of Adelaide
22 May, 1997

THE HONORABLE DOCTOR MICHAEL ARMITAGE

Mr Chancellor of the University of Adelaide, Mr. Lewis O'Brien, Elder of the Kaurna People, Professor Jean-Pierre Soubrier, President of the International Association for Suicide Prevention, Dr. David Clark, Professor Riaz Hassan, Professor Oivind Ekeberg, Mr. Alan Staines, Dr. Graham Martin, Professor Bob Goldney as the Convenor, delegates and distinguished guests. Thank you very much for inviting me to perform the opening ceremony of the 19th Congress of the International Association for Suicide Prevention.

I take the opportunity particularly to welcome interstate and the many international delegates to South Australia. On behalf of the government I sincerely hope that you will enjoy our hospitality, our good food and the lifestyle for which Adelaide is justly famed. I understand some of you have already enjoyed a good dose of our wines last night!

Suicide is obviously a blight on society which can affect any age group and can result in the loss of loved ones, partners, children, family and friends. In 1995 2,367 Australians committed suicide. Four times as many males approximately as females. This figure increased by 109 from the previous year. The questions "Why do people commit suicide" and "What can be done to prevent suicide" are complex issues that confront not only us here in South Australia, but also the rest of Australia and the world, as is evidenced by the broad international interest in this congress.

While the community ideally would like to see a swift and summary resolution of the issues, it is a fact that the very complexity of the issues involved demand a great deal of research and candid discussion to ensure that the strategies developed are effective and importantly that they achieve the desired outcome. Hence the formation of the International Association for Suicide Prevention (IASP)

In 1960, the late Professor Erwin Ringel founded the I.A.S.P. in Austria and during the ensuing 37 years professionals and volunteers from more than 50 different countries have joined this organisation, indicating a world-wide desire to address, to confront, and hopefully to conquer the challenge issued to society by suicide. The aims of the I.A.S.P. are to provide a common platform for the interchange of experience and ideas that will facilitate the wider dissemination of effective suicide prevention strategies to professional groups and the general public, and also to arrange specialised training in the area of suicide prevention. The aim as well is to provide a forum to encourage joint international research programmes. These aims are all certainly met in your congress.

The I.A.S.P. congress convenes every two years and in hosting this year's congress South Australia will hear from world leaders from more than 30 countries in the field of suicide prevention. Throughout the ensuing week your myriad of workshops will be a stimulating environment for professionals and volunteers alike and will provide an opportunity to learn more about suicide prevention and future research planning and clinical collaboration.

No doubt you will be offered insights into suicide within various socio-economic groups, insights into primary care issues, insights into prevention and intervention, into legislation and issues surrounding euthanasia and assisted suicide. All challenging issues.

Currently South Australia disperses more than three and a quarter million dollars on projects and services for the prevention or response to suicide or self harm each year. These projects include the Centalink Youth Suicide Prevention Project, Keep Yourself Alive, a project for general practitioners providing literature and audio visual material to doctors dealing with prevention of youth suicide, a Mood Disorders Unit, an early detection of emotional disorders project, and a health promotion in country schools project. Importantly, it also features an Aboriginal primary health care project. Whilst this is not an exhaustive list, the government is anxious to learn what more can be done to minimise the devastating impact on our society caused by this behaviour.

One of the initiatives of this government under the realignment of Mental Health Services has been the establishment of mobile Mental Health Service teams to deal with many people in need in a community setting within metropolitan and our far flung rural communities. Members of these teams and other mental health workers in the State will see your congress as an opportunity to review new strategies to help them meet the challenge of the suicide phenomenon. I believe that this is possibly the most important role of your international meeting: the flow-on effects to the workers in South Australia.

As Minister I thank you all for helping to provide this focus. I am sure everyone will benefit. It gives me great pleasure to declare open the 19th I.A.S.P. Congress entitled "Suicide Prevention - The Global Context" and to wish all delegates well in your deliberations, which hopefully will lead to a measurable reduction in the problem which is the focus of your worthy association. Thank you very much.

SUICIDE PREVENTION AS A MISSION

Jean-Pierre Soubrier

25 rue de la Faisanderie, Paris 75116, France
President Opening Lecture—XIX Congress of the International
Association for Suicide Prevention
March 23–27, 1997, Adelaide

At the last conference in 1995 in Venice, we had a special panel in memory of the founder of the IASP, Erwin Ringel, where I said that suicide prevention was our mission (1). So today I choose to present a complete reflection on this theme.

A mission can only be accomplished if one is not alone. I could refer to the history of religions or the discovery of continents. But the best example is taken from Chad Varah who wrote in 1970: *"Whenever I hear myself referred to as the Founder of the Samaritans, I want to protest: I did not found them — I did not even find most of them. The first of them found me, and without them the Samaritans would not exist (2).*

Suicide prevention achieved its developments by the constitution of teams: The opening of the Los Angeles Suicide Prevention Centre, the Suicide Prevention Centre in Vienna, polyprofessional staff in general, hospitals and of course telephone services. I have found my interest in suicidology as a resident at the bedside of patients just being resuscitated from an overdose of drugs or toxics, most of them helpless.

Suicide prevention must be understood as a collective mission with the main goal of preserving the life of people in despair with an ambiguous death-wish. The notion of solidarity has been again fairly well expressed by Chad Varah when he explained why he chose the name Samaritans: *"Because it implies a collection of people, in each of whom the purpose of the fellowship is to be fulfilled." (2).* However a dedicated group cannot speak only for itself and most integrate into society in order to break through resistances built or consolidated by taboos.

Did Captain Cook know after discovering Australia that bringing back to Europe and the Western hemisphere the notion of the sacred taboo, this some day would lead to a major discussion on suicide? This question has been studied in depth by Norman Farberow along with Edwin Shneidman in 1965. (3).

We had to wait nearly two centuries to perceive the taboo, originally understood as a sacred, religious, pagan, polynesian notion and thus is specific of a primitive ethnic group, which was indeed to be found in the contemporary western societies such as ours with well-structured religions and well-established ethics.

Taboos are ancient prohibitions directed against the deepest desires and wishes of human beings. A number of authors describe a taboo as a compromise between two conflictual tendencies: the need to obey the law and the persistant desire to transgress it.

Sigmud Freud taught us that the taboo of the dead is not only a sign of mourning but a mark of hostility towards the dead person.

I have recently been asked to see a 33 year old, West African woman. An intelligent attorney, she has been rescued from a severe suicide attempt, leaving an aggressive note filled with anger, explaining the reasons for her act. This was directed against her family and mainly towards her father, the apparent "significant other" and an important personality of her country. She had a double culture, European and African. Using classic therapeutics in crisis intervention, I suggested a meeting with members of her family. I was told that the father could not phone his daughter. Her sister said: *"Doctor, in my country, we do not talk to suicidal persons. In case of death by suicide, relatives do not attend the funeral. Sometimes they are even buried in another region or country."*

An important ambiguity is created by the resistance or opposition between intellectual evolution and tradition, which makes the therapeutic approach difficult, even though we have now efficient medications. To quote Farberow (4): *"Suicide is still a taboo topic, one that stigmatizes not only the suicidal victim but the survivors as well."*

The mission in suicide prevention includes the struggle against taboos. However, we recently found that this may be dangerous and confirms that finally a taboo could protect the individual as Farberow said: *"To protect against and, at the same time, to preserve the imputed spiritual force."* (5)

Meaning that primitive taboos, characterized by contact prohibitions and various every day life acts, were meant to protect and preserve, however, frustrating that protection might be.

Discussing taboo suicide may have unexpected results such as suicide promotion, a dramatic event.

Halbwachs (6), a French sociologist who continued Durkheim's work (7), said in 1930: *"Reasons for suicide are in ourselves as well as out of ourselves."* It reminds me also of what I declared in a report for WHO in 1974 in *"Modern Aspects of and Trends in Self-Destructive Behaviour"*: *".....modern society has provided additional means for the individual to proceed with the suicidal act, i.e. to mobilize his death wish and to permit a change in the balance between his primitive instincts of Eros and Thanatos."* (8)

Charles Darwin gave us an important message to preserve and observe human nature. "Struggle for life" could be the credo for those concerned with suicide prevention. We have learned that Charles Darwin was depressive, hypochondriac but not suicidal, and had had many panic attacks. (9). Apparently, in his "Theories on the Origin of Species" he understood the necessity of aggressivity between living creatures, but he was against suicide considered as an egoistic vision of oneself. Society is in danger if at least part of this taboo remains or if society is not homogeneous. (10)

What would Darwin say today when informed of the suicide promotion movement promoting assisted suicide for mental patients and even in cases of manic-depression psychosis? This is a strong obstruction to preservation of human life and to scientific research. It is an attack against suicide prevention, a task which, as we all know here today, is so difficult to conduct.

I do believe that Dr Cade, the Australian scientist, known for his major work on lithium salts for dysthymic disorders, would not be in favour of this deadly movement.

Finally, as above, I shall raise the question:

- Have we reached the limits of our mission in suicide prevention?
- Should we react or not?

THE MISSION OF IASP

In 1995 in Venice, I addressed Professor Ringel in these words: *Đear Honorary President, we have heard your message, we have accepted your mission...the mission will continue, however difficult........(1).* IASP was created for suicide prevention whatever the settings, countries, races. It led to the opening of suicide prevention centers, telephone services...and the emergence of research in the study of self-destructive behaviours, which then became known as Suicidology.

In the early 70's Ringel said that we should also focus on crisis intervention. This is why the Association Journal was named CRISIS. Crisis intervention means also emergency psychiatry and rescue of any psychiatric distress, including study of the many self-destructive behaviours. The suicide crisis can take many forms. I wish in 1995 that IASP was also present in the horrible necessity of emergency humanitarian assistance.

We have found out this included prevention of suicide among helpers, professional or not, dedicated to this mission. The future of IASP will have to be more concerned with various contemporary forms of human distress and despair. However interesting suicidiology is, we have to face the development of suicide promotion. That means suicidology has its limits, or suicide prevention is limited or obstructed by suicidology. We may say that some (so-called) suicidologists are ambivalent, divided by two different views, one towards death, the other towards life. Here we immediately think of Janus with his two different and opposite faces.

Unfortunately that means the new mission of IASP will be to oppose the suicide promotion movement even within our association.

In response to a paper published in CRISIS in 1994 on *"Assisted Suicide among Psychiatric Patients in the Netherlands,"* by Kerkhof. I had wished CRISIS to present an Editorial Comment with this paragraph which unfortunately was omitted for no reasons by the Editors: *"But the Executive Board of IASP do not hesitate to declare that IASP is an organization that should deal with suicide prevention and not with suicide promotion."* (11).

In France, in 1987, we started to act by creating a law against provocation to suicide. I said some time ago that book control is as urgent as gun control.

We initiated in 1996, in collaboration with the Ludeck Foundation and in two successive series of lectures, an educational program on suicide prevention for psychiatrists and reached 2400 of them (12). Most of them realized that suicidology has its own clinical language, different but not opposed to the traditional psychiatric clinical nosology.

We started within IASP a world-wide investigation on suicide that will be presented during the meeting, and I am pleased to have obtained a good feed-back for 34 national representatives of the association. Our goal is to define guidelines which can be used by physicians and to obtain more precise statistical data. We must help each other within IASP to obtain accurate statistical data, one more step towards understanding and preventing suicide all over the world. As Professor Debout, national representative for France, said: *"We must not be afraid of suicide rates."*

The poster of the National Day for Suicide Prevention held in Paris at the Congress Hall last February 1997, depicted two hands reaching for each other.

Let's show solidarity, openness: and awareness.

REFERENCES

JP Soubrier, *Souvenirs to remember and meditate,* Erwin Ringel. Memorial Session, 18th
IASP Congress, Venice, 1995.

C Varah, *The Samaritans in the 70's,* Constable, London, 1977.

E Shneidman, *Suicide, in Taboo Topics,* Ed. N. Farberow, Atherton Press, New York, 1966, p.42.

G Evans, N Farberow, *The Encyclopedia of Suicide,* Face on File, New York, 1988.

N Fareberow, Taboo Topics, Atherton Press, New York, 1966, p.8.

M. Halbwachs, *Les Causes du Suicide,* Paris, Alcan, 1930.

E. Durkheim, *Le Suicide,* Paris, Alcan, 1930.

JP Soubrier, *Modern Aspects of and Trends in Self-Destructive Behaviour,* in: *Suicide and Attempted Suicide in Young People,* published by World Health Association, Copenhagen, 1974.

TJ Barloon, R Noyes, *Charles Darwin and Panic Disorder,* in JAMA, Jan. 8, 1997, Vol, 277, No.2, p.138.

C Darwin, *On the Origin of Species,* London, 1859.

A Kerkhof, D Clark, *Editorial Independence,* CRISIS, 17/1, Hogrefe Huber Publishers, 1996.

12. JP Soubrier, *International Perspectives 1996—Reflections on Suicidology for 1997,* in Review of Suicidology, Ed R. Maris, M Silverman, S Canetto, chapter 11, p.271–279, Guildford Press, New York, 1977.

3

DURKHEIM ORATION

Durkheim and Australian Suicidology

Riaz Hassan

Flinders University
GPO Box 2100, Adelaide 5001 Australia

Let me begin by thanking the Organising Committee of the Congress for inviting me to deliver the Durkheim Oration and the Australian Sociological Association for supporting it. I feel greatly honoured by this invitation. I have been a student of Emile Durkheim's sociology for over thirty years and I am very pleased that the timing of this congress coincides with the hundredth anniversary of Durkheim's seminal publication, "Suicide: A Study in Sociology" (1897, 1966).

Durkheim's book was a landmark publication for two important reasons. Firstly, it firmly established sociology as an academic discipline in the Academy. Secondly, it was instrumental in initiating the scientific study of suicidal behaviour. Before the publication of Durkheim's book the social meaning and perception of suicide was largely shaped by religion and it was regarded as a moral problem. Durkheim's book was the first systematic sociological study which pierced through the moral indignation and philosophical defences surrounding suicide, thus pioneering systematic, scientific research on the subject. In this respect it represented a paradigm shift in the study of suicide.

Following the publication of Durkheim's book, suicide came to be regarded by many as a social problem which was fundamentally a product of the nature of the relationship between the individual and society. In the lexicon of Durkheim's theory, the relative degree of disturbance of regulation; isolation and oppression of individuals in society were among the primary causes of the suicide rates found in different counties.

By using official statistics on suicide from various European countries, including his native France, he demonstrated that the rate of suicide in a society was associated with the degree of social integration and not with race, heredity, cosmic or psychological factors. He viewed suicide as a product of the increasingly alienated and egoistic nature of the social milieu.

Durkheim brought together a number of sociological insights to identify the areas and growing points of social dissolution in contemporary societies, putting these within a general theoretical framework which stated that: suicide varies inversely with the degree

Suicide Prevention, edited by Kosky *et al.*
Plenum Press, New York, 1998

of social integration of the group of which the individual forms a part. Durkheim's concept of integration, as a general rule, refers to the strength of the individual's ties to society and the stability of social relations within that society.

While recognising the significance of a wide variety of psychological causes at the individual level such as apathy, melancholy, anger and weariness, Durkheim was emphatic that individual explanations cannot explain the variations in and within the overall suicide rates which he regarded as the proper object of sociological analysis. His approach was determined by his conceptualisation of suicide, which he defined as "all cases of deaths resulting directly or indirectly from a positive or negative act of the victim himself which he knows will produce this result." In short, the defining feature of suicide is the conscious renunciation of existence. The focus of sociological analysis was to determine the cause of this phenomenon and once causes were known, one could then deduce from them the nature of the effects, namely individual suicides.

In other words the starting point for Durkheim was in fact a causal social theory. He sought to verify this theory by establishing that suicide rates vary as a function of several social environments, such as religious, family, political society, or professional group. For him, individual suicide merely represented an echo of the moral state of society.

He believed in the existence of a 'collective force' which exerted pressure on individual members of society and determined the rate of voluntary deaths. Each social group possessed a 'collective inclination' for the act of suicide which became the source of all individual inclinations. These ideas were the underlying rationale of his now famous typology of suicide.

Durkheim's theory of suicide in summary amounts to this: that under adverse social conditions, when personal social context fails to provide the requisite sources of attachment and/or regulation at the appropriate level of intensity, then psychological or moral health is impaired, and a certain number of vulnerable individuals respond by committing suicide.

The major contribution of Durkheim's study was that it provided a new perspective from which to look at and understand suicide. Suicide was not an irredeemable moral crime or the result of unpredictable madness but a fact of society. It had social causes that were subject to discernible sociological laws, which in turn could be identified, discussed and analysed scientifically and rationally. Although the final structure of Durkheim's theory is somewhat confusing and at times unsystematic and inconsistent, his analysis of data is particularly illuminating and perceptive. The fundamental preoccupation of Durkheim throughout his work is the relationship between the individual and society. Durkheim took the act of suicide, which was by definition an individual action, and demonstrated the sociological aspect of it.

Since the publication of Durkheim's book exactly a century ago, numerous sociological studies have been published, most of which clearly reveal the impact of his pioneering study. Some of these studies have added significantly to the objectives which Durkheim had charted himself. Many studies have been concerned with operationalising concepts such as integration, others with explaining the causes of suicide in modern societies. Several studies have taken up the task of examining and refining Durkheim's typology of suicide. Some have criticised Durkheim's epistemological assumptions. They have argued that official statistics are unreliable because of the potential for concealment, misrepresentation and under-counting of suicides which may prevent the discovery of true social correlates. Some have suggested that in order to understand the social and cultural meanings and patterns of suicide it is necessary to start with intensive observations, descriptions and analyses of individual cases of suicide.

The sociological approach expounded by Durkheim has become a focus of two divergent developments. On the one hand, the changing patterns of suicidal behaviour in modern societies have led to a renewed interest in identifying the social correlates of suicide. This is evident in the papers which have appeared in the specialist journals on suicidology such as 'Crisis,' 'Archives of Suicide Research,' and 'Suicide and Life Threatening Behaviour,' over the past twenty years.

This interest has also been aided by cross-cultural sociological studies of suicide. These studies have become possible as a result of the availability of statistical data which has been produced through the application of uniform conceptual and technical standards under the aegis of the World Health Organisation and the United Nations. New advanced computing facilities and sophisticated statistical software have greatly facilitated the analysis of large sets of suicide data, thus enabling us to test sociological theories and hypotheses inspired by Durkheim's work.

Durkheim's work sought to establish the significance of the social factors in human behaviour. His preoccupation with social factors probably prevented him from fully recognising the role of psychological factors in suicide. We know from recent studies that biological factors may also play a critical role in some suicidal behaviour. It would probably be unfair, however, to criticise Durkheim on these accounts, as scientific research in biology, especially in genetics and human physiology, was not developed when Durkheim was writing on suicide.

My reading of Durkheim is that by highlighting the role of social factors he was not seeking to minimise the possible role of psycho-physiological factors in suicide. He was however sure that suicide was not a disease. He would have probably agreed with Edwin Schneidman that it was a malaise caused by social, cultural, psychological and economic factors.

Let me now turn to the issue of the impact of Durkheim on Australian suicidology .

While the scientific study of suicide in Australia is still developing, Australian studies on suicide display high scientific standards. In the Australasian region the state of Australian suicidology would rank very highly. One useful perspective from which to assess the impact of Durkheim's work on Australian suicidology is through its periodization.

In the first half of this century, most of the scientific studies were concerned with the statistical trends in suicidal behaviour. Most of these studies took a distinctly sociological approach and many of the findings were similar to those suggested by Durkheim. For example, the findings revealed a fall in the suicide rate during the two world wars, and a rise in the 1930's depression and during times of high unemployment and bankruptcy.

After the 1950's the studies of suicide have become more focussed and problem oriented. A number of important studies in the 1960's and 1970's examined the link between mental illness and suicide and found significant relationships between suicidal behaviour and depression, alcoholism and other mental illnesses.

With the advent of massive European migration to Australia in the post world war II period, a number of studies concentrated on the relationship between suicide and migration. These studies found significant differences in suicide rates and methods among various ethnic groups. Immigrants in general had significantly higher suicide rates than Australian born and this difference was attributed to disruption of established social ties and the prevalence and high incidence of mental illness and alcoholism among immigrants. The difference among the immigrant groups was generally found to be related to family cohesion, sponsorship of the immigrants, size of the group, cultural affinity with the host society, and downward occupational mobility.

In this period, studies also explored the spatial distribution of suicide as Australian cities began to grow rapidly under the impact of immigration. Inner cities were found to have higher suicide rates because of the concentration of more vulnerable groups in these areas. Another important problem addressed in some studies was the role of availability of sedatives and changes in the pharmaceutical provisions of the National Health Act and Suicide.

In the 1980's and 1990's the focus of suicide studies expanded to include topics such as: Are Australian youth becoming more suicidal?, prediction of suicide, management of suicidal behaviour, aboriginal suicide, methods of suicide, role of the media, and temporal variation in suicide. In these studies, two main foci appear to predict suicide and social factors in suicide. The psychiatric studies about the aetiology of suicidal behaviour have found significant and predictable relationships between depression, alcoholism, physical and mental illnesses. One general conclusion which seems to be drawn from this relationship is that suicide is symptomatic of psychiatric illness rather than anti-social behaviour.

This relationship has been questioned on methodological as well as on theoretical grounds in some studies which have emphasised the multi-faceted causality of suicide. The dominant view in Australian psychiatry is that while there is a causal link between pre-existing mental illness and suicide, there is also a recognition that there are many contributory factors which may interact with each other to form a complex matrix of biological, social and psychological causes.

Recent sociological studies have made important contributions to Australian suicidology by focusing on social factors in suicide which in particular highlight the role of economic cycles, the media, women's emancipation, social dependency, oppression and temporal variations in the occurrence of suicide.

In the course of preparing this presentation I reviewed 51 Australian studies of suicide which have appeared in national and international scientific journals over the past one hundred years. These studies varied in their objectives, scope, and underlying assumptions. Most of the studies, particularly those which have appeared since 1950, have been conducted by psychiatrists and physicians. They have appeared mostly in the medical journals. Some of the studies view suicide as a form of psychiatric illness but others acknowledge the role of social and environmental factors in suicide and clearly echo Durkheim' conceptualisation and analysis of suicide.

I asked myself the question, whether this would have been the case if the authors had not been informed by Durkheim's seminal work. I leave the final assessment of this question to you all. It is clear from these papers that Durkheim's work has become an integral part of the scientific discourse in Australian suicidology.

I think the essence of Durkheim's message is that some social groups are more vulnerable than others in terms of hopelessness, loneliness, alienation and anomie. In order to develop effective suicide prevention policies in Australia we will need to develop programs which address these issues and seek to reduce the problems of chronic hopelessness, alienation and loneliness which characterise more vulnerable groups such as found among youth and indigenous Australians.

If, through the incorporation of Durkheim's theoretical insight, suicide prevention programs can effect some reduction in the incidence of suicide, now the leading cause of death among young Australians, it would clearly signify the positive impact of Durkheim's work on Australian suicidology. For this we will be indebted to Durkheim's contributions, which we have chosen to celebrate as part of this World Congress.

REFERENCES

Durkheim, Emile [1897] (1966). *Suicide: A Study in Sociology*. Spaulding, John A. (trans) With an Introduction by George Simpson (Ed.). New York: Free Press.

Lukes, S. (1975). *Emile Durkheim, His Life and Work: A Historical and Critical Study*. Harmondsworth: Penguin Books.

Hassan, Riaz (1995). *Suicide Explained: The Australian Experience*. Melbourne: Melbourne University Press.

Schneidmann, E. S. (1985). *Definition of Suicide*. New York: John Wiley & Sons.

Evans, Glen. & Norman L. Farberow (1988). *Encyclopedia of Suicide*. New York, Oxford: Facts On File.

4

NORMAN FARBEROW

A Legend in Suicide Prevention

Robert D. Goldney

Department of Psychiatry
University of Adelaide
The Adelaide Clinic
33 Park Terrace
Gilberton, 5081

The definitive biography of Norman Farberow remains to be written, but when it is, it will chronicle a major contribution to suicide prevention covering half a century. For the present, a bare outline of his career must suffice here.

Norman Farberow was born in Pittsburgh, Pennsylvania and graduated from the University of Pittsburgh with a Bachelor of Arts degree in psychology in 1938. He completed his Master of Science degree in psychology in 1940.

During the second World War between 1941 and 1945 Norman Farberow saw service as a Captain in the United States Air Force. His assignment was as an intelligence officer with a medium bomber group in the European theatre of operations. After the cessation of hostilities he commenced work with the Veteran's Administration Graduate program with the University of California at Los Angeles and pursued research in suicidal behaviour for his PhD. It was there that he first co-operated with Ed Shneidman and in fact he used Shneidman's Make a Picture Story Test as one of the personality tests in his doctoral dissertation. That dissertation entitled "Personality patterns of suicidal mental hospital patients" was published in 1950 in the Genetic Psychology Monographs series.

It is pertinent to quote the initial few words of the "Statement of the Problem" in Norman Farberow's thesis. He wrote: "The primary purpose of this study is to describe, by means of certain psychological tests, various personality characteristics of patients in a mental hospital who have been classified as suicidal. The secondary purpose is to determine whether such patients are different, not only from other patients who have not been so judged, but also from each other, when they are divided in terms of major, local categories, such as Attempts and Threats, or Serious and Non-Serious." This is a succinct statement of a problem with which we are still grappling fifty years later.

Suicide Prevention, edited by Kosky *et al.*
Plenum Press, New York, 1998

Following the completion of his doctorate, Farberow moved to an out-patient mental hygiene clinic, and with Ed Shneidman began collaborative work on the status of suicide in a major American city, Los Angeles. Indeed, that work led to the development of the Los Angeles Suicide Prevention Centre with Ed Shneidman, Bob Litman, Micky Heilig, Michael Peck and others.

The need to establish a Suicide Prevention Centre arose from work which Farberow and Shneidman had done examining the clinical management of those who had attempted suicide. It appeared to them that the psychological problems, which had led to the suicidal behaviour, were not being addressed.

The Centre began to receive calls from those who were suicidal but who had not yet carried out their actions. That gave a window of opportunity for the prevention of suicide and attempted suicide. The operation of the Centre demonstrated that a community based agency could provide a useful emergency service. It also demonstrated that professionals, and other community members, such as teachers, police and probation officers, coroners and volunteers, could participate.

Farberow's work and that of his colleagues was recognised in 1961 when he was awarded a "Resolution of Commendation" by the Los Angeles City Council for his outstanding accomplishments with the Los Angeles Suicide Prevention Centre.

Besides their clinical work, Farberow and Schneidman produced pioneering research studies into suicidal behaviour. It was an era when it was still taboo to speak openly about suicide, and it is of interest that their Central Research Unit was set up in the Veterans Administration, ostensibly for the "Study of Unpredicted Deaths." Farberow is open in acknowledging that this was a pragmatic way to study suicidal behaviour. During those early years the psychological autopsy was developed, a methodology which has been utilised for suicide studies in many different countries.

In 1961, in collaboration with Edwin Shneidman, Farberow wrote the seminal book, "The Cry for Help." This had a profound impact upon clinicians and researchers. "The Cry for Help" was a distillation of the work of Farberow and a number of his colleagues. Even then they were actuely aware of the dilemma that sometimes arises between researchers and clinicians in the area of suicidal behaviour. He quoted of Ruth Tolman, to whom the book was dedicated, who noted that there were problems between the "pure" and "applied" scientist; the "theoretician" and the "professional practitioner." These words were prescient, and they apply now just as they did forty years earlier. An organisation such as the International Association for Suicide Prevention can provide an umbrella under which clinicians, researchers and volunteers and those from other disciplines, can meet and share their experience and wisdom. An important part of the book, "Cry for Help" was the extensive bibliography on suicide, a bibliography which extended from 1897, the year of Durkheim's pioneering work, to 1957.

It is interesting that the most prominent of the founding fathers of the I.A.S.P., Erwin Ringel, Erwin Stengel, and Norman Farberow, published some of their most significant work within a few years of each other, in the early 1950's. Ringel's classic work on "Practical Suicide Prevention" was published in 1951 in Vienna, and Stengel's influencial article on suicide was publlished in a volume on Recent Progress in Psychiatry in 1950.

Farberow's work in the last thirty five years has covered many aspects of suicidal behaviour. Titles of some of his papers include "Suicide and the police officer"; "Suicide and the aged"; "Suicide among schizophrenic mental hospital patients"; "The nurses role in the prevention of suicide"; "Suicide among general medical and surgical hospital patients with malignant neoplasms"; "Suicide prevention telephone services"; and many others in a wide ranging field.

In the last few years, he has focused more on those who have been bereaved through suicide. His research and clinical expertise in this hitherto neglected, but important, area has been recognised by the International Association for Suicide Prevention with the establishment of the Farberow Award for those who have contributed significantly in the area of bereavement after suicide.

In addition to the above research, he has also pursued a lifelong interest in suicide in art and has observed representations of suicide in the visual arts, over the centuries, has changed along with the changing attitude of society to suicide. He has noted that the Greek artists portrayed suicide as acceptable; the Romans were more legalistic in their views; and in the Dark Ages there was a sinful, moralistic portrayal of suicide. In more recent centuries, changes have also been documented, until in our present century the focus on ambivalence and the cry for help has been apparent. Farberow has generously donated his art collection to the American Association of Suicidology.

One of Norman Farberow's most important achievements has been his role in the establishment of the International Association for Suicide Prevention. During a sabbatical year in Vienna in 1961, Farberow, with Erwin Ringel, developed the constitution of the International Association for Suicide Prevention. Farberow has remarked on the compromises needed to blend the American as opposed to European concepts of how an international organisation should be set up, and it is testimony to his work that the Association has stood the test of time. There are now National Representatives from over 50 different countries and there have been 19 bi-annual conferences over the last 37 years.

Farberow's contributions to the field of suicidal behaviour have probably obscured the fact that he has also contributed in other areas of mental health. For example, his contribution to the management of mental health problems following major disasters has been considerable.

Farberow has published 13 books, he has contributed over 50 book chapters, and he has also written over a hundred other articles in the international literature. He has been a consultant and participant on ten films dealing with suicide and suicide prevention, and he has been a consulting Editor for at least a dozen journals. Even now, fifty years on from when he commenced his research into suicidal behaviour, he is still contributing to the international literature with innovative ideas and rigorous research projects.

In common with many others when I met Farberow, I found him a gentle and unassuming man, although he had a firm sense of purpose. In fact, it is easy to see why he is a superb therapist, as he is able to win over the friendship and trust of all who come into contact with him. I was delighted to have spent time with him and to have discussed issues of suicidal behaviour with him.

In short, Farberow has contributed significantly to suicide prevention in a number of ways. He has been a pioneer in introducing rigorous scientific research projects in this most challenging field; he was a co-founder of the first professionally organised suicide prevention centre in the United States; he has investigated the impact of indirect self-destructive acts in our lives; he has encouraged cross-cultural research using the psychological autopsy methodology; he has firmly focused attention on the needs of those who have been bereaved through suicide; and he was instrumental in the establishment of the International Association for Suicide Prevention. He has also provided wisdom and support to countless researchers, clinicians, volunteers and survivors through his work, not only nationally in the United States, but also in many other countries through the International Association for Suicide Prevention. All those who have had the privilege of contact with him would share the view that he is truly a legend in suicide prevention.

REFERENCES

Farberow, N. L. (1997) My legacy in suicide: professional and personal. Manuscript prepared for presentation at A.A.S. meeting in memphis.

Farberow, N. L. (1950) Personality patterns of suicidal mental hospital patients. Genetic Psychology Monographs, 42: 3–79.

Farberow, N. L. And Shneidman E. S. (1961) The Cry for Help. McGraw-Hill Book Company Inc., New York.

5

2. MEET THE LEGEND

Who Is the Norman L. Farberow?

Onja T. Grad

Centre for Mental Health
University Psychiatric Hospital
Zaloska 29, 1000 Ljubljana, Slovenia.

What is a legend? Webster's dictionary describes a legend as a "notable person whose deeds or exploits are much talked about in his own time." We hear, read, talk and fantasise about legends; but do we usually know them? I don't think so. No, usually they are too important, distant and unreachable in our life, people whom we admire and humbly honour or glorify. They may shape the subtleties of our personalities, but they remain in the haze of fiction or imagination.

Yet, when we know a living legend we feel a tremendous burden of our own limitations as to how to express our feelings about them. Dear Norman, allow me to humbly try to put into words the impact of the fact that I was privileged enough to have known you for years. Let me talk about the seal you have put not only on my professional growing, but how you have also touched me at the personal level. The prism through which I can see you, is of course, totally subjective; the perspective is only mine and is hardly reliable; but I'll try hard to reflect the feelings built in me over 20 years of our — may I say — friendship. I hope people that know Norman will at least partly agree with my thoughts.

I first came across the name of Norman Farberow in 1977, while preparing a student research project on suicide. There were many references to be found under his name and I soon learnt that he was one of the contemporary founders of modern suicidology.

When I first met Dr. Norman Farberow in person in 1978, I was a Fulbright scholar, who was accepted to spend three months at the Suicide Prevention Center in Los Angeles. It was the leading contemporary institution of its kind, founded and led by Norman Farberow and Bob Litman, while the third partner of the famous three, Ed Shneidman, had already moved to UCLA. It was Norman who agreed that a young psychologist from an unknown European country should come to study there, in order to learn how crisis lines operated and how a crisis center should function. I sat in with his patient groups, I watched him lead staff meetings, I listened to his lectures, I experienced his benevolent nature easing team conflict, I observed the supervision process with junior clinicians. I was obviously amazed by his enormous knowledge, but more so by his gentle and charismatic personality. Being quite young at that time, Norman's natural father-figure role had a deep influence on my professional and personal forming.

He and his staff gave me a very good basic knowledge for organising and starting the first crisis line in our country. I perceived him not only as a very good clinician and leader, but as a good colleague and friend as well. Norman attracted people from all over to come, observe and discuss. I met colleagues from Finland, Holland, Austria, Hungary and from many places in the United States, all of whom were influenced by the well-organised and productive institution and its staff.

When I went home, there were many good friends and close liaisons left behind, but the most important one of them survived all these years. I have never lost touch with Norman Farberow.

In 1981, at the time of the Paris I.A.S.P. meeting, which I couldn't attend because of my first pregnancy, Norman and Pearl came to Ljubljana to visit us and stay a few days. We enjoyed their visit and strengthened our friendship. When I got my sabbatical and an American grant for the academic year 1987/88, I knew I wanted to spend it with Norman again. I came to Los Angeles with my family and again it was Norman who was the first person to greet us there.

At that time I thought I was professionally quite grown up, but when Norman and I started to write protocols for research projects, there I was again — the old feeling was back — I was a learning student again, as there was such an enormous discrepancy in knowledge, skills, wisdom and know-to-how between us. He was persistent, demanding, incredibly precise and meticulous and he insisted in rewriting and re-doing the paper as many times as necessary.

In the meantime Norman's activities broadened. He followed the new stream of the needs that relatives and friends bereaving suicide had been showing and demanding. He started the 8-week program for suicide survivors at the Los Angeles Suicide Prevention Center, initiated the monthly meetings and supervised them, and educated and prepared professionals, volunteers, and suicide survivors themselves to work in those groups. He also supervised colleagues who worked with suicide survivors, and instituted the first evaluation and research projects in the field. It was his irresistible and contagious enthusiasm that made us follow his path. In Slovenia we have been working with suicide survivors systematically for nine years now and this was inspired by Norman Farberow.

I was always impressed by his reliability for patients, students and colleagues alike. I remember Linda, an obese, chronic, marginalised schizophrenic lady, who had been coming to the open group, led by Drs. Katharine Marmor and Norman Farberow in the year 1978 and was still around on a regular basis in 1988. As was Norman. He was there — he didn't provide all the answers always, but he was there: wise, well balanced, sensitive and honest.

When I am talking about Norman, there is someone else who should be more than just mentioned. Pearl Farberow. She is a fascinating lady, extremely unconventional and special. Not just Norman's wife, but his soul mate, his companion, his inspirer and his stimulator. Never did I see Norman not taking care of Pearl in the most noble manner a husband should have. They are inseparable for — I wouldn't mention how many — but many many years. The fruits of their togetherness are David — the lawyer, and Hillary — a homeopathic physician and, most important, a grand-daughter Ariana — Norman's present joy and sunshine of life.

Norman and I are living 7,000 miles apart. I am aware of the fact that many facets of his rich life are hidden to my eyes. We write letters—seldom, but on a regular basis. He is still very active in research, which everybody can judge by his publications. I know that he is still doing therapy, supervision and some teaching and consulting. He plays tennis with Bob Litman regularly and enjoys his grand-daughter's charm. He and Pearl are a good life-team.

Let me finish this brief overview with an anecdote that explains and reflects Norman's "joie de vivre." When we celebrated his 70th birthday, he told us that he had visited some friends somewhere south of LA, where there was a nice village prepared for older people, where they could be independent but still taken care of. Norman obviously liked the setting very much and was quite enthusiastic about it. So his secretary at that time, Nancy, asked him: "Well, Norman, are you and Pearl considering moving down there soon?" He looked at her in his gentle, non-offensive way and said very seriously: "Yes, we thought we should be preparing ourselves to think about this sort of arrangement in 15, 20 years, when the time comes for us."

This is Norman. Full of an incredible charm and life force. To many more fruitful and happy years!

SOME RECOLLECTIONS OF ERWIN STENGEL DURING HIS SHEFFIELD YEARS

Issy Pilowsky

University of Adelaide

I had the good fortune to have Professor Erwin Stengel as my mentor during my early training in psychiatry between 1959 and 1966, at Sheffield. I began as a 'Senior House Officer' there, and progressed to being a lecturer in the university department when I left to take up a position as Senior Lecturer in Psychiatry in the University of Sydney.

Stengel came to the UK as a refugee from Nazi Austria in 1938. He described how he and his wife were billeted in the palace of the Bishop of Bath and Wells for a short period. The palace had a moat with a draw-bridge. This Bishop showed Stengel a letter from the local 'Home Guard' with instructions on how to destroy the draw-bridge in the event of a German invasion. Stengel commented in his typical way: 'It would have held up the progress of the German army by a full two minutes."

In Austria, Stengel was a neurophsychiatrist associated with people such as Schilder, Gerstmann, Hartmann, Wagner-Jauregg, Sakel, Redlich and others. On one occasion, during his psycho-analytic training, he was treating a young man who was the fiance of a woman in Freud's household. He received a message that Professor Freud would like a word with him.

When he arrived Freud asked him how the treatment was progressing. After listening to what Stengel had to relate, he said "Stengel, you must show the patient more warmth'. Taken aback Stengel said 'But Professor Freud, I have been reviewing your writings on technique for my study group, and you empahsize the importance of presenting the patient with a blank screen, a neutral attitude'. Freud expostulated: 'Ah, no-one will ever understand me!"

Stengel's interest in suicide began when he was asked to write a review of the subject for a volume on recent advances in s]psychiatry edited by GW Fleming, then editor of the Journal of Mental Science (forerunner to the British Journal of Psychiatry). He once pointed out to me that, in keeping with the times, he had not made a distinction between attempted and completed suicide. Thereafter he became more interested in, and conducted a clinical study which resulted in, a 'Maudsley Monograph' on attempted suicide and later a Penguin paperback 'Suicide and Attempted Suicide'. He showed that there were two separate, but overlapping populations involved. He emphasized that attempted suicide

Suicide Prevention, edited by Kosky *et al.*
Plenum Press, New York, 1998

should be studied as an independent phenomenon and that it was the result of mixed and complex motivations.

When asked whether it was not reasonable for very old people to take their lives because they saw no future, he replied: 'Ask other people of the same age, they rarely think it is reasonable'.

Statistical studies were not his forte. He spoke despairingly of studies involving 'the scrupulous analysis of data unscrupulously gathered'. Nonetheless, he was impressed by epidemiological studies, and quoted them in his work.

The achievements of Erwin Stengel resulted in suicidal patients being accorded greater respect and was doubtless an important factor in attempted suicide being decriminalised in Britain. (He thought that most of the patients did not know this had happened. Prior to the change, he thought half did not know it was a crime).

Stengel was an extremely hard worker with very high professional standards. Although in England he was a foreigner with an Austrian accent, his attitude to the British seemed to suggest that *they* were the foreigners and they should improve their diction so that he could understand them better.

He was a grand man and a wonderful clinician.

BEYOND THE TOWER OF BABEL[*]

A Nomenclature for Suicidology

Patrick W. O'Carroll, Alan L. Berman, Ronald Maris, Eve Moscicki, Bryan Tanney, and Morton Silverman

School of Public Health
University of Washington
Seattle, Washington

Suicidology finds itself confused and stagnated for lack of a standard nomenclature. This paper proposes a nomenclature for suicide-related behaviour in the hope of improving the clarity and precision of communications, advancing suicidological research, knowledge and improving the efficacy of clinical interventions.

1. INTRODUCTION

Consider the following scenarios:

- A liaison psychiatrist is called to the hospital emergency room to interview a newly admitted patient. The patient, a 44 year old, married female with diagnoses of Dysthymic Disorder (Axis I) and Borderline Personality Disorder (Axis II), had been brought to the hospital, confused and dissociative, after taking an overdose (estimated eight pills) of her prescribed antidepressants on the evening her therapist was to leave for vacation. Her chart noted the following: (a) "patient admitted to ER following suicide attempt by overdose..." (ER psychiatric nurse), (b) "patient referred to ER following suicide gesture..." (patient's psychopharmacologist), and (c) "patient engaged in manipulative self-harm behavior..." (patient's therapist). Since none of the clinicians explicitly stated what they meant by the terms they used, the liaison cannot determine whether or not the patient did in

---

[*] First published in the Journal of Suicide and Life Threatening Behaviour, Volume 26(3), Fall 1996. © 1996 The American Association of Suicidology

fact try to end her life by suicide. He prepares to start his interview from scratch, essentially disregarding the input of the three clinicians who preceded him.

• A medical sociologist wishes to conduct research to refine and clarify existing findings regarding the relative efficacy of several common treatment approaches for suicide attempters. Unfortunately, in her review of the literature she finds that, although numerous studies have been done in this area, none are directly comparable. She determines that the equivocal nature of the combined results of these studies is due largely to the fact that (1) some researchers included all cases of overdose in their studies of "suicide attempters," regardless of intent, whereas others did not; (2) some did not distinguish suicidal ideation from suicidal acts; (3) some indiscriminately mixed first and third person reports of attempts in identifying study subjects; (4) others did not control for various methods of attempting; and (5) few used any operational definition of "lethality" (or other method for discriminating "serious" from "non-serious" attempts)--and those that did, used methods unique to their studies. Frustrated, she is forced to design a study based on a case definition of her own choosing--a study which, although well conceived, will yield results which are, in turn, not directly comparable to previous research efforts.

• A new state epidemiologist determines from vital statistics data that suicide is a leading cause of death in her state. To estimate the morbidity associated with suicidal behavior, and to establish a baseline incidence of attempted suicide by which the effectiveness of new prevention activities could be monitored, she seeks to institute suicide attempt surveillance based in emergency departments. Unfortunately, she discovers from a record review that clinicians seem to use widely varying terms to refer to patients with suicide attempt-related injuries, and terms such as "suicide attempt" and "gesture" seem to mean different things to different clinicians. Faced with the daunting task of trying to interpret such widely varying medical records in a consistent manner, she eventually abandons the idea of statewide emergency department-based suicide attempt surveillance.

These scenarios have two things in common. First, the problems they illustrate are not theoretical. They represent real, ubiquitously encountered barriers to understanding and preventing suicide. Second, all three scenarios devolve from this basic, almost incredible reality: despite hundreds of years of writing and thinking about suicide, and many decades of focused suicide research, there is to this day no generally accepted nomenclature for referring to suicide-related behaviors--not even at the most basic, conversational level. If one clinician says to a second, "I admitted a suicide attempter last night," the second clinician does not know whether that patient was injured in any way, whether the patient actually engaged in any self-harm behavior, or even whether that patient was actually trying to end his or her life. All that can be strictly inferred from the statement is that a person was admitted for engaging in thinking, speaking, or behaving in ways somehow related to the idea of self-killing. Because the term "attempted suicide" potentially means so many different things, it means almost nothing at all.

The absurdity of our current situation can be illustrated by a final scenario, in which we imagine ourselves called to testify before a subcommittee of the United States Senate that is interested in the problem of suicide. We are asked, "How many attempted suicides occur in the U.S. each year?" We respond, "What do you mean by 'attempted suicide'?" Rephrasing the question, the Chair replies, "How many people tried to kill themselves?" We respond, "Do you mean, how many came to the hospital? Or how many were injured? Or how many were injured who were serious about ending their lives? Or how many made some effort to kill themselves, even if they didn't mean it, or even if they were not injured?" After several more such exchanges, we might finally admit that, not only do we not know the answer to the Senator's question, but there is no way anyone *can* know, since the information we need to answer this question is not recorded in any uniform manner.

It is hard to imagine a similar state of affairs for other clinical maladies, and we assert that it is past time to take concrete (if incremental) steps to rectify this state of affairs. In this paper we propose a nomenclature, or set of terms, for the most basic epiphenomena of suicidology. This nomenclature evolved from discussions held over the years among the authors and many of their colleagues, as well as two workshops specifically called to explore this idea of developing a commonly defined set of terms. The first of these workshops was held in conjunction with the annual meeting of the American Association of Suicidology in New York City in April 1994; the second, held in November 1994 in Washington, DC, was jointly sponsored by the Center for Mental Health Services and the National Institute of Mental Health.

Our goal in proposing this nomenclature is very simple: to facilitate communication and minimize confusion among those who work to understand and prevent suicide. We contend that, should this or some similar nomenclature for suicide-related behaviors be accepted, operationalized, and widely used, it would improve and streamline communication among clinicians; facilitate suicide research by establishing at least a core set of case definitions (thus fostering valid cross-study comparisons); and permit valid epidemiologic surveillance of nonfatal suicide-related phenomena. It would also foster communication not only within the clinical, research, and public health communities, but also across these disciplines.

We make no effort to *operationalize* the nomenclature at this stage. Rather, we seek to clearly and unambiguously define a set of basic terms for suicidology, based on a logical and minimum set of necessary component elements. If, upon review and debate among our colleagues, the conceptual underpinnings of our approach are considered sound, then we will proceed to the next stage of the process: developing standard, operational means for applying these definitions in clinical practice, research, and public health. Disseminating and encouraging the use of an operationalized nomenclature would constitute a third stage in this process.

2. BACKGROUND

Of course, we are not the first to note the problem of conflicting or ambiguous definitions of suicide-related phenomena, nor to make efforts to resolve it. Pokorny (1974) reviewed several classification schemes that have been proposed for suicide-related thoughts and behaviors, including those of Durkheim (1951), Schneidman (1966, 1969), Schmidt, O'Neal, and Robins (1954), Dorpat and Boswell (1963), Farrar (1951), and Raines (1950). In 1972–1973, sixty-two medical and behavioral suicidologists met in Phoenix, Arizona under the sponsorship of the National Institute of Mental Health to consider various aspects of suicide prevention (Pokorny 1974). One of the six committees, the "nomenclature committee" chaired by Aaron T. Beck, developed another classification scheme for suicidal behavior (See Table 1). Beck still regards the scheme as basically appropriate even today (1995). In this scheme, suicidal phenomena are considered either as completions, as nonfatal suicide attempts, or as suicide ideas. Each of these three types is further specified by (A) certainty of the rater (0–100%), (B) lethality or medical danger to

Table 1. Classification of suicidal behaviors

I. Completed Suicide (CS)
   A. Certainty of rater (1–100%)
   B. Lethality (medical danger to life) zero, low, medium, high
   C. Intent (to die) zero, low, medium, high
   D. Mitigating circumstances (confusion, intoxication etc.) zero, low, medium, high
   E. Method (not an ordinal scale)
II. Suicide Attempt (SA)
   A. Certainty (1–100%)
   B. Lethality (medical danger to life) zero, low, medium, high
   C. Intent (to die) zero, low, medium, high
   D. Mitigating circumstances, zero, low, medium, high
   E. Method (not an ordinal scale)
III. Suicidal Ideas (SI)
   A. Certainty (1–100%)
   B. Lethality (medical danger to life)
      Undertermined, low, medium, high; refers to consequences, if life-threatening plan were to be carried out.
   C. Intent (to die) zero, low, medium, high
   D. Mitigating circumstances zero, low, medium, high
   E. Method (Multiple methods may be listed. In some cases the method may be unknown. Not an ordinal
      scale)

Source: Beck, A.T., Resnik, H.L.P., & Lettieri, D.J. (Eds). (1974) *The prediction of suicide.* Bowie, mD: Charles Press Publishers (p.41)

life (zero, low, medium, or high), (C) intent to die (zero, low, high), (D) mitigating circumstances (zero, low, medium, high), and method used.

After reviewing these classification efforts, Maris (1992) offers a further classification scheme (Table 2), involving two axes--outcome and "type" of suicide. On Axis I, the rater first has to decide whether a suicidal outcome (the focus is on just one outcome at a time) is a completion (code I), nonfatal suicide attempt (code II), suicide ideation (code III), or a mixed or uncertain mode or outcome (code IV). Second, Maris assumes based on his review of the suicide literature that suicidal phenomena are fundamentally either (A) escape, (B) revenge, (C) altruistic, (D) risk-taking, or (E) mixed types. Each type is elaborated to be as broad as possible and still relatively homogeneous, and yet to be reasonably exclusive with other basic types of suicidal behaviors.

Unfortunately, at this writing, neither these nor any other classification efforts have been widely adopted. Several explanations might account for this, not the least of which is that our current understanding of suicide causation may be insufficient to establish a valid classification scheme that reflects established biological and etiological pathways relevant to clinical practice and prevention.

However, quite apart from any consideration of the validity of these or other classification schema, we assert that wider adoption of any set of terms has been fundamentally hampered by a persistent confusion between the goal of developing a conceptually clear and compelling *nomenclature* for suicidology (a set of commonly defined terms) and the goal of developing an etiologically and/or therapeutically valid (or at least theory-based) *classification* scheme. In Pokorny's (1974) review, for example, the terms nomenclature and classification are treated as either interchangeable or inextricable. We assert, however, that the goals of a nomenclature and a classification scheme are different, if overlapping. Even if we grant, for the sake of argument, that the development of a valid, operational classification scheme is not currently possible given our understanding of suicide, we nevertheless can and should develop a basic nomenclature that facilitates communication among clinicians, researchers, and public health practitioners about at least the basic epiphenomena of suicide.

Table 2. Maris Multiaxial Classification of Suicidal Behaviours and Ideation, 1992 Scheme

Suicidal behaviour/ideas	Check (√)	1 Primary type	2 Certainty	3 Lethality	4 Intent	5 Circumstances	6 Method	7 Sex	8 Age	9 Race	10 Marital status	11 Occupation
I Completed suicides												
A Escape, egotic, alone, no hope												
B Revenge, hate, aggressive												
C Altruistic, self-sacrificing, transfiguration												
D Risk-taking, ordeal, game												
E Mixed												
II Nonfatal suicide attempts												
A Escape, catharsis, tension reduction												
B Interpersonal, manipulation, revenge												
C Altruistic												
D Risk-taking												
E Mixed												
F Single vs Multiple												
G Parasuicide												
III Suicidal ideation												
A Escape etc												
B Revenge, interpersonal etc.												
C Altruisitc etc												
D Risk-taking etc												
E Mixed												
IV Mixed or uncertain mode												
A Homicide-suicide												
B Accident-suicide												
C Natural-suicide												
D Undertermined, pending												
E Mixed												
V Indirect self-destructive behaviour (not an exclusive category)												
A Alcoholism												
B Other drug abuse												
C Tobacco abuse												
D Self-mutilation												

Table 2. (*Continued*)

E   Anorexia-bulimia
F   Over or under weight
G   Sexual promiscuity
H   Health management problem,
    medications
I   Risky sports
J   Stress
K   Accident proneness
L   Other (specify)

Source: Maris, RW, Berman, AL...Maltsberger, JT., & Yufit, RI (Eds) (1992) *Assessment and prediction of suicid* New York: Guilford Press (p. 82) *Note:* Certainty: Rate 0–100%

Lethality (medical danger to life): Rate zero, low, medium, high (O, L, M, H)

Intent: Rate zero, low, medium, high

Mitigating circumstances (psychotic, impulsive, intoxicated, confused): Rate zero, low, medium, high

Method: firearm (F); poison (solid and liquid) (P); poison (gas) (PG); hanging (H); cutting or piercing (C); jumping (J); drowning (D); crushing (CR); other (O); none (N).

Sex: Male (M); Female (F)

Age: Record actual age at event

Race: white (W); Black (B); Asian (A); other(O)

Marital status: Married (M); single (S); divorced (D); widowed (W); other (O)

Occupation: Manager, executive, administration (M); professional (P); technical workers (T); sales worker (S); clerical worker (C); worker in precision production (mechanic, construction) (PP); service worker (SW); operator, laborer (OL); worker in farming, forestry, fishing (F); other (O); none (N)

3. NOMENCLATURE VS. CLASSIFICATION

It is critical that the reader understand the distinction we make between the terms "nomenclature" and "classification." Far from splitting hairs, an understanding of this distinction is central to an appreciation of what we propose in this paper. By nomenclature, we mean a set of commonly understood, logically defined terms. The terms of any nomenclature may be considered a type of short-hand by which communication about classes of more subtle phenomena is facilitated. For example, consider the phrase "human being" This term doesn't begin to capture the richness, depths, and ambiguities of what it means to be human. Yet, despite its inadequacy for subtle discussions about philosophy (or, for that matter, taxonomy), the term "human being" is neither ambiguous nor imprecise when it comes to the needs of basic communication. In contrast, a classification scheme typically implies several elements that go beyond a mere nomenclature, including comprehensiveness; a systematic arrangement of items in groups or categories, with ordered, nested subcategories; scientific (e.g., biologic or etiologic) validity; exhaustiveness; accuracy sufficient for research or clinical practice; and an unambiguous set of rules for assigning items to a single place in the classification scheme.

The concepts of nomenclature and classification overlap, of course. Every classification scheme necessarily has a nomenclature (i.e., a set of unambiguous definitions for all its categories and subcategories). Further, a basic nomenclature can (and whenever possible, should) be elaborated into a valid and useful classification scheme, given the development of a sufficient understanding of the causal or other salient relationships between the various elements involved. However, a basic nomenclature is always the *sine qua non* of meaningful communication, even in the absence of a scientifically valid, widely accepted classification scheme.

Consider: if someone informed you that their relative died from breast cancer, you would understand what they meant. Yet the words "breast cancer" *do not appear anywhere* in the International Classification of Diseases (ICD) [ref to ICD9]. The closest ICD classification to "breast cancer" as the term is commonly used is **Malignant neoplasm of female breast** *(174)*. This ICD code is further sub-classified according to the anatomic area affected by the neoplasm (e.g., code 174.5, **Malignant neoplasm of lower-outer quadrant of female breast**). There are still other ICD codes for breast cancer in males (175), and for skin cancers affecting the breast (e.g., ICD codes 172.5 and 198.2). The classification must be precise so as to eliminate any possibility of *mis*classification. Yet daily interpersonal communication demands more direct, if necessarily less specific terms. Despite the fact that the term "breast cancer" is insufficiently specific and elaborate for a classification scheme relevant to research or clinical practice, it is entirely clear and sufficiently precise for most communication.

Further, a set of widely accepted, comprehensible, commonly understood terms for clinical phenomena is not valuable merely for conversation. A physician notating a patient's record during a review of systems might scribble "positive family history of breast cancer." Another physician reviewing that chart would know what is meant by the term, though he or she would not know the histology, course, or treatment given to the patient's relative with the breast cancer, much less the etiology of that neoplastic event. Under certain circumstances, it would be important to know whether the breast cancer was responsive to estrogen therapy; whether it was primary or metastatic; whether it was surgically removable; or whether the patient used oral contraceptives. All kinds of information might be needed to adequately describe--and thereby meaningfully classify-- a given patient with breast cancer. But that does not obviate the utility of a simple, parsimonious, uniformly understood term for such cases. Similarly, in a research article, an investigator might report the number of deaths due to breast cancer in the U.S. in a given year, without listing the number specifically attributable to each type of breast cancer listed in the ICD.

4. CONCEPTUAL BASES OF OUR PROPOSED NOMENCLATURE

4.1. OCDS as a Basis for a Nomenclature

In the mid-1980's, the Centers for Disease Control convened a multidisciplinary workgroup to develop a set of criteria to aid coroners and medical examiners in their task of certifying manner of death, specifically in cases of apparent or possible suicide. Prior to this work, in the absence of any consensus criteria, each coroner and medical examiner simply used their own internal set of rules and criteria for what did and did not constitute evidence of suicide. In 1988, the results of the CDC workgroup's deliberations were published as the Operational Criteria for the Classification of Suicide (OCDS) (Rosenberg et al. 1988). Despite this moniker, the OCDS as published were not in fact operationalized, nor did they constitute a classification scheme. Rather, they established a clear definition of the component evidential elements that are necessary to a certification of suicide, thus guiding coroners and medical examiners as to the kind of death-scene evidence to be sought and considered in cases of possible suicide.

The OCDS defined completed suicide as death from injury, poisoning, or suffocation where there is evidence (either explicit or implicit) that the injury was self-inflicted *and* that the decedent intended to kill himself/herself. Suicide is thus defined in terms of just three components: (1) *death* as the result of injury of some sort which is both (2) *self-inflicted* and (3) *intentionally* inflicted.

These are the essential elements which distinguish suicide from the other three modes of death in the so-called "NASH" classification (death due to Natural causes, Accidental death, Suicide, and Homicide). Table 3 illustrates schematically how the mechanism of death (diseases vs. injuries), intentionality, and source of the intentional act (self, others) combine to define four manners of death.

There are several subtle but important attributes inherent in OCDS. First, it is clear from the reference to evidence that someone's *judgement* is necessarily involved in determining death from suicide. This judgement is to be based on explicit or implicit evidence, both as regards whether the injury was self-inflicted and whether it was *intentionally* self-inflicted. Second, whereas the element of intent is necessary in order to rule any death a suicide, no mention is made of the *level* of the decedent's intent, the decedent's motivation for suicide, or any other element that bears on how much or how seriously the decedent wished to end their life by suicide. By implication, the question of intent is one of *any* intent vs. *no* intent whatsoever.[†]

Two other aspects of OCDS are important to this discussion. First, the application of OCDS is left to professionals who are specifically trained to make manner of death determinations. The idea that these criteria could be mechanically applied to death determination by untrained personnel was explicitly rejected by the developers of these criteria

---

[†] In practice, the decedent's ability to *form* intent, i.e., to understand the consequences and finality of suicide, is also taken into account. By convention for example, children less than five years of age who seem to intentionally take their lives are not coded as suicides (O'Carroll, 1988).

Table 3. Schematic of "NASH" classification used by coroners
and medical examiners in certifying manner of death

Manner of death	Due to injuries, Poisoning or Suffocation?	Intentionally inflicted? (if so, by whom?)
Natural Causes	No	—
Accidents	Yes	No
Suicide	Yes	Yes, by self
Homicide	Yes	Yes, by others

(Rosenberg et al. 1988). Both the element of judgment already discussed and the tremendous range of circumstances and human behavior associated with suicide necessitate that these criteria be thoughtfully and carefully applied by knowledgeable persons in each case.

Having said that, however, there is a final, critical aspect of OCDS relevant to this discussion: neither ambiguity of evidence (as to self-infliction and intentionality) nor evidence of ambiguity (on the part of the decedent) relieves those certifying manner of death from their responsibility to make a categorical determination: a certifier must rule that a given death either was or was not due to suicide. Although ambiguous cases can be classified (generally temporarily) as undetermined, no option is given for partial determinations--that a person died "partly from suicide," and "partly by accident" for example. We believe that the societal and medicolegal reasons for this are self-evident, and need not be reviewed here. The important point is that, despite the fact that human mortality clearly does not fall unambiguously into four neat manners of death, the requirements of communication, civil government, and public health are such that clear, categorical judgements regarding manner of death simply must be made on the best evidence available.

4.2. Elaborating a Broader Nomenclature

We assert that from the central elements inherent in OCDS (outcome, self-infliction, and intent to kill oneself) we can elaborate a broader nomenclature which encompasses much of the epiphenomenological panorama of suicide and life-threatening behavior, while retaining the simplicity necessary for a clear, comprehensible, unambiguous nomenclature. Additional terms must also be defined to encompass suicidal thinking (as opposed to behavior).

There is perhaps only one aspect of the application of OCDS which presents no challenge to coroners and medical examiners: in the case of manner of death determinations, the person in question is dead. Obviously, any broadly useful nomenclature for suicidology must encompass nonfatal outcomes of suicidal behavior, including outcomes which involve no injury whatsoever. For example, some clear term is needed to denominate suicide-related acts which result in nonfatal injuries; another, different term is needed to refer to all suicide-related acts of whatever outcome (death, injury, or no injury); yet another term is needed to refer to nonfatal suicide-related acts (with or without injury). So one expanded axis of our proposed nomenclature is that of immediate outcome--death, injury, or no injury.

An important distinction must be made as regards intent. Unlike the manner of death question, the full spectrum of suicide includes persons whose behavior is clearly suicide-related, *but who have no intention of killing themselves.* Terms such as "suicide gesture" and "instrumental suicidal behavior" have been used to refer to such behavior. This determination of underlying motivation is often of enormous clinical importance, and may be of great importance from a research perspective as well (for example, if one wishes to study a reasonably homogeneous group of persons who have truly tried to take their own lives). The distinction is also important from a public health surveillance perspective. If a man who has no intention of dying stands on a ledge to invoke the attention that the fear of suicide predictably engenders, and then he *unintentionally* falls to his death, the manner of death should be certified as accident, not suicide--despite the fact that his behavior was clearly related to suicide, i.e., to the *idea* of intentional self-killing.

To avoid confusion, it is important that we not use the same word--intent--both to refer to the person's intent to kill himself/herself, and to the person's intent to use the idea of suicide to cry for help, etc. In our proposed nomenclature, the word "intent" always refers to the intention to take one's own life; other terms are used to denominate instrumental, suicide-related behavior.

Our example of the "accidental" fall from the ledge raises, of course, the question of whether such a man might have been *slightly* suicidal despite being, even in his own mind, primarily interested in the hoped-for instrumental effects of his behavior. We propose to follow the OCDS model: for practical purposes, we propose a nomenclature that distinguishes between zero intent to kill oneself on the one hand, and *any* level of intent, however trivial or intense, on the other. In our example, if a certifier judged that the decedent in question had some slight suicidal intent, then we propose that this death should be ruled a suicide. And we propose to elaborate our nomenclature for nonfatal suicide-related behavior along the same lines.

5. PROPOSED TERMS AND DEFINITIONS

With this background, we submit the following nomenclature for consideration by our colleagues. Several terms are defined as supersets of other terms; for example, "suicidal acts" are those which are either "suicide attempts" or "completed suicides." For several of our proposed terms, an understanding of the subsidiary (component) terms is logically necessary to an understanding of the umbrella term. For this reason, we first present the definitions for subsidiary terms, then progress to the more inclusive. The component elements that uniquely define each suicide-related behavior are illustrated in Figure 1, whereas the relationships between the proposed terms for suicide-related thoughts and behaviors may best be understood by reference to Table 4.

Again, it is of great importance that the reader understand that Table 1 is not meant as a clinically applicable classification of suicide (which it clearly is not), nor is it meant to reflect causal or behavioral pathways. Rather, it is simply meant to do what outlines traditionally do: to clarify which terms represent logical (definitional) subsets or supersets of other terms.

Suicide: Death from injury, poisoning, or suffocation where there is evidence (either explicit or implicit) that the injury was self-inflicted *and* that the decedent intended to kill himself/herself (OCDS definition). (Note: The term "completed suicide" can be used interchangeably with the term "suicide.")

Table 4. An outline indicating superset/subset relationships of the proposed nomenclature for suicide and self-injurious thoughts and behaviors

I. *Self-injurious thoughts and behaviors*
  A. *Risk-taking thoughts and behaviors*
    1. with immediate risk (e.g., motocross, skydiving)
    2 with remote risk (e.g., smoking, sexual promiscuity)
  B. *Suicide-related thoughts and behaviors*
    1. Suicidal Ideation
      a. Casual ideation
      b. Serious ideation
        (1) persistent
        (2) transient
    2. Suicide-related Behaviors
      a. Instrumental suicide-related behavior (ISRB)
        (1) Suicide Threat
          (a) passive (e.g., ledge-sitting)
          (b) active (e.g., verbal threat, note writing)
        (2) Other ISRB
        (3) Accidental death associated with ISRB
      b. Suicidal Acts
        (1) Suicide attempt
          (a) with no injuries (e.g., gun fired, missed)
          (b) with injuries
        (2) Suicide (Completed Suicide)

Terms for suicide-related behaviors		Intent to die from suicide[¶]	Instrumental thinking	Outcome		
				No injury	Non-fatal injury	Death
INSTRUMENTAL BEHAVIOUR	Instrumental suicide-related behavior					
	-with injuries	No	Yes		x	
	-without injuries	No	Yes	X		
	-with fatal outcome[§]	No	Yes			X
SUICIDAL ACTS	Suicide attempt					
	-with injuries	Yes	+/-			
	-without injuries	Yes	+/-	X		
	Completed suicide	Yes	+/-			X

[¶]Conscious intent to ends one's life through the suicidal behavior.
[§]Note that a fatal outcome of instrumental behavior is properly considered accidental death, since by definition there is no intent to die from suicide.

Figure 1. An illustration of the proposed nomenclature for suicide-related behavior, in terms of outcome and intent to die from suicide.

Suicide Attempt with injuries:	An action resulting in nonfatal injury, poisoning, or suffocation where there is evidence (either explicit or implicit) that the injury was self-inflicted *and* that the decedent intended at some (non-zero) level to kill himself/herself.
Suicide Attempt:	A potentially self-injurious behavior with a nonfatal outcome, for which there is evidence (either explicit or implicit) that the person intended at some (non-zero) level to kill himself/herself. A suicide attempt may or may not result in injuries.
Suicidal Act:	A potentially self-injurious behavior for which there is evidence (either implicit or explicit) that the person intended at some (non-zero) level to kill himself/herself. A suicidal act may result in death (completed suicide), injuries, or no injuries.
Instrumental Suicide-related Behavior:	Potentially self-injurious behavior for which there is evidence (either implicit or explicit) that (a) the person did not intend to kill himself/herself (i.e., had zero intent to die), **and** (b) the person wished to use the *appearance* of intending to kill himself/herself in order to attain some other end (e.g., to seek help, to punish others, to receive attention)
Suicide-related Behavior:	Potentially self-injurious behavior for which there is explicit or implicit evidence **either** that (a) the person intended at some (non-zero) level to kill himself/herself, **or** (b) the person wished to use the *appearance* of intending to kill himself/herself in order to attain some other end. Suicide-related behavior comprises suicidal acts and instrumental suicide-related behavior.
Suicide Threat:	Any interpersonal action, verbal or non-verbal, stopping short of a directly self-harmful act, which a reasonable person would interpret as communicating or suggesting that a suicidal act or other suicide-related behavior might occur in the near future.
Suicidal Ideation:	Any self-reported thoughts of engaging in suicide-related behavior.

6. DISCUSSION

We believe the nomenclature we have here proposed has several advantages. First, by defining our terms with an absolute minimum set of logically distinguishing elements (outcome, evidence of self-infliction, and evidence of intent to die from suicide), this nomenclature may be clear and conceptually compelling to clinicians, researchers, public health practitioners, and laymen alike. Second, the nomenclature addresses only the most general classes of suicide-related thoughts and behaviors. For the purposes of basic communication, this minimum nomenclature probably meets the vast majority of needs. Further, this parsimony will hopefully encourage critics to focus on the concepts underpinning our nomenclature, rather than on distracting arguments about the specification and definition of narrow subclasses of suicide-related epiphenomena. Third, as an elaboration on the OCDS, this nomenclature incorporates a great deal of thought-work and conceptual synthesis and simplification that went before it. Fourth, by avoiding the temptation to base our nomenclature on current etiologic theories or standards of clinical practice, our terms are relatively "agnostic." In other words, regardless of future developments in our understanding of the etiology of suicide and treatment of suicidal persons, this set of terms (based as it is on fundamental definitional elements that constitute suicidality) may remain valid and useful.

6.1. Terms vs. Definition of Terms

There are implicitly two components inherent in each element of a standard nomenclature: the terms themselves and the definitions of those terms. We strongly believe that the primary consideration at this juncture should be on the *definitions*, and on the conceptual structure demarcating the set of terms we have defined. That is what we have focused on here. We have used the concepts of outcome, self-infliction, and intent to die to identify a matrix of terms, and we have offered definitions for those terms. At this stage, we would rather focus the readers' attention on those concepts and definitions than on the terms themselves. For example, if a fundamental objection is raised to the way we have structured and defined our matrix of terms, it is relatively unimportant whether we use the term (for example) "suicide attempt" vs. "attempted suicide" vs. "nonfatal suicidal behavior."

Of course, the terms themselves are also important, and--assuming we come to some consensus on concepts and definitions for our nomenclature--we will need to address ourselves to the choice of the most appropriate terms. Choosing the terms will likely present its own controversies. An example: Canetto and Lester (1995) suggest the use of the term "nonfatal suicidal behavior" as preferable to "attempted suicide," since the latter term implies that the goal of all suicidal behavior is death by suicide. Canetto (1992) further argues that the term "attempted suicide" is inherently sexist, since it defines typically female behavior (surviving a suicidal act) as a "failure" and typically male behavior (killing oneself), as "success." Another example: In the European literature the term "parasuicide" is commonly used in preference to"attempted suicide," because it is simply descriptive of potentially self-destructive behavior, and therefore doesn't require the (often impossible) assessment of intent toward self-destruction for its valid application.

Although we welcome further input on the choice of the terms for our nomenclature, we have been guided in our current choice of terms by the primary considerations of *intelligibility* and *practicality*. For better or worse, in the English language the terms "suicide" and "attempted suicide" are common parlance. If we fail to define and use these terms--choosing instead to define newly-invented, clumsy, or uncommon terms that we suicidologists find philosophically more appealing--then we run the risk of dooming the acceptance of our nomenclature from the start. If one must be schooled in the lore of suicidology to understand the terms we use for our most basic outcomes of interest, then we will have failed to meet our goal of a cross-disciplinary, intelligible, conceptually clean and appealing nomenclature.

In any case, again, we would rather defer this discussion until after we have first reached consensus on the underlying concepts that demarcate our matrix of terms. To do otherwise could lead to lengthy discussions that might later prove to have been needless. Consider again, for example, the argument by Canetto et al. that the term "attempted suicide" implies that the goal of all suicidal behavior is death from suicide. This is not true under our proposed nomenclature: we reserve the term "attempted suicide" for cases in which there is indeed at least some level of intent to die from suicide. Thus the first issue to be debated is whether our definition of this particular entity--regardless of what we call it--seems a valid and useful one. If it is, then we can proceed to select a term for it which seems reasonable, practical, and clear.

6.2. Next Steps

For this nomenclature to become both useful and applied, several things must happen in sequence. First, this set of terms and the concepts by which they are defined must be thoroughly scrutinized and critiqued by our colleagues. Second, assuming that the ideas presented here are both improved upon and ultimately accepted as useful, more work is needed to *operationalize* the final set of terms. Finally, assuming that practical means can be developed for applying these terms in real-life situations, efforts must be undertaken to *market* these terms, so that they can in fact become part of a standard lexicon of suicidology. To begin this process, let us briefly address each of these three steps.

6.2.1. Critiquing the Proposed Nomenclature. We strongly encourage readers of this article to respond in some way to our proposed nomenclature, whether to indicate support, suggest refinements, or explain why our proposal is inadequate, wrong-headed, or unnecessary. Indeed, this response is critical to the improvement of these ideas and to building consensus. Personal communication with the authors is, of course, always welcome. However, we recommend instead that interested readers write letters to the editor of this Journal, so that other readers will have the opportunity to consider your views.

To begin this dialogue, we here review the most common criticisms encountered in discussing this nomenclature with our colleagues, and present our responses to those criticisms.

> *The "perfect nomenclature" objection:* We shouldn't adopt this or any other set of definitions until we know more about how to do so along truly etiological or at least therapeutically relevant lines.

We would respond that real or potential inadequacies in any proposed nomenclature can easily prevent us from ever getting started, which prevents us from making any progress whatsoever. All really useful nomenclatures had to begin somewhere, even with syndromatic descriptions that seem arbitrary in retrospect. These early "case definitions" were revised as science and circumstances permitted. Consider, for example, the various surveillance definitions that have been used for acquired immunodeficiency syndrome (AIDS) (see, for example, CDC 1992 and 1994). Early definitions at least permitted rational public health surveillance and the beginnings of rational medical research. But those definitions, in retrospect, were far from perfect.

> *The "binary reality" objection:* We shouldn't adopt this nomenclature because, in real life, people simply do not fall into such neat, "yes/no" categories.

Of course, any discrete set of terms inevitably fails to capture all shades of gray, but again, this should not become a barrier to developing a nomenclature. Consider the word "snow," which utterly fails to capture the rich and varied types of snow that exist. Yet the question "Is it snowing?" is rarely met with the retort, "Define your terms." We understand the question, while at the same time understanding the difference between heavy snow, wet snow, sticky snow, snowstorm, etc. *Any* nomenclature is a short-cut meant to broadly summarize a set of generally distinct if somewhat overlapping phenomena, so as to permit communication. A nomenclature necessarily trades precision for intelligibility. We should not confuse an admittedly and deliberately simplified model (our nomenclature) for reality. We are not trying to define reality in all its nuance, we are trying to define workable constructs.

> *The "universal consensus" objection:* we should not accept this or any nomenclature until is found acceptable by everyone who has a stake in this area.

First, no nomenclature, even one found to be broadly useful by many clinicians, researchers, and public health practitioners, will satisfy everyone's needs. Departures from a standard nomenclature are inevitable, even desirable--they may enable us to modify or otherwise enrich the original nomenclature. But such departures from standard terminology should be explicitly acknowledged and explained, so as to avoid confusion.

Second, it may be that researchers, clinicians, and epidemiologists will each need to expand a standard nomenclature in ways that are unique to their field--but cross-field communication is still critical, making it desirable that we agree whenever possible upon the definitions of the most common suicide-related phenomena.

> *The "measured approach" objection:* We should not simply accept this or any other nomenclature; rather, we should continue to work to improve it, and in so doing, will eventually define a set of terms that is not only acceptable, but also etiologically and therapeutically valid.

Certainly, we believe our proposed nomenclature may be improved with further input. However, we must also recognize that people have now been writing about suicide for thousands of years, and have been interested in suicide classification for dozens of years-- yet we do not agree upon the meaning of basic suicidologic terms. Endlessly discussing this will not lead gradually and inexorably to a perfect system. As noted, any nomenclature is an artificial construct that can never perfectly represent reality. As suicidologists, we ought to be able to come to some agreement in the near term as to what we mean by such basic, commonly used terms as "suicide attempt." Any nomenclature can be changed and improved over time. We would argue that it is time to identify a reasonable set of terms, try to incorporate their usage in our professional practices, and see how it works.

Again, this is not to minimize the need or opportunity for further input at this stage. Indeed, this paper is submitted to some extent as a "straw man" document, to begin a fruitful discussion. But our hope is that, with this as a beginning, we can agree upon a basic nomenclature within a relatively short span of time.

6.2.2. Operationalizing the Proposed Nomenclature. Specific operational techniques will vary from setting to setting, but this need not violate the fundamental precepts or spirit of the nomenclature. Consider, for example, our liaison psychiatrist from the scenario with which we opened this article. After interviewing the patient regarding her overdose, using our nomenclature, he must record his assessment as either a "suicide attempt" or as "instrumental suicide-related behavior." The latter is defined as involving zero intent to die. However, given that it is impossible to determine another person's intent with perfect accuracy, our clinician might operationalize the definition of "instrumental suicide-related behavior" as behavior for which there is "no substantial evidence" of intent to die.

This departure from the strict definition of "zero intent" towards "no substantial evidence of intent" does not violate the spirit of the nomenclature. It is rather a recognition of the need to adapt the conceptually clear definition to the practical limitations of clinical evidence. What constitutes "substantial evidence" may, of course, vary from clinician to clinician, as judgements about what constitutes satisfactory evidence of completed suicide varies from among medical examiners. Nevertheless, it would be an important step toward intelligibility and communication if various clinicians were at least *trying* to employ the same definitional elements and entities in describing their patients' suicide-related behaviors.

6.2.3. Marketing the Proposed Nomenclature. Assuming, for the sake of discussion, that a basic nomenclature eventually receives some substantial acceptance among suicidologists, concrete efforts will yet be needed to ensure that this set of terms becomes common parlance among clinicians, researchers, public health practitioners and others. Without this last step, the benefits which we believe would accrue from having defined a standard nomenclature would remain merely theoretical. While is premature to explore this last step in great detail at this juncture, several possible mechanisms for speeding the adoption of this nomenclature may be mentioned here.

First, the final results of our deliberations should be published widely, certainly in the suicidological, psychiatric, and psychological literature, but also in general clinical and public health journals and ancillary publications (newsletters, etc.). Professional journals might be encouraged to require (or at least encourage) the standard application of these terms by those submitting articles, except in those cases where the nature of particular scientific inquiry dictates otherwise. Similarly, funding agencies (like NIMH and CDC) ought to require applicants to use the standard nomenclature, again with appropriate exceptions. Third, schools of medicine, psychology, and public health should be encouraged to incorporate this nomenclature in their teaching of students and residents.

Who would do this work? Those who wish to advance the understanding and prevention of suicide. The American Association of Suicidology would seem the natural organization to take the lead in this effort, obviously enlisting key partners (e.g., the American Psychological Association, the National Institute of Mental Health) in that process. Much work remains to be done before we can begin to dismantle suicidology's Tower of Babel. The sooner we start, the better.

ACKNOWLEDGMENTS

We are indebted to our many colleagues who have helped us conceptualize the ideas presented in this paper. We particularly thank those attending the 1994 AAS workshop and the 1994 CMHS/NIMH workshop on suicide nomenclature and classification.

REFERENCES

Beck, A.T., Davis, J.H., Frederick, C.J., Perlin, S., Pokorny, A.D., Schulman, R.E., Seiden, R.H., Wittlin, B.J. (1973). Classification and nomenclature. In: Resnik, H.L.P. and Hathorne B.C. (Eds.), Suicide Prevention in the Seventies (pp. 7–12). Washington, D.C.: U.S. Government Printing Office.
Beck, A.T. (1995). [referred to by Maris--Ron, please supply the ref.]
Canetto, S.S. (1992). Gender and suicide in the elderly. Suicide and Life-Threatening Behavior, 22, 80–97.
Canetto, S.S. and Lester, D. (1995) Women and suicidal behavior: issues and dilemmas. In: Canetto, S.S. and Lester, D., eds. Women and suicidal behavior. New York: Springer Publishing Company, 3–8.
CDC. (1992). 1993 Revised classification system for HIV infection and expanded surveillance case definition for AIDS among adolescents and adults. MMWR, 41 (no. RR-17).
CDC. (1994). Update: Impact of the Expanded AIDS Surveillance Case Definition for Adolescents and Adults on Case Reporting -- United States, 1993. MMWR, 43(09), 160–161,167–170.

Dorpat, T., and Boswell, J. (1963). An evaluation of suicide intent in suicide attempts. Comprehensive Psychiatry 4:117–125.

Durkheim, E. (1951). Suicide. Glencoe, IL: The Free Press.

Farrar, C.B. (1951). Suicide. Journal of Clinical and Experimental Psychopathology 12:79–88.

Maris (1992) [Ron, please supply the ref.]

O'Carroll, P.W., Smith J.C. (1988) Suicide and homicide. In: Wallace, H.M., Ryan, G., Oglesby, A.C., eds. Maternal and Child Health Practices. Oakland, CA: Third Party Publishing.

Pokorny, A.D. (1974) A scheme for classifying suicidal behaviors. In: Beck, A.T., Resnik, H.L.P., Lettieri, D.J., eds. The prediction of suicide. Phildaelphia, PA: The Charles Press.

Raines, G. (1950). Suicide: some basic considerations. Digest of Neurology and Psychiatry 18:97–107.

Rosenberg, M.L., Davidson, L.E., Smith, J.C., Berman, A.L., Buzbee, H., Gantner G., Gay, G.A., Moore-Lewis, B., Mills, D.H., Murray, D., O'Carroll, P.W., Jobes, D. (1988) Operational criteria for the determination of suicide. Journal of Forensic Sciences, 32(6), 1445–1455.

Schmidt, E., O'Neal, P., and Robins, E. (1954). Evaluation of suicide attempts as guide to therapy. JAMA 155:549–557.

Schneidman, E. (1966). Orientation toward death: a vital aspect of the study of lives. Int. Journal of Psychiatry 2:167–200.

Schneidman, E. (1968). Classifications of suicidal phenomena. Bulletin of Suicidology. No. 2, p.1–9.

Schneidman, E. (1969). Prologue in "On the nature of suicide." San Francisco: Jossey-Bass, inc.

USDHHS. (1991). *International classification of diseases* (9th revision, 4th ed.). Washington, DC: US Department of Health and Human Services, Public Health Service.

8

FAMILIAL RISK FACTORS FOR ADOLESCENT SUICIDE[*]

A Case-Control Study[1]

David A. Brent,[1] Grace Moritz,[1] Laura Liotus,[1] Joy Schweers,[1] Lisa Balach,[1] Claudia Roth,[1] and Joshua A. Perper[2]

[1]Western Psychiatric Institute and Clinic
3811 O'Hara Street, Pittsburgh, Pennsylvania
[2]Allegheny County Coroner
542 Fourth Avenue, Pittsburgh, Pennsylvania

1. INTRODUCTION

In the search for risk factors for adolescent suicide, many investigators have posited that familial contributions to suicidal risk are among the most potent. This view has included that of the "expendable child," in which the family environment is so strife-laden and rejecting that the child commits suicide (1). Others have noted high rates of parent-child discord in adolescent suicide attempters and completers, and have frequently cited such occurrences as precipitants for suicide and suicidal behavior (2–6). Factors affecting the quality of the family environment such as those of parental loss, separation, and divorce have been cited as contributors to suicidal risk (4,5,7). Still other lines of research have suggested that among the most potent risk factors for adolescent suicide and suicidal behavior are parental psychopathology and family history of suicidal behavior (8–12). Clearly, these views are not mutually exclusive or conclusive. However, their emphases differ sufficiently, so that an understanding of the relative contributions of these different components of familial risk could have important implications for the formulation of a hierarchy of prevention strategies.

[*] We are grateful to the Munksgard International Publishers Ltd, Copenhagen, Denmark for permission to publish this paper (Familial Risk Factors for Adolescent Suicide: A Case Control Study) which was originally published in the Acta Psychiatrica Scandinavica, 1994:89:52–58.

Previous studies of familial risk factors in adolescent suicide have been few and only two have been controlled (11,12). Shafii et al. (11), in a comparison of 20 suicide victims and 17 close friends, found higher rates of parental "emotional problems," "parental absence," and abuse. Shaffer et al. (12) noted higher rates of suicide and suicidal behavior in the families of suicide victims compared to those of community controls. Neither study reported on rates of parental psychopathology, nor were multiple familial and non-familial risk factors examined simultaneously.

Controlled studies of suicide attempters have noted the role of parental loss, parental psychopathology, and family discord. Garfinkel et al. (7), in a consecutive series of suicide attempters matched to non-suicidal admissions to an urban emergency department, found that the former had higher familial rates of substance abuse and suicidal behavior, as well as an increased frequency of parental loss or separation. In a community sample, Kashani et al. (13) found that the parents of suicidal ideators, compared to non-ideators, showed a greater prevalence of psychiatric symptomatology. Joffe et al. (14), reporting from the Ontario Child Health Study, found that suicidal ideation and attempts in 12–16 year olds were related to parental conditions of criminality, psychopathology, substance abuse, as well as overall family dysfunction. In a school-based survey, Hibbard et al. (15) found that sexual and physical abuse were frequent accompaniments of adolescent suicidality. Studies of clinically referred suicide attempters contrasted to non-suicidal psychiatric controls have found increased intrafamilial discord and decreased familial support associated with youthful suicidal behavior (5,6,16,17).

To address these issues, we report on a comparison of a consecutive series of 67 adolescent suicide victims and 67 demographically matched community controls. On the basis of our previous work, and a review of the literature, we hypothesized that suicide completers, compared to community controls, would show:

1. greater familial loading for affective disorder, conduct/antisocial disorder, substance abuse, and suicidal behavior.
2. greater number of familial stressors, including parent-child discord, loss and separation, physical and sexual abuse, and residential instability.
3. lower likelihood to be living with both biologic parents. However, we also hypothesized that family constellation would be related to parental psychopathology and increased number of life stressors, and that familial loading for psychopathology would be more closely associated with suicide than family constellation.

2. MATERIAL AND METHODS

2.1. Cases

The suicide completer sample was drawn from a consecutive series of adolescent suicide victims over a period from July 1986 to August 1990 in the 28 counties of Western Pennsylvania, and has been described in other reports (18). This is a new sample and does not overlap with our previous study (3). The greatest number of suicides came from Allegheny County (35.8%), an area that includes Pittsburgh and its suburbs, and is much more densely populated than the other counties in Western Pennsylvania. Only families of adolescents aged 19 and under who received a definite verdict of suicide were identified for study. The families of the suicide victims were contacted by mail three months after the death, and then by telephone one week later to schedule an interview. Of 91 suicides that occurred over this time period, the families of 67 agreed to participate (73.6%), whereas 8 (8.8%) could not be traced, and 16 (17.6%) refused the interview. Interviews took place a median of five months after the death (M=5.1 months, SD=2.9, range one to 19 months). Primary informants consisted of parents, or a parental figure. Additionally, siblings, and friends were interviewed in a majority of cases. The median number of informants per suicide was four (range one to 14). The majority of interviews took place in the homes of the informants, and the remainder were conducted at Western Psychiatric Institute and Clinic. The completers were older adolescents (age in years, M=17.1; SD=69), mostly white (95.5%), mostly male (85.1%), with median SES (Hollingshead, 1975) of III, and had high lifetime rates of major depression (46.3%), substance abuse (30.3%), and conduct disorder (32.8%).

2.2. Community Controls

Controls were obtained by geographic cluster sampling of communities with similar median income, population density, racial composition, and age distribution to those of suicide victims from October 1989 through March 1991 (19). Nearly complete ascertainment of 38 randomly targeted housing tracts (number of homes assessed = 7,721) was obtained (98%), and 73% of controls approached for the interview agreed to participate. The 67 community controls for this study were drawn from a pool of 129 controls obtained through this sampling procedure, and were individually matched to suicides on age, gender, socioeconomic status (SES; using the Hollingshead Four Factor Scale) (20), and county of residence. The 67 controls who were utilized were representative of the entire sample with respect to age, race, SES, proportion that lived with both biologic parents, and mean Child Behavior Checklist scores (21). Both the community control and at least one parent served as informants. With respect to lifetime diagnoses at the time of interview, community controls showed much lower rates, compared to suicide victims of major depression (13.4%), substance abuse (10.6%), and conduct disorder (13.4%).

Informed consent was obtained from all informants in both groups in accordance with the guidelines of the Psychosocial Institutional Review Board of the University of Pittsburgh.

2.3. Assessment

Family constellation was obtained using a standardized demographic questionnaire (3), and was based on the living arrangement for the previous year. Family stressors were assessed using a standardized interview format about stressful life events (3,19).

Family history of psychiatric disorder was assessed by use of Family History-Research Diagnostic Criteria (FH-RDC) (22), with criteria modified for DSM-III (23). Usually the caretaking parent was directly interviewed and served as the informant; a median of two first-degree relatives (usually father or a sibling in addition to the mother) were directly interviewed. There were no differences in the ages of first- (31.8 [SD=13.5] vs. 31.9 [SD=15.0] years) or second-degree relatives (50.1 [SD=18.2] vs. 52.1 [SD=16.0] years) between groups, nor was there a difference in the proportion of missing data on relatives (2.2% vs. 0.5%, for first degree relatives; 7.7% vs. 3.5% for second-degree relatives). Family histories were obtained by experienced interviewers who were blind to proband diagnosis, but not to proband suicidal status. Diagnoses were reviewed in a diagnostic conference using the best-estimate procedure (24). For the purposes of this study, only psychiatric disorders that were present before the suicide were counted. Inter-rater reliability for diagnoses was monitored throughout this project and remained high (κ=0.98, SD=0.06).

2.4. Data Analysis

The two groups were compared using paired statistics, either McNemar's χ^2, paired t-test, or Wilcoxon's paired sign rank test. The morbid risk of psychiatric disorder in the families of each of the two groups was obtained by the Kaplan-Meier product-limit method (25). The morbid risks were compared between the two groups using the Mantel-Cox and the Generalized Wilcoxon χ^2. For convenience, only Mantel-Cox χ^2 are reported in Table 1, although the Wilcoxon χ^2 gave quite similar results. Log-linear analyses were employed to test for three-way interactions between groups and pairs of familial stressors. The relative contribution of family history, family constellation, and life events was tested by use of paired logistic regression (26). Analyses were performed using BMDP software (27).

3. RESULTS

3.1. Family History

The morbid risks of the following psychiatric disorders were substantially greater in the first-degree relatives of suicide completers than community controls; for any affective disorder (p<0.0001), major depression (p<0.0001), alcohol abuse (p=0.006), drug abuse (p=0.0004), and suicide attempt (p=0.01).

Similar trends were found for the second-degree relatives of completers vs. controls (data available upon request).

3.2. Family Stressors

Suicide victims experienced considerably more familial stress than did community controls within the previous 12 months. Completers were more likely to have experienced

Table 1. Demographic characteristics of suicide probrands and community controls

Characteristics	Suicide probrands (n=58)	Community controls (n=55)
Age mean: ± 95% CL, y	17.2 ± 0.5	17.4 ± 0.5
Gender: M:F	51:7	48:7
Race: white: African American	57:1	55:0
Socioeconomic status, % ± 95% CL		
I	8.6 ± 7.2	1.8 ± 3.5
II	24.1 ± 11.0	20.0 ± 10.6
III	20.7 ± 10.4	30.9 ± 12.2
IV	32.8 ± 12.1	38.2 ± 12.8
V	13.8 ± 8.9	9.1 ± 7.6
From Allegheny County, % ± 95% CL		
Lives with both biological parents	41.4 ± 12.7	38.2 ± 12.8
% ± 95% CL	32.8 ± 12.1	65.5 ± 12.6

conflict with parents (p=0.01), a medically ill parent (p=0.05), parental legal difficulties (p=0.06), physical abuse (p=0.06), and a move from the neighborhood (p=0.02).

In the time before 12 months prior to the suicide, completers also appeared to have experienced many of the same stressors at a greater frequency than did controls: conflict with parents (p=0.02), parental legal trouble (p=0.02), physical abuse (p=0.0002), and a move from neighborhood (p=0.02). Additionally, parents of completers were more likely to have experienced unemployment (p=0.02). Completers experienced more of these events than did controls in the previous year (1.7 [1.4] vs. 1.1 [1.2], Wilcoxon's W=305.0, p=0.001), before the past year (3.5 [2.0] vs. 2.7 [1.6], Wilcoxon's W=432.0, p=0.007), and over their entire lives (4.1 [2.0] vs. 3.1 [1.6], Wilcoxon's W=413.5, p=0.001).

3.3. Family Constellation

A significantly lower proportion of suicide completers lived with both biological parents than did community controls (43.3% vs. 64.2%, χ^2=7.00, p=0.01). In both completers and controls, *not* living with both biological parents was associated with trends towards higher rates of psychiatric disorder in the parents. Completers who did *not* live with both biologic parents, compared to those who did, showed trends towards having fathers with higher rates of any psychiatric disorder (63% vs. 39%, χ^2=3.35, p=0.07) and alcohol abuse (37% vs. 19%, χ^2=2.32, p=0.1), and mothers with higher rates of drug abuse (14% vs. 0%, Fisher's Exact Test, [FET], p=0.07). For controls, not living with both biologic parents was associated with higher rates in fathers of any disorder (33% vs. 12%, χ^2=4.17, p=0.04), alcohol abuse (19% vs. 5%, χ^2=3.44, p=0.06), and suicide attempts (13% vs. 0%, FET, p=0.02) and higher rates among mothers of any disorder (54% vs. 23%, χ^2=6.53, p=0.01), affective disorder (35% vs. 14%, χ^2=3.89, p=0.05), and bipolar spectrum disorder (bipolar I, II, or cyclothymia; 9% vs. 0%, FET, p=0.05).

Family constellation was also related to stressful life events in both completers and controls. Among completers, those who did not live with both parents had more stressful life events in the last 12 months (2.1 [1.5] vs. 1.1 [1.0], Mann Whitney U=762.5, p=0.006), and prior to that (4.3 [2.0] vs. 2.4 [1.5], Mann Whitney U = 849.0, p=0.0003). Among controls, those who did not live with both biological parents had more life events prior to the 12 months before interview (3.6 [1.8] vs. 2.2 [1.2], Mann Whitney U =769.0, p=0.001), with no difference in the number of stressors in the 12 months before assessment (1.3 [1.3] vs. 1.0 [1.2], NS).

3.4. Logistic Regression

Those familial variables that differentiated suicide completers from community controls were examined using log-linear models. No three-way interactions among group, family history variables, and any familial stressor were noted. Therefore, all the familial stressors and family history variables that differentiated completers and controls upon univariate analyses were entered into paired logistic regression equations, without any additional interaction terms, using backwards stepping. Significant familial risk factors for completed suicide include family history of depression (OR=11.0, 95% CI=1.7–70.8), family history of substance abuse (OR=10.4, 95% CI=1.1–100.0), and lifetime history of parent-child discord (OR=5.1, 95% CI=1.2–21.0). A lifetime history of parent-child discord was a more significant risk factor than parent-child discord over just the last 12 months (for the latter, OR=2.7, 95% CI=0.8–8.4).

Family history of psychiatric disorder or other familial stressors might very well be associated with suicide by simply increasing the risk for the development of psychopathology in the suicide victim. Three psychopathological variables: depression, conduct disorder, and substance abuse have been found to be increased in suicide victims vs. controls (3,11,12,18,28). Therefore, these three proband psychopathological variables were entered first into a paired logistic regression, and the additional explanatory power of each of the above-noted familial variables was examined. In separate logistic regressions, family history of depression (OR=14.4, 95% CI=1.5–147.0), and family history of substance abuse (OR=5.1, 95% CI=0.8–34.3), each contributed to risk for suicide, above and beyond proband psychopathology, whereas parent-child discord did not (OR=0.9, 95% CI=0.2–3.5).

4. DISCUSSION

In this study, we have demonstrated a significant association between several familial risk factors and completed suicide in adolescents. Family histories of depression, substance abuse, and suicidal behavior were more common in completers than in controls. Also, family constellation of not living with both biological parents, parent-child discord, parental chronic medical illness, parental legal difficulties, physical abuse, and a move during the past year were related to suicidal risk. When both family history of psychiatric disorders and familial stressors were examined simultaneously, family history of depression and of substance abuse were both closely associated with risk for completed suicide, as was parent-child discord, whereas family constellation was non-contributory. Furthermore, both family history of depression and family history of substance abuse added significantly to risk for completed suicide, even *after* controlling for proband psychopathology.

How does familial loading for psychopathology contribute to the risk of suicide? The most obvious possibility is that familial loading for a given disorder increases the risk of that disorder in the proband, which in turn increases the risk of suicide. In a separate set of analyses, we have shown that a family history of the above-noted disorders is specifically associated with its respective condition in the suicide victim probands (29). Several high-risk and adoption studies show that parental diagnoses of affective illness, substance abuse, conduct disorder, and suicidal behavior are associated with increased risks of these same disorders in offspring (30–38). However, in the present study, familial loading for depression and substance abuse were associated with suicide, even after controlling for proband diagnoses of depression, conduct disorder, and substance abuse. This suggests that familial psychopathology may add to suicidal risk by mechanisms other than simply increasing the risk for similar psychopathology in the proband. For example, Cadoret et al. (34), in an adoption study, noted that a family history of alcohol problems in the adopted fathers increased the risk of depression in the proband. Moreover, in another adoption study, parental affective illness conveyed a 15-fold increased risk of suicide on offspring, which was not explainable simply by concordance of biological relatives for psychopathology (37).

Our data does not allow us to determine how familial psychopathology increases the risk for suicide. Parental psychopathology could decrease the amount of social support available to the proband, and increase the amount of discord in the home, thereby modifying the presentation and course of psychopathology in probands (39). Prospective studies of offspring of depressed parents suggest that the chronicity and degree of exposure to depression or an event such as divorce may alter the course of depressive illness in offspring

(33,40). Furthermore, there is a considerable body of evidence that familial factors influence the course of affective illness in adults (41).

Our findings of an association between parent-child discord and suicide has extensive support in the literature. Parent-child discord may differentiate those who actually attempt suicide from those who merely have ideation or from non-suicidal psychiatric controls (5,6,16). In their longitudinal, high-risk study of offspring of psychiatrically ill parents, Rutter and Quinton (42), found that parent-child hostility was a critical mediating variable between parent and child psychopathology. Moreover, parent-child discord is the most common precipitant for suicide and suicidal behavior (2,3). In the present study, parent-child discord was related to suicide, even *after* controlling for elevated rates of familial psychopathology in the suicide victims relative to controls. Lifetime history of parent-child discord was more closely associated with suicide than was more recent discord, which suggests that parent-child discord exerts its most pernicious effects when it is chronic. However, after controlling for proband psychopathology, parent-child discord made no significant contribution to suicidal risk. It is possible that discord may play an etiological role in psychiatric disorder among youth, and, alternatively, that discord could be the consequence of psychopathology in both youth and their parents.

One important negative finding to emerge is the lack of relationship between family constellation and risk for suicide, after controlling for family history of psychopathology. Much has been made of the role of marital separation and divorce in the genesis of suicidal behavior, and the relationship between the secular trends in divorce and in adolescent suicide (43). However, as we demonstrate in this study, for both suicides and controls, not living with both biological parents is associated with higher rates of parental psychopathology and a greater exposure to stressful life events. Furthermore, after controlling for family history of psychopathology, family constellation did *not* load into the logistic regression equation. Previous studies of assortative mating among affectively disordered patients support the view that marital separation can be a *consequence* of spousal psychiatric illness, and that having a psychiatrically ill spouse may be associated with greater functional impairment in affectively ill patients (44). In our analyses, it would appear that parental psychopathology was a much more significant risk factor for adolescent suicide than was family constellation. This is consistent with other high-risk studies of child and adolescent development that indicate that *quality* of family life is more significant than is family constellation (42,45).

It is important to consider these findings in the context of the strengths and limitations of this study. The strengths of this study include the representativeness of the samples of completers and controls, standardized assessments of familial psychopathology and family stressors, and pairing of closely matched subjects. Limitations of the study include the use of family history method for ascertaining familial psychopathology rather than direct interview, lack of detailed assessment of family environment, and the limitations of a retrospective, case-control study. While the family history approach is not as sensitive as the family study method, it is specific, and is an acceptable alternative to direct interviews of all relatives (46). While we acknowledge that the lack of detailed assessment of the family environment is a weakness of this study, we felt that only the most global aspects of family environment could be assessed retrospectively, especially after a suicide. This leads to the final limitation, that of design. A case-control study can only point to associations, but can never determine the direction of causality. A high-risk prospective study of offspring of psychiatrically ill parents is required to illuminate how family history, intra-familial discord, and proband psychopathology are related to suicidal risk.

These findings have important implications for the prevention of suicide, the clinical management of youth at risk for suicide, and for further research. First, the children of depressed or substance abusing parents appear to be at substantially increased risk for completed suicide. It is vital that the offspring of adults with these psychiatric disorders be screened because their risk of mental disorder and impairment is so high (30–33,35,39). Second, these data highlight the importance of assessing, and referring for treatment if necessary, psychiatrically ill parents of suicidal youth. If psychiatric illness in parents increases the risk of suicide above and beyond proband psychopathology, then failure to treat the psychiatrically impaired parents of clinically referred ill youth could undercut even the most ostensibly effective individually-oriented treatment. Third, parent-child discord must be addressed in the context of the treatment of youth at risk for suicide. Family-based treatments designed to reduce parent-child discord and parental psychopathology are likely to be essential components of effective treatments for youth at high risk for suicide. These results also suggest that such family interventions may be effective in attenuating the impact of parental psychiatric illness on youthful offspring, and may serve as useful forms of preventive intervention (47). Finally, prospective studies of offspring of substance abusing and affectively ill parents are likely to be helpful in precisely formulating the mechanisms whereby risk for suicide is familially transmitted, and thereby enabling the development of more precise and effective preventive interventions.

ACKNOWLEDGMENTS

This work was supported in part by the William T. Grant Foundation, #86-1063, and two awards from the National Institute of Mental Health: MH:44711 "Youth Exposed to Suicide," and MH#43366, "Adolescent Family Study." The authors gratefully acknowledge the assistance of Karen Rhinaman in preparing this manuscript. A special thanks to Satish Iyengar, Ph.D. for his helpful editorial comments and statistical consultation.

REFERENCES

1. Sabbath JC. The role of the partents in adolescent suicidal behaviour. Acta paedopsychiatr 1971: 38: 211–220
2. Hawton K, Cole D, O'Grady J, Osborn M. Motivaltionbal aspects of deliberate self-poisoning in adolescents. Br J Psychiatry 1982: 141: 286–291
3. Brent DA, Perper JA, Goldstein CE et al. Risk factors for adolescent suicide: a comparison of adolescent suicide victims with suicidal inpatients. Arch Gen Psychiatry 1988: 45: 581–588.
4. Cohen-Sandler R, Berman AL, King RA. Life stress and symptomatology: determinants of suicidal behaviour in children. J Am Acad Child Psychiatry 1982: 21: 178–186.
5. Kosky R, Silburn S, Zubrick SR. Are childre and adolescents who have suicidal thoughts different from those who attempt suicide? J Nerv Ment Dis 1990" 178: 38–43
6. Taylor EA, Stansfeld SA. Children who poison themselves. I. A clinical comparison with psychiatric controls. Br Psychiatry 1984: 145: 127–135.
7. Garfinkel BD, Froese A, Hood J. Suicide attempts in children and adolescents. Am J Psychiatry 1982: 139: 1257–1261.
8. Friedman RC, Corn R, Hurt SW, Fibel B, Schulick J, Swirksky S. Family history of illness in the seriously suicidal adolescent: a life-cycle approach. Am J Orthopsychiatry 1984: 54: 390–397.
9. Brent DA, Kolko DJ, Goldstein CE, Allan MJ, Brown RV. Suicidality in affectively disordered adolescent inpatients. J Am Acad Child Adolsc Psychiatry 1990: 29:586–593.
10. Pfeffer CR. The suicidal child. new York: Guilford Press, 1986.

11. Shafil M, Carrigan S, Whittinghill JR, Derrick AM. Psychological autopsy of completed suicide in children and adolescents. Am J Psychiatry 1985: 142: 161–1064
12. Shaffer D, Garland A, Gould M, Fisher P, Trautman P. Preventing teenage suicide: a critical review. J Am Acad Child Adolesc Psychiatry 1988: 27: 675–687
13. Kashani JH, Goddard P, Reid JC. Correlates of suicidal ideation in a community sample of children and adolescents. J Am Acad Child Adolesc Psychiatry 1989: 28: 912–917.
14. Joffe RT, Offord DR, Boyle MH. Ontario child health study: suicidal behaviour in youth age 12–16 years. Am J Psychiatry 1988: 145: 1420–1423
15. Hibbard RA, Brack CJ, Rauch S, Orr DO. Abuse, feelings, and health behaviours in a student population. Am J Dis Child 1988: 142: 326–330
16. Asarnow JR, Carlson G. Suicide attempts in preadolescent child psychiatry inpatients. Syuicide Life Threat Behav 1988: 18: 129–136
17. Topol P, Reznikoff M. Perceived peer and family relationships, hopelessness and locus of control as factors in adolescent suicide attempts. Suicide Life Threat Behav 1982: 12: 141–150
18. Brent DA, Perper JA, Moritz G et al. Psychiatric risk factors for adolescent suicide: a case control study. J Am Acad Child Adolesc Psychiatry 1993: 32: 521–529
19. Brent DA, Perper JA, Moritz G et al. Psychiatric effects of exposure to suicide among the friends and acquaintances of adolescent suicide victims. J Am Acad Child Adolesc Psychiatry 1992: 31: 629–640
20. Hollingshead A. Four-factor index of social status. New Haven: Yale University, 1975
21. Achenbach TM, Edelbrock CS. Manual for Child Behaviour Checklist and revised Child Behaviour Profile. Burlington, VT: Department of Psychiatry, University of Vermont, 1983.
22. Andreasen NC, Endicott J, Spitzer RL, Winokur G. The family history method using research diagnostic criteria: reliability and validity. Arch Gen Psychiatry 1977: 34: 1229–1235
23. American Psychiatric Association. Diagnostic and statistical manual of mental disorders. 3rd edn. Washington, DC: APA, 1980
24. Leckman JF, Sholomskas D, Thompson D, Belanger A, Weissman MM. Best estimate of lifetime diagnosis: a methodological study. Arch Gen Psychiatyr 1982: 39: 879–883
25. Kaplan EL, Meier P. Nonparametric estimation from incomplete observations. J Am Statist Assoc 1958: 53: 457–481
26. Breslow NE, Day N. Statistical methods in cancer research: the analysis of case-control studies. Vol 1. Lyon: IARC Scientific Pulbications No 32, 1980: 248–279
27. Dixon WJ. BMDP statistical software manual. Berkeley: University of California Press, 1990
28. Shafii M, Steltz-Lenarsky J, Derrick AM, Beckner C, Whittinghill JR. Comorbidity of mental disorders in the post-mortem diagnosis of completed suicide in children and adolescents. J Affective Disord 1988: 15: 227–233
29. Brent DA, Perper JA, Moritz G et al. The validity of diagnoses obtained through the psychological autopsy procedure: use of family history. Acta Psychiatr Scand 1993: 87: 118–122
30. Weissman MM, John K, Merikangas KR et al. Depressed parents and their children: general health, social and psychiatric problems. Am J Dis Child 1986: 140: 801–805
31. Weissman MM, Gammon D, John K et al. Children of depressed parents: increased psychopathology and early onset of major depression. Arch Gen Psychiatry 1987: 44: 847–853
32. Hammen C, Burge D, Burney E, Adrian C. Longitudinal study of diagnoses in children of women with unipolar and bipolar affective disorder. Arch Gen Psychiatry 1990: 47:1112–1117
33. Keller MB, Beardslee WR, Dorer DJ et al. Impact of severity and chronicity of parental affective illness on adaptive functioning and psychopathology in children. Arch Gen Psychiatry 1986: 43: 930–937
34. Cadoret RJ, O'Gorman TW, Heywood E, Troughton E. Genetic and environmental factors in major depression. J Affective Disord 1985: 9: 155–164
35. Orvaschel H, Walsh-Allsi G, Ye W. Psychopathology in children of parents with recurrent depression. J Abnorm Child Psychol 1988: 16: 17–28
36. Schulsinger F, Kety SS, Rosenthal D, Wender PH. A family study of suicide. In: Schou M, Stromgren E, ed. Origin, prevention and treatment of affective disorders. London: Academic Prtess, 1979: 277–287
37. Wender PH, Kety SS, Rosenthal D, Schulsinger F, Ortmann J, Lunde I. Psychiatric disorders in the biological and adoptive families of adopted individuals with affective disorders. Arch Gen Psychiatry 1986: 43: 923–929
38. Beardslee WR, Keller MB, Lavori PW, Klerman GK, Dorer DJ, Samuelson H. Psychiatric disorder in adolescent offspring of parents with affective disorder in a non-referred sample. J Affective Disord 1988: 15: 313–322
39. Downey G, Coyne JC. Children of depressed parents. An integrative review. Psychiatr Bull 1990: 108: 50–76

40. Warner V, Weissman MM, Fendrich M, Wickramaratne P, Moreau D. The course of major depression in the offspring of depressed parents: incidence, recurrence and recovery. Arch Gen Psychiatry 1992: 49: 795–801

41. Keitner G, Miller I. Family functioning and major depression: an overview. Am J Psychiatry 1990: 147: 1128–1137

42. Rutter M, Quinton D. Parental psychiatric disorder: effects on children. Psychol Med 1984: 14: 853–880

43. McAnarney ER. Adolescent and young adult suicide in the United States: a reflection of societal unrest? Adolescence 1979: 14: 765–774

44. Merikangas KR, Bromet EJ, Spiker DG. Assortive mating, social adjustment and course of illness in primary affective disorder. Arch Gen Psychiatry 1983: 40: 795–800

45. Rutter M,. Resilience in the face of adversity: protective factors and resistance to psychiatric disorder. Br J Psychiatry 1985: 147: 598–611

46. Andreasen NC, Rice J, Endicott J, Reich T, Coryell W. The family history approach to diagnosis: how useful it is? Arch Gen Psychiatry 1986: 43: 421–429

47. Beardslee WR, Salt P, Porterfield K, Clark-Rothbert P et al. Comparison of preventive interventions for families with parental affective disorder. J Am Acad Child Adolesc Psychiatry 1993: 32: 254–263

9

SUICIDAL BEHAVIOR RUNS IN FAMILIES

A Controlled Family Study of Adolescent Suicide Victims

David A. Brent, Jeff Bridge, Barbara A. Johnson, and John Connolly

Western Psychiatric Institute and Clinic
Pittsburgh, Pennsylvania

1. BACKGROUND. While previous studies have shown an increased rate of suicidal behavior in the relatives of suicide victims, it is unclear if this is attributable merely to increased familial rates of psychiatric disorder. Therefore, we conducted a family study of adolescent suicide victims (suicide probands) and community control probands (controls) to determine if the rates of suicidal behavior were higher in the relatives of adolescent suicide probands even after adjusting for differences in the familial rates of psychiatric disorder.

2. METHOD. The relatives of 58 adolescent suicide probands and 55 demographically similar controls underwent assessment as to Axis I and II psychiatric disorders, lifetime history of aggression, and history of suicidal behavior (attempts and completions) using a combination of family study and family history approaches.

3. RESULTS. The rate of suicide attempts was increased in the first-degree relatives of suicide probands, compared to the relatives of controls, even after adjusting for differences in rates of proband and familial Axis I and II disorders (OR=4.3, 95% CI, 1.1–16.6). On the other hand, the excess rate of suicidal ideation found in the relatives of suicide probands was explained by increased familial rates of psychopathology disorders. Among suicide probands, higher ratings of aggression were associated with higher familial loading for suicide attempts.

4. CONCLUSION. Liability to suicidal behavior might be familially transmitted as a trait independent of Axis I and II disorders. The transmitted spectrum of suicidal behavior includes attempts and completions, but not ideation, and the transmission of suicidal behavior and aggression is related.

1. INTRODUCTION

The aggregation of suicide and suicide attempts in the families of suicide victims is well known, and has been demonstrated in the relatives of both adolescent (1,2) and adult suicides.(3,4,5) Adoption and twin studies have also demonstrated a concordance between biological relatives for suicide (6,7).

The familial clustering of suicidal behavior also extends to the relatives of prepubertal children,(8) adolescents,(9) and adults (10,11) who attempt suicide. Furthermore, those who make the most lethal attempts are most likely to have a positive family history of suicide,(9,10) suggesting a shared familial liability for suicide attempts and completions.

Family history of substance abuse, depression, antisocial and other personality disorders, and assaultive behavior have also been linked to suicidal behavior (8,12–14) Two reports support the view that the familial transmission of suicide is independent of the transmission of either affective illness[5] or "endogenous psychosis"(4,5). However, no published study has examined the familial aggregation of suicidal behavior while controlling for all of these psychopathological conditions. Therefore, we undertook a family study of adolescent suicide victims (suicide probands) and demographically similar community control probands (controls) to test the following hypotheses:

1. The relatives of suicide probands, compared to the relatives of community controls, will show a greater prevalence of suicide and suicidal attempts, even after controlling for an expected increased rates of Axis I disorders.
2. The familial aggregation of suicidal behavior in the relatives of suicide probands will be explained by the familial aggregation of impulsive-aggressive (Cluster B) personality disorders, and tendency to aggressive behavior.
3. The prevalence of suicide and suicidal behavior will be higher among the relatives of suicide probands with high intent completions, violent completions (i.e., firearms, hanging, jumping), and high levels of aggression.

2. METHODS

2.1. Sample

The sample consists of the first degree reatives (mothers, fathers, siblings) and second-degree relatives (grandparents, uncles, aunts, half-siblings) of adolescent suicide probands victims and demographically matched adolescent community controls.

2.2. Suicide Victims

The fifty-eight adolescent suicide probands were a consecutive series who died within a 28-county region of Western Pennsylvania, and were assigned a definite verdict of suicide. They represent 78% of all those available during the recruitment period, from July 1989 through May 1994. The suicide probands whose families accepted participation in the study did not differ from refusers with respect to age, gender, race, county of origin, or method of suicide.

2.3. Controls

Fifty-eight controls were recruited from an original pool of 173 adolescents obtained by geographic cluster sampling that matched control communities to those of suicide probands with respect to age, gender, median income, population density, racial composition.

Almost all controls 59 of 60, (98%) consented to the interview and of these 55 of 59 (93%) of all available controls agreed to participate in the family study. Subsequently, it was found that 3 controls had made serious suicide attempts and we eliminated these subjects from the control cell, leaving 55 controls. No differences were found between accepters and refusers with respect to age, race, gender, county of origin, family constellation, and socioeconomic status (15).

2.4. Relation of Sample to Other Reports

Forty-three suicide probands and (40) controls have been described previously, but no data on relatives were reported (16). Family history data have previously been reported on (16) suicide probands and (34) controls, but no family study data have been reported on this sample (13).

2.5. Comparison of Suicide Victims and Controls

As noted on Table 1, the two groups were similar with respect to age, gender, race, socioeconomic status, and county of origin, but fewer of the suicide probands than controls lived with both biological parents (p=0.002). As has been previously reported, (19) suicide probands showed higher rates than did controls on a broad range of psychiatric disorders (Table 2).

2.6. Relatives

The sample under study in this report are the first and second-degree relatives of the probands: 203 first-degree and 607 second-degree relatives of 58 suicide probands and 207 first-degree relatives and 558 second-degree relatives of 55 controls. As noted in Table 3, there were no differences between the groups in mean pedigree size, number of direct interviews per family, gender or age distribution of the relatives, or proportion with missing data with two exceptions; the proportion of missing data from the first-degree

Table 1. Demographic characteristics of suicide probands and community controls*

Characteristics	Suicide probands (n-58)	Community controls (n=55)
Age mean ± 95% CL,y	17.2–0.5	17.4–0.5
Gender—M:F	51:7	48:7
Race—White:African American	57:1	55:0
Socioeconomic status, % ± 95%CL[†]		
I	8.6–7.2	1.8–3.5
II	24.1–11.0	20.0–10.6
III	20.7–10.4	30.9–12.2
IV	32.8–12.1	38.2–12.8
V	3.8–8.9	9.1–7.6
From Allegheny County, % ± 95%CL	41.4–12.7	38.2–12.8
Lives with biological parents, % ± 95%CL	32.8–12.1	65.5–12.6[‡]

*CL indicates confidence limit
[†]Defined in Hollingshead[15]
[‡]P<.005

Table 2. Diagnostic and clinical characteristics of adolescent completers and community controls (% 95% CI)

Diagnosis	Suicide probands (n=58)	Controls (n=55)
Axis I disorder	77.6–10.7	18.5–10.4[†‡]
Any affective disorder	36.2–10.0	0.0–0.0[†‡]
Major depressive disorder	29.3–11.7	0.0–10.0[†‡]
Dysthymia	12.1–8.4	0.0–0.0[§]
Substance abuse	36.8–12.5	5.6–6.1[†‡]
Alcohol abuse	32.8–12.1	5.6–6.1[†‖]
Other drugs	14.3–9.2	0.0–0.0[‖]
Conduct disorder	38.6–12.6	5.5–6.0[†‡]
Any anxiety disorder	17.2–9.7	1.9–3.6
Any personality disorder (PD)	19.0–10.1	0.0–0.0[†‖]
Cluster A[#]	1.7–3.3	0.0–0.0
Cluster B**	8.6–7.2	0.0–0.0
Cluster C[††]	10.5–8.0	0.0–0.0[§]
Assaultive behavior	28.1–11.7	10.9–8.2[§]
Brown-Goodwin Lifetime History of Aggression (M ± 95% CI)	13.2 2.7	4.9–1.6[†‡]
Buss-Durkee Hostility Inventory–Assault (M ± 95% CI)	15.9 0.9	14.5–0.7[§]
Buss-Durkee Hostility Inventory–Irritability (M ± 95% CI)	16.6 0.9	14.4–0.8[†‖]

*Unless otherwise indicated, data are given as % ± 95% confidence limit (CL)
[†]Significant at the alpha <.05 level with Bonferroni correction
[‡]$P \leq .001$
[§]<.05
[‖]<.005
[¶]<.01
[#]Includes paranoid, schizoid and schizotypal
** Includes antisocial, borderline, histrionic and narcissistic
[††]Includes avoidant, passive-aggressive, obsessive-compulsive and dependent

relatives of suicide probands was greater than from the relatives of controls (5.0% vs. 0.5%, p=.005) and the second-degree relatives of controls were slightly older (p=0.02).

3. RECRUITMENT AND INTERVIEW PROCEDURE

3.1. Assessment of Suicide Probands and Controls

Approximately one to two months after the suicide, the families of suicide probands were sent a letter expressing our condolences and inviting family members to participate in the study. This letter was followed up one week later by a telephone call from the project clinician responsible for the interview. Families who did not have a telephone were sent an additional postcard to be returned to the clinician that indicated their willingness to participate and how they were to be contacted. On average, the interview took place 5–3 months after the suicide (range = 1.8–15.0 months). For each of the suicide probands, the primary caretaking parent (or parental figure, e.g., grandparent or older sibling) served as the main informant. In addition, siblings, friends, other relatives, and professional contacts were interviewed, with a median of five informants per subject (range 1 to 9). Pre-

Table 3. Demographic characteristics of relatives of completers and community controls

Characteristics	Suicide probands (n=58)	Controls (n=55)
Pedigree size, No. of members (M 95% CI)	14.1–1.2	13.9–1.1
Direct interviews per family (M 95% CI)	5.0–0.8	4.3–0.5
Direct interview (% 95% CI)		
Father	53.4–12.8	58.2–13.0
Mother	81.0–10.1	92.7–6.9
Sibling	72.4–9.4	72.2–8.9
First-degree relatives		
Number of relatives	203	207
Gender number M:F	98:105	100:107
Age (Mean=95% CI; years)	31.8–2.2	31.9–2.1
Father	44.0–2.2	45.9–1.9
Mother	42.1–1.7	43.0–1.5
Sibling	17.2–1.5	17.8–1.0
Missing data (% 95% CI)	4.7–3.0	0.5–1.0[‡]
Father	5.2–5.7	0.0–0.0
Mother	5.2–5.7	0.0–0.0
Sibling	4.2–4.5	1.1–2.2
Second-degree relatives No.	607	558
Gender M:F	304:303	276:282
Age (M 95% CI; years)	49.9–1.4	52.1–1.4[†]
Missing data (%)	7.5–2.1	8.6–2.4

M mean
CI confidence interval
[†] p0.05
[‡] p0.01

vious work has indicated that the diagnoses obtained by the psychological autopsy procedure are both reliable, valid, and unaffected by state of bereavement of the informant (18,19). Psychiatric and demographic data were obtained on the controls from the caretaking parent and by self-report proband.

3.2. Interview Procedure with Relatives

Upon agreeing to participate in the family study, the caretaking parent provided the names, telephone numbers, and addresses of all first- and second-degree relatives, and gave permission for an interviewer to contact them.

3.3. Diagnostic Procedure

All interviewers were master's level clinicians who had been given extensive training in the administration of semi-structured interviews. Best-estimate diagnoses were made by consensus and utilized all available sources in diagnostic conferences chaired by two of the authors (Drs. David Brent or Barbara Johnson) (20). Discrepancies between informants were resolved by reinterview of all informants until consensus could be obtained. Diagnostic assessment and best-estimate conferences were conducted without knowledge of the subject's diagnostic status. Interrater reliability for direct and family history interviews for Axis I and Axis II were high throughout the study (k's 0.79–0.95).

Informed consent for all interviews was obtained as approved by the Psychosocial Institutional Review Board of the University of Pittsburgh.

4. ASSESSMENT

4.1. Axis I Psychiatric Diagnoses

The School Age Schedule for Affective Disorders and Schizophrenia, Epidemiologic and Present versions (K-SADS-E and P) (21,22) were used to assess lifetime and current symptoms and corresponding DSM-III diagnoses (23) for all suicide probands, controls, and for directly interviewed relatives younger than 18 years. All directly interviewed adult first- and second-degree relatives underwent assessment for the presence of past and current psychiatric disorder by use of the Schedule for Affective Disorders and Schizophrenia-Lifetime Version (SADS-L) (24). The Family History-Research Diagnostic Criteria (FH-RDC) method (25) was used to obtain information from those relatives directly interviewed regarding all other first and second-degree relatives, with diagnostic criteria modified from Research Diagnostic Criteria to DSM-III criteria. Because it is known that loss of a family member can increase the risk of subsequent depression, (26,27) we only report disorders in relatives of suicide probands that had a clear onset prior to the suicide.

4.2. Axis II Psychiatric Disorder

The Structured Clinical Interview for the DSM-III-R Diagnosis of Personality Disorders (SCID-II-R) (28) was utilized to assess DSM-III-R29 personality disorders in all suicide probands, controls, and directly interviewed relatives older than 13 years. A subset of questions on the interview was modified to make them more appropriate for adolescents. Reliability and validity for this interview have been established previously for adults (29) and for adolescent (16,30). Based on previous analyses, personality disorder assessment in relatives was restricted to avoidant, antisocial, and borderline personality disorder (16,31) In addition, questions from the informant version of the SCID-II-R about these three personality disorders were added to the FH-RDC interview, allowing us to obtain information about personality disorders on all relatives in the pedigree.

4.3. Suicidal Intent

The Beck Suicidal Intent Scale was used to assess suicidal intent among the suicide victims (32,33) We report on only the first nine items, relevant to observable behavior, which were administered to the completer informant(s).

4.4. Definition of Suicidal Behavior

A suicide attempt was defined as intentional self-harm that is not self-mutilatory in nature. On both the K-SADS and SADS-L, this corresponds to a rating of at least "2" on the medical lethality question of Suicide Attempt section. Data were also gathered on history of suicidal ideation, which for the purposes of this study refers to suicidal thoughts or threats. All relatives were classified on the basis of their most serious suicidal episode.

4.5. Measures of Aggression

The Brown-Goodwin Assessment for Lifetime History of Aggression (BG-LHA), a 12-item interview was administered to suicide proband and control proband informants and directly interviewed relatives older than 13 years (34,35) In this study, internal consistency of the BG-LHA was acceptable (Cronbach's a = 0.78). The Assault and Irritability subscales of the Buss-Durkee Hostility Inventory, (36) a self-report measure of aggressive personality traits, was filled out by the same informants as received the BG-LHA. Internal consistency was adequate for both the Assault and Irritability subscales (a's=0.66, and 0.69, respectively). These measures are associated with suicidal behavior and changes in central serotonergic metaboliSM (34,35,37). These self-report questionnaires (filled out by parents) were missing for more suicide probands than controls (33% vs. 9%, c2=9.45, p=0.002), and more first-degree relatives of suicide probands than for relatives of controls (25% vs. 9%, c2 = 12.08, p=0.0005). We were concerned that these data might not be "missing at random." Therefore, we modelled substitution of extreme scores (>75th percentile) for all missing data with no substantial change in the results. Therefore, data are reported without the substitution.

4.6. History of Assaultive Behavior

History of assaultive behavior on suicide probands, controls, and directly interviewed pedigree members was obtained through the assessment of behavioral indicators taken from all available sources (BG-LHA, K-SADS, SADS-L, SCID-II-R, FH-RDC). For all other relatives, history of assaultive behavior was obtained from the FH-RDC.

5. DATA ANALYSES

All dependent measures were compared between the relatives of suicide probands and those of the community controls using standard univariate parametric and non-parametric methods. For dichotomous outcomes, Pearson's c2 test was employed. When any one cell had an expected value of <5 or when there was a zero cell, Fisher's exact test was used. For continuous outcomes, either a two-sample t-test or, when the distribution was skewed, the non-parametric equivalent, the Mann-Whitney U test, was utilized.

The rate suicide of attempts and completions for first and second-degree relatives was compared between groups using either Pearson's c2 or Fisher's exact test. The age-corrected lifetime rates of attempts and completions between the two groups of relatives were compared using Kaplan-Meier analyseS (38). The results using both c2 and Kaplan-Meier analyses were similar, so that only the former are reported, although both approaches are displayed in Table 4. To determine whether rates of attempts/completions differed between relatives after adjustment on other psychopathological variables (e.g., rates of Axis I disorder, assaultive behavior etc.), logistic regression was used. Adjusted hazard ratios were derived from Cox proportional hazards regression models, using the same analytic scheme as was used for the logistic regression analyse (39).

The familial rate of a disorder was determined by taking the ratio of the number of affected relatives over the total number of relatives (i.e. "pooled" data). In addition, we conducted analyses using the family as the unit of analysis, wherein if at least one first-degree relative had attempted suicide, that family was considered positive for suicide attempt. Comparisons between groups using the family as the unit of analysis yielded

Table 4. Lifetime psychiatric diagnosis in first-degree and second-degree relatives of completers and controls*

Diagnosis	Rate % ± 95% CL		MR ± 95% CL	
	Completers (N = 58)	Controls (N = 55)	Completers (N = 58)	Controls (N = 55)
Any axis I disorder				
1st degree	63.6 ± 6.9	52.7 ± 6.9[†]	0.81 ± 0.08˙	0.76 ± 0.10
2nd degree	48.8 ± 4.2	37.9 ± 4.3[‡]	0.57 ± 0.06	0.45 ± 0.06[§]
Any affective disorder				
1st degree	34.8 ± 6.8	25.5 ± 6.0[†]	0.43 ± 0.10	0.32 ± 0.08
2nd degree	20.8 ± 3.4	12.9 ± 2.9[‡]	0.21 ± 0.04	0.13 ± 0.04[§]
Major Depressive disorder				
1st degree	24.5 ± 6.1	18.0 ± 5.3	0.29 ± 0.08	0.21 ± 0.06
2nd degree	14.7 ± 3.0	10.4 ± 2.7[†]	0.14 ± 0.04	0.11 ± 0.04
Dysthymia				
1st degree	12.7 ± 4.7	6.3 ± 3.3[†]	0.17 ± 0.08	0.09 ± 0.06[†]
2nd degree	6.3 ± 2.0	2.8 ± 1.4[§]	0.07 ± 0.02	0.03 ± 0.02[†]
Mania				
1st degree	1.1 ± 1.5	0.5 ± 1.0	0.01 ± 0.02	0.01 ± 0.02
2nd degree	0.7 ± 0.7	0.2 ± 0.4	0.00 ± 60.007	0.002 ± 0.005
Hypomania				
1st degree	2.1 ± 2.0	1.0 ± 1.4	0.02 ± 0.02	0.01 ± 0.01
2nd degree	0.7 ± 0.7	0.2 ± 0.4	0.00 ± 50.006	0.00 ± 0.00
Any anxiety disorder				
1st degree	20.8 ± 5.9	18.6 ± 5.3	0.30 ± 0.10	0.32 ± 0.12
2nd degree	12.7 ± 2.8	4.9 ± 3.0[‡]	0.15 ± 0.04	0.07 ± 0.02[‡]
Alcohol abuse				
1st degree	26.5 ± 6.3	21.5 ± 5.6	0.29 ± 0.08	0.31 ± 0.10
2nd degree	20.5 ± 3.4	16.9 ± 3.3	0.21.04	0.16 ± 0.04
Other drug abuse				
1st degree	5.9 ± 3.4	2.4 ± 2.1	0.06 ± 0.04	0.02 ± 0.02[†]
2nd degree	6.2 ± 2.0	2.6 ± 1.4[§]	0.06 ± 0.02	0.03 ± 0.02[†]
Conduct disorder				
1st degree	16.8 ± 5.4	7.4 ± 3.6[∥]	0.19 ± 0.08	0.13 ± 0.08
2nd degree	8.5 ± 2.4	3.7 ± 1.7[∥]	0.09 ± 0.04	0.05 ± 0.04[†]
Any personality disorder (PD)				
1st degree	11.5 ± 4.6	5.1 ± 3.1[†]		
2nd degree	8.6 ± 2.3	2.4 ± 1.3[‡]		
Antisocial PD_				
1st degree	3.8 ± 2.8	0.0 ± 0.0[§]		
2nd degree	3.3 ± 1.5	0.8 ± 0.8[∥]		
Avoidant PD_				
1st degree	6.0 ± 3.5	4.6 ± 2.9		
2nd degree	4.6 ± 1.8	1.6 ± 1.1[§]		
Borderline PD_				
1st degree	2.2 ± 2.1	0.5 ± 1.0		
2nd degree	1.8 ± 1.1	0.4 ± 0.6[†]		
Suicide attempt				
1st degree	10.6 ± 4.4	2.4 ± 2.1[‡]	0.14 ± 0.06	0.03 ± 0.02[∥]
2nd degree	4.6 ± 1.8	1.4 ± 1.0[∥]	0.04 ± 0.02	0.01 ± 0.01[§]
Suicide completion				
1st degree	1.1 ± 1.5	0.0 ± 0.0	0.01 ± 0.02	0.00 ± 0.00
2nd degree	0.4 ± 0.5	0.0 ± 0.0	0.00 ± 40.01	0.00 ± 0.00
Suicide ideation				
1st degree	14.7 ± 5.0	8.2 ± 3.7[†]	0.22 ± 0.14	0.09 ± 0.04
2nd degree	7.6 ± 2.2	4.5 ± 1.8[†]	0.07 ± 0.02	0.04 ± 0.02

Table 4. (*Continued*)

Diagnosis	Rate % ± 95% CL		MR ± 95% CL	
	Completers (N = 58)	Controls (N = 55)	Completers (N = 58)	Controls (N = 55)
Assaultive behavior				
1st degree	24.5 ± 6.1	15.5 ± 4.9[†]	0.30 ± 0.08	0.18 ± 0.06[†]
2nd degree	17.2 ± 3.2	7.5 ± 2.3[‡]	0.15 ± 0.04	0.05 ± 0.02[‡]
Brown-Goodwin Lifetime History Measures of Aggression[¶]				
1st degree	5.9 ± 1.1	4.8 ± 0.8		
2nd degree	3.8 ± 0.8	4.2 ± 1.2		
Buss-Durkee Hostility Inventory, Assault Subscale[¶]				
1st degree	14.4 ± 0.5	14.0 ± 0.4		
2nd degree	13.0 ± 0.5	12.7 ± 0.5		
Buss-Durkee Hostility Inventory, Irritability Subscale[¶]				
1st degree	15.6 ± 0.6	15.3 ± 0.4		
2nd degree	14.6 ± 0.5	13.8 ± 0.5		

*Data on mothers, fathers, and siblings are available upon request.
CL indicates confidence limit; PD Personality disorder.
[†]$P \leq .05$
[‡] $P < .001$
[§]$P < .01$
[‖]$P < .005$
[¶]Morbid risk not applicable
#Measured as mean ± 95% CL

essentially the same results as the polled data strategy. Therefore, we report only the "pooled" approach to assessing familial rates. Analyses were computed using the 1990 version of the BMDP software (40).

6. RESULTS

6.1. Suicidal Behavior

The rate of suicide attempts or completions (almost all were attempts, see Table 4) was significantly higher in the first-degree relatives of suicide proband than in the first-degree relatives of controls (11.6% vs. 2.4%, $c2 = 13.1$, $p = 0.0003$, odds ratio [OR]=5.3, 95% confidence interval [CI], 2.0–14.3). The familial rates of attempts or completions were significantly elevated in mothers (18.2 vs. 3.6, $c2=5.99$, $p=0.01$), and siblings (11.0 vs. 2.1, $c2=6.12$, $p=0.01$), with a non-significant trend in the same direction for fathers (5.7 vs. 1.8, $c2=1.12$, $p=0.29$). The rate of suicidal ideation was also higher in relatives of completers than controls (14.7% vs. 8.2%, $c2=4.20$, $p=0.04$).

Second-degree relatives of suicide probands were also found to have higher rates of suicide attempts and completions than relatives of controls: (4.9% vs. 1.4%, $c2 = 10.81$, $p = 0.001$, OR=3.7, 95% CI = 1.6–8.7). The rate of suicidal ideation was higher in relatives of suicide probands than controls (7.6% vs. 4.5%, $c2=4.63$, $p=0.03$).

6.2 Axis I and II Disorders in Relatives

First-degree relatives of suicide probands reported similar rates of most Axis I and II disorders but significant differences between these two groups were found for any Axis I disorder (p=0.03), affective disorder (p=0.45), dysthymia (p=0.03), conduct disorder (p = 0.004), and antisocial personality disorder (p=0.006), largely in keeping with our original hypotheses. Directly interviewed relatives of suicide probands and controls did not differ on any of the three measures of impulsive aggression (the BG-LHA, or the two Buss-Durkee Hostility Inventory subscales), although relatives of suicide probands showed significantly higher lifetime rates of assaultive behavior (p=0.02).

Among second-degree relatives, higher rates of disorder were also found in families of suicide probands vs. controls, with increases in any affective disorder (p=0.001), substance abuse disorder (p=0.05), conduct disorder (p=0.001), anxiety disorder (p<0.001), antisocial (p=0.005), avoidant (p=0.006), and borderline personality disorders (p's=0.03–0.005), and assaultive behavior (p<0.001).

7. RISK OF SUICIDAL BEHAVIOR IN FIRST-DEGREE RELATIVES ADJUSTING FOR OTHER PSYCHIATRIC CONDITIONS

7.1. First-Degree Relatives

A greater risk of attempts/completions persisted in the relatives of suicide probands even after controlling for differences between the relatives with respect to lifetime Axis I psychopathology (i.e., affective and conduct disorder; [OR = 5.2, 95%, CI = 1.7 - 15.8]). The increased odds of suicidal behavior in the relatives of suicide vs control probands persisted after controlling for differences in rates of Axis I disorder (i.e., affective and conduct disorder, Axis II disorder, and assaultive behavior [OR=4.5, 95% CI = 1.5–14.1]). Inclusion of proband psychiatric disorder and other traits as additional covariates did not substantially change any of these analyses (OR=4.3, 95% CI = 1.1 to 16.6). On the other hand, when controlling for these variables, the rate of suicidal ideation was no longer significantly increased in the relatives of suicide probands (OR=1.6, 95% CI = 0.5–5.1). Parallel analyses, using Cox proportional hazards regression, showed similar results (suicidal behavior in relatives, OR=5.3, 95% CI, 1.4–21.0; for suicidal ideation in relatives OR=1.1, 95% CI, 0.4–3.1).

7.2. Second-Degree Relatives

Among second-degree relatives, greater risk of attempts and completion in relatives of suicide probands persisted after controlling for familial Axis I covariates (i.e., affective, substance abuse, conduct, and anxiety disorders [OR=2.4, 95% CI = 1.0 - 5.8]). When logistic regression included Axis I and II disorders (avoidant, borderline, and antisocial) and assaultive behavior as covariates, the risk of suicidal behavior in relatives of suicide probands was increased but the CI included unity (OR=2.3, 95% CI, 0.9–5.7). The rate of suicidal ideation was not different between the two groups when adjusting for the above-noted familial and proband differences (OR=1.0, 95% CI 0.4–2.3). Parallel analyses, using Cox proportional hazards regression showed similar results (for suicidal behavior in relatives, OR=2.2, 95%CI, 0.5–10.9; suicidal ideation in relatives, OR=1.3, 95%CI, 0.6–2.9).

8. CHARACTERISTICS OF SUICIDE PROBANDS AND FAMILIAL LOADING FOR SUICIDAL BEHAVIOR

There was no relationship between the presence of high suicidal intent or violent method in the suicide probands and familial loading for suicide attempts and completions. Suicide probands who scored above the median on the BG-LHA, compared with those who scored below the median, had much greater familial loading for suicide attempts and completions in first-degree relatives (15.6+ 8.1% vs. 2.9 +3.9% [c2=6.89 p<0.009]), with a trend in the same direction even after controlling for BG-LHA scores (OR=4.1, 95% CI, 0.8–21.4) in relatives.

9. DISCUSSION

In this family study of adolescent suicide and community control probands, we found increased rates of suicide attempts in relatives of the former, compared to relatives of the latter. This increased familial aggregation of suicide in suicide probands persisted, even after controlling for the increased prevalence of Axis I and II disorders in their relatives. Furthermore, familial aggregation of actual suicidal behavior was demonstrated, whereas the excess rate of suicidal ideation in relatives of suicide probands was explained by an increased familial prevalence of psychopathology conditions. While the familial aggregation of suicidal behavior is not completely mediated by the transmission of aggressive behavior, a relationship between familial rates of suicidal behavior and aggression in suicide probands was demonstrated. The implications of these findings will be discussed, after placing them in the context of the limitations of this study.

Most of these limitations are inherent to family studies. In this type of study, family aggregation can be demonstrated, and familial transmission can be inferred, but clear demonstration of familial transmission and its mechanisms require different and more powerful designs. For example, familial aggregation could be due to genetic, environmental, or artifactual causes. The genetic etiology of familial aggregation is best demonstrated by adoption or twin studies (6,7) Family studies are often a precursor to these more powerful designs, because they help to more sharply define the phenotype under investigation. The familial transmission of suicidal behavior can also involve non-genetic mechanisms, such as exposure to family violence, hostility and discord, separation and loss, low parental involvement, or imitation of parental suicidal behavior (41–52). A prospective high-risk design would be best suited to examine the genetic and environmental components of the familial transmission of suicidal behavior. Artifact may also explain the familial aggregation of suicidal behavior, insofar as suicide may affect the report, recall, and actual psychiatric status of relatives (26,27). However, it has been demonstrated previously that the psychiatric status of parents does not appear to affect their recall or report of psychopathology in suicide victims (18) and that their report appears valid (19). Furthermore, our estimation of the familial morbid risk included only those conditions in relatives of suicide probands that had their onset prior to death of the suicide victim, so as not to confound preexisting rates of disorder with new-onset conditions precipitated by the stress of the suicide. One further limitation of this particular family study was the relatively low rate of direct interviews for fathers. Although the rate of direct paternal interviews was similar in both groups, we may have underestimated the contribution of familial impulsive aggression on suicidal risk, given that those fathers who were not available for interview may have been more aggressive.. However, we did statistically model the substitution of extreme scores of aggression for all missing data without any substantial alteration in the results.

To our knowledge, this study is the first demonstration of the familial aggregation of suicide attempts in the families of suicide victims, while controlling for the increased rate of a broad range of Axis I and II psychopathology conditions in relatives. These results strongly suggest that the tendency to suicidal behavior is familially transmitted by a mechanism distinct from the familial transmission of other psychiatric conditions. This finding is consistent with previous reports that the familial aggregation of suicide is distinct from that of either affective illness (5) or endogenous psychose (4).

However, distinct the familial transmission of liabilities to suicidality and psychopathology conditions are from one another, it appears likely that these two sets of liabilities intersect to result in attempted or completed suicide, since the vast majority of those who attempt and complete suicide suffer from at least one major psychiatric condition (1,2,17,45,46,50,53). Conversely, if liability to suicidal behavior alone was sufficient to trigger a suicide attempt or completion, then it would be highly unlikely that such an overwhelming proportion of suicide probands would show evidence of major psychiatric conditions.

What is the spectrum of suicidal behavior that appears to be familially transmitted? Our data suggest that the "phenotype" for the familial liability to suicidality includes suicide attempts and completions, and does not include suicidal ideation. These findings are consistent with those of Pfeffer et al., (8) who reported increased rates of suicide attempts in the relatives of prepubertal suicide attempters, but not in the relatives of suicidal ideators. Similarly, in our study, the familial aggregation of attempts persisted after controlling for the increased rate of familial psychopathology condition in the relatives of suicide probands, whereas the familial aggregation of suicidal ideation was explained by the excess rates of Axis I and II disorders among relatives. The view that suicide attempts and completions represent the expression of a specific liability, whereas ideation is a manifestation of underlying psychopathology condition, is supported by research showing similar changes in serotonergic function in attempted and in completed suicide, but not in suicidal ideation (37,54–56). In addition, our finding that the relatives of adolescent suicide probands showed a familial excess of suicide attempts, supports the view that attempts and completions are part of the same clinical and familial spectrum. The continuity between suicide attempts and completions is also supported by other family studies, (2,9–11) as well as both retrospective, (2,17) and prospective studies (57).

The "phenotype" of suicidal behavior that is familially transmitted may also include aggressive behavior. Among suicide probands, higher familial loading for suicide attempts was associated with higher ratings of aggression in the probands, even after adjustment for family loading of aggression. Therefore, family transmission of the liability for suicidality also involves the transmission of liability to aggression. Numerous other studies have reported a relationship between suicidal and aggressive behavior (1,2,16,17,58,59). Our particular set of findings showing greater family loading for suicide attempts in more aggressive suicide probands is consistent with that of a recent report showing a relationship between a polymorphism of the tyrosine hydroxylase allele and repeated suicide attempts, in violent attempters (60). Since, in our study, familial aggregation for suicidal behavior occurred even after controlling for impulsive aggressive personality disorders, assaultive behavior, and other measures of aggression, familial transmission of suicidal behavior appears at least partially independently of the familial transmission of aggression.

These results support further investigations into the familial transmission of suicidal behavior. A high risk study examining the offspring of attempted suicide victims and a comparison group may be useful in clarifying mechanisms of familial transmission, particularly those mechanisms that may be mediated by non-genetic mechanisms. Genetic investigations using an allele-sharing approach may also be a fruitful avenue of inquiry. Research should focus on clarifying the unique genetic and non-genetic contributions to the familial transmission of suicidal behavior. With a better understanding of familial transmission of suicidal behavior comes the hope of prevention of youthful suicide and suicidal behavior.

ACKNOWLEDGEMENTS

We are very grateful to the Americah Medical Associateion for permission to publish this paper, Suicidal Behaviour Runs in Families, which was originaly published in the journal of General Psychiatry, Volume 53, December 1996, Pages 1146–1152.

REFERENCES

1. Shafii M, Carrigan S, Whittinghill JR, Derrick, AM. Psychological autopsy of completed suicide in children and adolescents. Am J Psychiatry. 1985;142:1061–1064.
2. Shaffer D, Garland A, Gould M, Fisher P, Trautman, P. Preventing teenage suicide: A critical review. J Am Acad Child Adolesc Psychiatry. 1988;27:675–687.
3. Tsuang MT. Risk of suicide in the relatives of schizophrenics, manics, depressives, and controls. J Clin Psychiatry. 1983;44:396–400.
4. Mitterauer B. A contribution to the discussion of the role of the genetic factor in suicide, based on five studies in an epidemiologically defined area (Province of Salzburg, Austria). Comprehensive Psychiatry. 1990;31:557–565.
5. Egeland JA, Sussex JN. Suicide and family loading for affective disorders. J Amer Med Assoc. 1985;254:915–918.
6. Schulsinger F, Kety SS, Rosenthal D, Wender PH. A family study of suicide. In: Schou, M. and Stromgren, E. eds. Origin, Prevention and Treatment of Affective Disorders. London: Academic Press; 1979; 277–287.
7. Tsuang MT. Genetic factors in suicide. Dis Nerv Syst. 1977;38:498–501.
8. Pfeffer CR, Normandin L, Tatsuyuki K. Suicidal children grow up: Suicidal behavior and psychiatric disorders among relatives. J Am Acad Child Adolesc Psychiatry. 1994;33:1087–1097.
9. Garfinkel BD, Froese A, Hood J. Suicide attempts in children and adolescents. Am J Psychiatry. 1982;139:1257–1261.
10. Linkowski P, de Maertelaer V, Mendlewicz J. Suicidal behaviour in major depressive illness. Acta Psychiatr Scand. 1985;72:233–238.
11. Roy A. Family history of suicide. Arch Gen Psychiat. 1983;40:971–974.
12. Buydens-Branchey L, Branchey MH, Noumair D. Age of alcoholism onset: I. Relationship to psychopathology. Arch Gen Psychiat. 1989;46:225–230.
13. Brent DA, Perper JA, Moritz G, Liotus L, Schweers J, Balach L, Roth C. Familial risk factors for adolescent suicide: A case-control study. Acta Psychiatr Scand. 1994;89:52–58.
14. Wender PH, Kety SS, Rosenthal D, Schulsinger F, Ortmann J, Lunde, I. Psychiatric disorders in the biological and adoptive families of adopted individuals with affective disorders. Arch Gen Psychiat. 1986;43:923–929.
15. Hollingshead A. Four Factor Index of Social Status. New Haven, CT: Yale University Sociology Department; 1975.
16. Brent DA, Johnson BA, Perper J, Connolly J, Bridge J, Bartle S, Rather C. Personality disorder, personality traits, impulsive violence, and completed suicide in adolescents. J Am Acad Child Adolesc Psychiatry. 1994;33:1080–1086.
17. Brent DA, Perper JA, Moritz G, Allman C, Roth C, Schweers J, Balach L, Baugher M. Psychiatric risk factors of adolescent suicide: A case control study. J Am Acad Child Adolesc Psychiatry. 1993;32:521–529.

18. Brent DA, Perper JA, Kolko DJ, Zelenak JP. The psychological autopsy: Methodological considerations for the study of adolescent suicide. J Am Acad Child Adolesc Psychiatry. 1988;27:362–366.

19. Brent DA, Perper JA, Moritz G, Allman C, Roth C, Schweers J, Balach L. The validity of diagnoses obtained through the psychological autopsy procedure: Use of family history. Acta Psychiatr Scand. 1993; 87:118–122.

20. Leckman JF, Sholomskas D, Thompson WD, Belanger A, Weissman MM. Best estimate of lifetime psychiatric diagnosis: A methodological study. Arch Gen Psychiat. 1982;39:879–883.

21. Orvaschel H, Puig-Antich J, Chambers W, Tabrizi MA, Johnson R. Retrospective assessment of prepubertal major depression with the Kiddie-SADS-E. J Am Acad Child Psychiatry. 1982;21:392–397.

22. Chambers WJ, Puig-Antich J, Hirsch M, Paez P, Ambrosini PJ, Tabrizi MA, Davies M. The assessment of affective disorders in children and adolescents by semistructured interview: Test-retest reliability of the Schedule for Affective Disorders and Schizophrenia for School-Age Children, Present Episode Version. Arch Gen Psychiat. 1985;42:696–702.

23. American Psychiatric Association, Diagnostic and Statistical Manual of Psychiatric Disorders, DSM-III. Washington,DC: American Psychiatric Association; 1980.

24. Endicott J, Spitzer RL. A diagnostic interview: The Schedule for Affective Disorders and Schizophrenia. Arch Gen Psychiat. 1978;35:837–844.

25. Andreasen NC, Endicott J, Spitzer RL, Winokur G. The family history method using diagnostic criteria: Reliability and validity. Arch Gen Psychiat. 1977;34:1229–1235.

26. Brent DA, Perper JA, Moritz G, Liotus L, Schweers J, Roth C, Balach L, Allman D. Psychiatric impact of the loss of an adolescent sibling to suicide. J Affect Disord. 1993;28:249–256.

27. Brent DA, Moritz G, Bridge J, Perper J, Canobbio R. The impact of adolescent suicide on siblings and parents: A longitudinal follow-up. Suicide Life-Threat Behav; in press.

28. Spitzer RL, Williams JBW, Gibbon M, First MB. The Structured Clinical Interview for DSM-III-R (3rd ed.-revised). New York: New York State Psychiatric Institute; 1989.

29. American Psychiatric Association, Diagnostic and Statistical Manual of Psychiatric Disorders, DSM-III-R. Washington, DC: American Psychiatric Association; 1987.

30. Johnson BA, Brent DA, Connolly J, Bridge J, Matta J, Constantine D, Rather C, White T. The familial aggregation of adolescent personality disorders. J Am Acad Child Adolesc Psychiatry. 1995;34:789–804.

31. Brent DA, Johnson B, Bartle S, Bridge J, Rather C, Matta J, Connolly J, Constantine D. Personality disorder, tendency to impulsive violence, and suicidal behavior in adolescents. J Am Acad Child Adolesc Psychiatry. 1993;32:69–75.

32. Beck AT, Schuyler D, Herman I. Development of suicidal intent scales. In: Beck AT, Lettieri DJ, Resnick HLP eds. The Prediction of Suicide. Maryland: Charles Press; 1974:45–55.

33. Pierce DW. The predictive validation of a suicide intent scale: A five year follow-up. Brit J Psychiatry. 1981;139:391–396.

34. Brown GL, Goodwin FK, Ballenger JC, Goyer PF, Major LF. Aggression in humans correlates with cerebrospinal fluid amine metabolites. Psychiatry Res. 1979;1:131–139.

35. Brown GL, Ebert MH, Goyer PF, Jimerson DC, Klein WJ, Bunney WE,Goodwin FK. Aggression, suicide, and serotonin: Relationships to CSF amine metabolites. Am J Psychiatry. 1982;139:741–746.

36. Buss A, Durkee A. An inventory for assessing different kinds of hostility. J Consulting Psych. 1957;21:343–349.

37. Coccaro E, Siever L, Klar HM, Maurer G, Cochrane K, Cooper TB, Mohs RC, Davis KL. Serotonergic studies in patients with affective and personality disorders. Arch Gen Psychiat. 1989;46:587–599.

38. Kaplan EL, Meier P. Nonparameteric estimation from incomplete observations. J Am Stat Assoc. 1958;53:457–481.

39. Cox DR. Regression models and life-tables. J Royal Stat Society. 1972;34:187–220.

40. Dixon WJ. BMDP Statistical Software Manual. Berkeley, CA: University of California Press; 1990.

41. Asarnow J, Carlson G. Suicide attempts in preadolescent child psychiatry inpatients. Suicide Life Threat Behav. 1988;18:129–136.

42. Taylor EA, Stansfeld SA. Children who poison themselves. I. A clinical comparison with psychiatric controls. Brit J Psychiatry. 1984;145:127–132.

43. Kosky R, Silburn S, Zubrick SR. Are children and adolescents who have suicidal thoughts different from those who attempt suicide? J Nerv Mental Disease. 1990;178:38–43.

44. Kienhorst CWM, deWilde EJ, Van Den Bout J, van Groenou MIB, Diekstra RFW, Wolters WHG. Self-reported suicidal behavior in Dutch secondary education students. Suicide Life Threat Behav. 1990;20:101–112.

45. Lewinsohn PM, Rohde P, Seeley JR. Psychosocial risk factors for future adolescent suicide attempts. J Cons Clin Psychol. 1994;62:297–305.

46. Garrison CZ, Jackson KL, Addy CL, McKeown RE, Waller J.L. Suicidal behaviors in young adolescents. Am J Epidem. 1991;133:1005–1014.

47. Joffe RT, Offord DR, Boyle MH. Ontario child health study: Suicidal behavior in youth age 12–16 years. Am J Psychiatry. 1988;145:1420–1423.

48. Kashani JH, Goddard P, Reid JC. Correlates of suicidal ideation in a community sample of children and adolescents. J Am Acad Child Adolesc Psychiatry. 1989;28:912–917.

49. Fergusson DM, Lynskey MT. Childhood circumstances, adolescent adjustment, and suicide attempts in a New Zealand birth cohort. J Am Acad Child Adolesc Psychiatry. 1995;34:612–622.

50. Reinherz HZ, Giaconia RM, Silverman AB, Friedman A, Pakiz B, Frost AK, Cohen E. Early psychosocial risks for adolescent suicidal ideation and attempts. J Am Acad Child Adolesc Psychiatry. 1995;34:599–611.

51. Brent DA, Kolko DJ, Goldstein CE, Allan MJ, Brown RV. Suicidality in affectively disordered adolescent inpatients. J Amer Acad Child Adol Psychiatry. 1990;29:586–593.

52. Harkavy-Friedman JM, Asnis GM, Boeck M, Difiore J. Prevalence of specific suicidal behaviors in a high school sample. Am J Psychiatry. 1987;144:1203–1206.

53. Marttunen MD, Aro HM, Henriksson MM, Lonnquist JK. Mental disorders in adolescent suicide: DSM-III-R Axis I and II diagnoses in suicide among 13- to 19-year-olds in Finland, Arch Gen Psychiat. 1991;48:834–839.

54. Asberg M, Traskman-Bendz L, Thoren P. 5HIAA in the cerebrospinal fluid: A biochemical suicide predictor? Arch Gen Psychiat. 1976;33:1193–1197.

55. Mann JJ, McBride PA, Brown RP, Linnoila M, Leon AC, DeMeo M, Mieczkowski T, Myers JE, Stanley M. Relationship between central and peripheral serotonin indexes in depressed and suicidal psychiatric inpatients. Arch Gen Psychiat. 1992;49:442–446.

56. Mann J, Stanley M, McBride A, McEwen BS. Increased serotonin and b-adrenergic receptor binding in the frontal cortices of suicide victims. Arch Gen Psychiat. 1986;43:954–959.

57. Otto U. Suicidal acts by children and adolescents: A follow-up study. Acta Psychiatr Scand. 1972;233(supp):entire.

58. Virkkunen M, DeJong J, Bartko J, Linnoila M. Psychobiological concomitants of history of suicide attempts among violent offenders and impulsive fire setters. Arch Gen Psychiat. 1989;46:604–606.

59. Pfeffer CR, Newcorn J, Kaplan G, Mizruchi MS, Plutchik R. Suicidal behavior in adolescent psychiatric inpatients. J Am Acad Child Adolesc Psychiatry. 1988;27:357–361. 60. Nielsen DA, Goldman D, Virkkunen M, Tokola R, Rawlings R, Linnoila M. Suicidality and 5-hydroxyindoleacetic acid concentration associated with a tryptophan hydroxylase polymorphism. Arch Gen Psychiat. 1994;51:34–38.

10

SUICIDES IN AUSTRALIA

Pierre Baume and Philippa McTaggart

Australian Institute for Suicide Research and Prevention
Griffith University
Nathan QLD, 4111

1. INTRODUCTION

Suicide is now the leading cause of death by injury in Australia ahead of car accidents and homicide (Australian Bureau of Statistics (ABS), 1996). Suicide is always a tragic and unique event that has profound personal effects on those associated with the loss. Many families and friends are often affected by suicides and the impact of that loss is often heightened when the suicide is of a young person. Although Australia is not alone in having witnessed an increase in rates of suicide among young people, this major public health concern warrants further investigation. There is never one single reason for why a person may choose to end their life as the reasons are multiple and are different for each individual. This chapter provides a broad epidemiological background, discussing the suicide trends in Australia as well as comparisons between states and with overseas countries. Geographical location and methods of suicide are also described. It is not the intent of this chapter to provide comprehensive information about the epidemiology of suicide, but rather to highlight some of the more relevant issues which may be used by policy makers and other interested parties in the context of suicide prevention.

2. DIMENSIONS OF THE PROBLEM

Over the last 20 years nearly 50,000 Australians have lost their lives by suicide and as many again will die in the next two decades. While this figure is likely to be an under estimation of the true picture, it is known that suicide is now a leading cause of death from all external causes for all age groups, in some states, ahead of motor vehicle accidents and well ahead of homicides (ABS 1996). The most disturbing trends which have emerged over the last 30 years are in young people, especially males aged 15 to 24 years for whom the suicide rate has increased nearly four fold. In 1960, 50 males (a rate of 6.8 per 100,000) died by suicide and 35 years later this figure had risen to 374 deaths, or 27 per 100,000 (ABS,1996). This increase in suicide rates has not been reflected in the same way

Suicide Prevention, edited by Kosky *et al.*
Plenum Press, New York, 1998

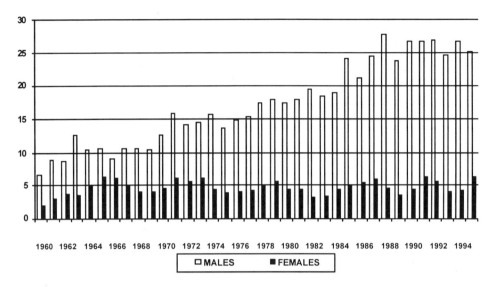

Figure 1. Rates of suicide for Australia. Males and females, 15–24 years. 1960–1995. Source: ABS.

for young females whose rate, although fluctuating, has remained relatively constant (see Figure 1). For young people, mortality from suicide now represents 25% of all deaths for males and 17% for females (see Figure 2) with the highest frequency occurring around 24 years of age (see Figure 3).

3. AUSTRALIA'S TRENDS

Suicide trends since 1881 for all ages are described in Figure 4. Apart from some occasional, but nonetheless significant variations, the rates for both males and females have remained stable. These variances can be explained in a number of ways. The significant

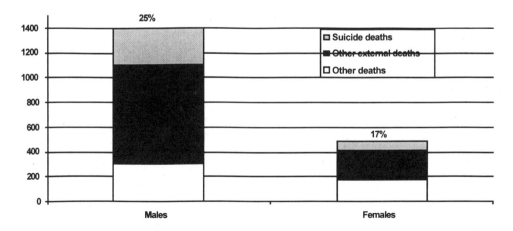

Figure 2. Causes of death at ages 15–24 in Australia, 1995. Source: AIHW National Injury Surveillance.

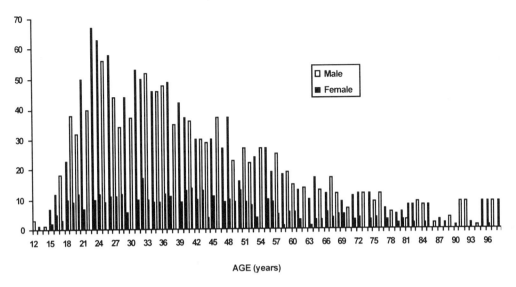

Figure 3. Suicide cases registered in Australia, 1995 by single year of age. Source: AISRAP.

increase before the war years during the depression, for example, can be seen in males but not seen in females. The following decline in rates for males began during the Second World War and continued for several years after. The increases observed for both males and females in the 1960s to the mid 1970s reflect primarily the increased prescription of barbiturates. When prescriptions of Benzodiazepines, became more prevalent as a safer sedative alternative, in the early 1970s, and limitations were placed on barbiturates, a sig-

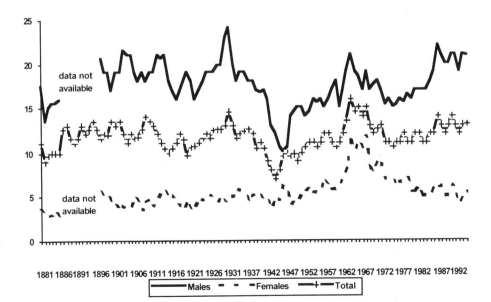

Figure 4. Rates of suicide, Australia. Males, females and total, all ages, 1881–1995. Source: ABS.

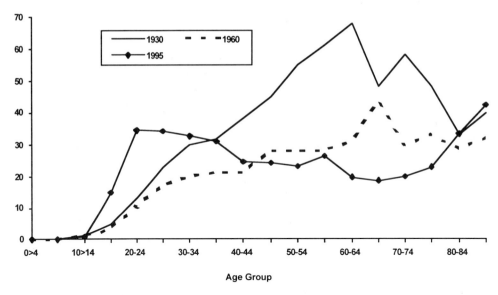

Figure 5. Rates of suicide by age group, males in Australia. 1930, 1961 and 1995. Source: ABS.

nificant decline followed for both genders. These trends were not, however, reflected in the 15–24 years age group.

Regardless of these fluctuations, the overall Australian suicide rates today are similar to those seen at the end of last century (ie: in 1887 the male rate per 100,000 was 20.6 as compared to 21 in 1995, and female rates were 5.5 per 100000 in 1887 and remain at the same level in 1995). What has changed, however, is the age distribution of those who complete suicide. The rising rate of suicide in young males for example, has been offset by declines in rates in the older males. In the earlier part of this century the rate of suicide in Australia was observed to increase as a function of age (see Figure 5) but in the last two decades or so the rates for older people aged over 65 have nearly halved (ABS 1996). Whilst the rates for the elderly aged over 80 years remain the highest of all age groups, the numbers of deaths in this age group are small when compared with those aged under 30 years (Baume, Cantor & McTaggart, 1997).

4. DISTRIBUTION OF SUICIDE

4.1. Comparisons between States and Territories

Australia is a large country almost the size of Europe but with a population of only 18 million. The country is divided into 7 states and territories. Table one describes the suicide rates for each state and territory for a 32 year period from 1964 to 1995. These data demonstrate that some states continuously have higher rates above the National average. While suicide rates will always vary between states, it is notable that Queensland and Tasmania have consistently had rates significantly above the national average. Interestingly both of these states have the lowest concentration of migrants from southern Europe of any states and one (Queensland) has the second highest proportion of indigenous people living in rural areas (Baume et al, 1997).

Table 1. Suicide rates by state and territory, 1964–1995 (all ages)

	NSW	VIC	QLD	SA	WA	TAS	NT	ACT	TOTAL
1964	15.3	10.6	20.1	16.0	15.3	11.5	9.1	10.0	14.6
1965	17.5	11.0	18.1	12.5	13.6	12.0	25.6	11.3	14.8
1966	16.0	10.9	17.0	12.4	15.1	9.2	7.1	10.4	14.0
1967	16.9	13.2	16.8	12.9	13.9	12.8	9.7	8.7	15.0
1968	13.5	11.3	14.1	11.8	12.8	14.0	11.8	8.9	12.7
1969	13.2	10.1	14.6	12.2	11.2	13.3	5.5	14.0	12.2
1970	12.7	11.0	15.2	12.0	11.1	12.9	14.0	9.9	12.4
1971	13.1	14.0	15.1	10.2	14.3	11.8	4.7	7.9	13.3
1972	13.3	11.8	12.4	10.5	12.1	10.7	9.8	5.6	12.2
1973	12.2	9.7	12.8	9.8	11.3	13.6	12.4	9.8	11.3
1974	12.1	10.0	13.3	10.6	10.7	12.8	11.7	8.1	11.4
1975	11.7	9.7	13.9	11.8	7.3	9.8	8.6	8.5	11.0
1976	11.3	8.8	12.1	11.5	10.9	11.2	17.3	10.1	10.7
1977	10.5	11.8	11.5	10.0	11.6	10.1	5.8	12.2	11.0
1978	10.8	9.8	14.5	11.9	10.4	11.7	7.3	9.2	11.1
1979	10.5	11.9	13.4	13.7	9.3	13.3	9.6	8.6	11.6
1980	10.6	11.2	12.1	11.2	10.0	10.6	12.7	5.8	10.9
1981	10.4	10.9	12.8	12.1	10.6	15.2	13.0	9.7	11.2
1982	11.0	11.7	12.3	13.0	12.8	13.7	5.4	7.3	11.7
1983	10.1	12.7	11.2	10.3	10.6	15.9	11.8	11.7	11.2
1984	9.4	11.5	12.4	11.0	12.7	11.7	7.7	13.5	11.0
1985	11.7	10.2	13.3	10.0	12.1	15.8	10.8	11.1	11.6
1986	11.2	12.5	14.7	13.2	11.2	15.5	9.1	12.7	12.4
1987	11.6	15.5	15.7	13.5	13.6	15.1	10.1	15.1	13.8
1988	12.8	12.6	14.9	13.1	13.5	16.0	17.6	11.4	13.3
1989	11.8	11.6	14.5	14.2	11.7	13.0	14.9	12.7	12.5
1990	11.6	11.4	14.6	14.9	13.3	15.1	18.3	12.4	12.7
1991	13.0	13.7	14.3	16.0	12.9	14.4	11.5	11.8	13.6
1992	12.3	12.5	14.1	14.6	12.9	20.4	13.7	10.5	13.1
1993	11.7	11.1	11.8	11.3	12.9	17.6	13.0	9.0	11.8
1994	12.9	11.4	14.2	11.5	12.8	14.8	11.1	12.0	12.7
1995	12.5	12.6	15.1	13.6	12.6	14.0	13.2	11.2	13.1

SOURCE - ABS, 1996.

4.2. Rural and Urban Comparison

A number of studies have reported significant increases in young people aged 15–24 in rural areas (Baume & Clinton, 1997; Dudley, Waters, Kelk & Howard, 1993; Dudley, Kelk, Florio, Howard, Waters, Haski & Alcock, 1996) (see Figure 6). These increases, however, are predominantly in young males, especially for those aged 15 to 19 years. The largest numbers of suicides continue to be recorded in urban centers, especially for those aged 20 to 24 years (Dudley et al 1996). The rate of increase in young females is once again less in country areas, except in smaller towns with populations of less than 4000 people (ABS 1996). Research from the third largest state, Queensland, has found few overall urban/rural differences in suicide rates. These observations are partly explained by the fact that small rural regions have both the lowest and highest suicide rates in that state. For example, low rates were found in more affluent rural areas and high rates in more isolated and less resourced areas, especially those with high concentration of indigenous people. (Baume, Cantor & McTaggart, 1997). Hence whilst there is general agreement on the

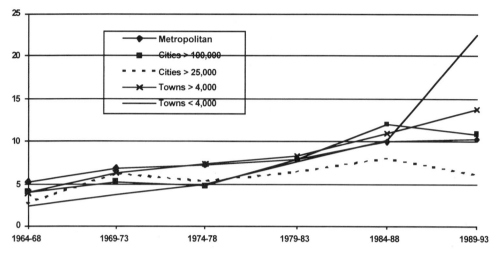

Figure 6. Suicide rates by residence. Both sexes. 10–24 years. 1964–1993. Source: AISRAP.

findings that rural areas have experienced severe upturns in their suicide rates, these cannot always be generalised to all regions.

5. COMPARISON WITH OTHER COUNTRIES

A number of western nations have reported significant increases in the suicide of young people (Diekestra, 1985). Whilst Australia does not have the highest rate of suicide among young people (see Figure 7), it is significant that in terms of western nations, only New Zealand has higher rates. It is also interesting to note that the Japanese rates for

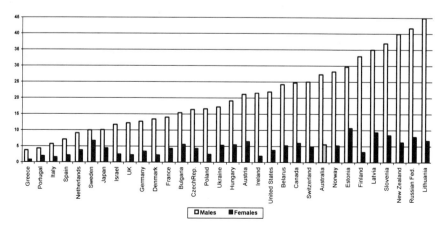

Figure 7. Deaths by suicide — international data 1991–1993. 15–24 years (rates per 100,000). Source: UNICEF.

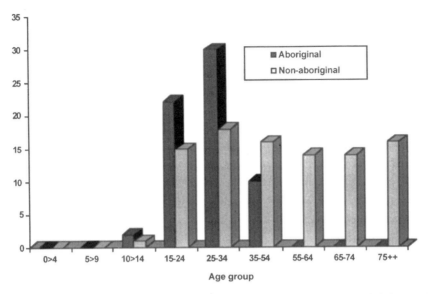

Figure 8. Indigenous and non-indigenous rates of suicide, Australia (except Qld) 1990–1992. Source: AIHW.

young men are less than half of that of Australia. Traditionally, countries which form part of southern Europe, have had lower rates of suicide than those of eastern and northern Europe which have had much higher rates. Migrants coming to Australia from those countries usually carry the rates of their mother country, but their off-springs have tended towards Australian rates.

6. INDIGENOUS SUICIDES

The rate of suicide among the indigenous population of Australia is substantially higher than the non-indigenous population (see Figure 8). Suicide was reported to be uncommon in Indigenous communities until recently (Hunter 1993) but young indigenous Australians now have an alarming rate of mortality by suicide with rates peaking at over 30 per 100,000 for both genders. This is nearly twice the national average for the non-indigenous population and a recent study in Queensland suggests that the rate may be as high as four times that of the non-indigenous population in that state (Baume et al 1997). Although suicide rates in older Indigenous persons remain low, the older age group rates may increase as the current cohort of young indigenous people age.

7. METHODS USED FOR SUICIDE

The most commonly used methods of suicide in Australia in 1995 for males were hanging, poisoning by motor vehicle exhaust, and firearms (together accounting for around 80% of male suicides). For females the most commonly used methods were poisoning by solids and liquids and hanging (together accounting for around 57% of female suicides) (Australian Institute for Suicide Research and Prevention (AISRAP), 1996). Taken together, these four methods account for more than 90% of all suicides (see Figures 9 & 10). Addi-

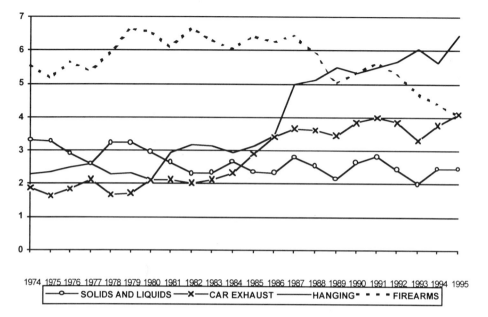

Figure 9. Rates of suicide by selected methods, Australia — males all ages. 1974–1995. Source: ABS.

tionally there are other suicides by jumping, lying in front of moving vehicles, drowning, self-burning and the use of a vehicle. For males, deaths by hanging and poisoning by motor vehicle exhaust gases have risen dramatically while in the Australian female population the rates of suicide by hanging and motor vehicle exhaust are increasing, but these increases have been partly offset by a decline in suicides by poisoning by overdoses.

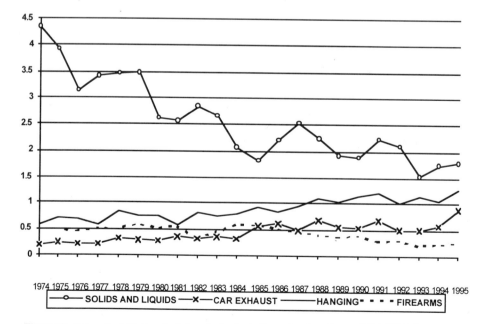

Figure 10. Rates of suicide by selected methods, Australia — females all ages. 1974–1995. Source: ABS.

Age seems to play no role in the selection of methods of suicide, but rather gender and culture are crucial determinants. Moreover, the distribution of methods used varies according to geographical location. There is a tendency, for example, for firearm suicides to be more likely to occur in rural areas where access to firearms is more prominent.

Changes in method selection have been noted over the last two decades. Deaths by drug overdoses, after a peak in the 1960s for male and females, primarily associated with barbiturate overdoses, have declined. Much of this reduction has been associated with a change in prescribing and resuscitation practices. Self poisoning, either in terms of attempts or completed suicides, remains a concern. It is clear that this method is an important cause of hospitalisation as well as death for both gender. Substances, particularly under the categories of tranquillisers and analgesics are still very problematic (Buckley, Whyte, Dawson, McManus & Ferguson, 1995a; Buckley, Whyte, Dawson, McManus & Ferguson, 1995b). In terms of analgesics, paracetamol is usually associated with very serious liver damage even if death does not occur (Vale & Proudfoot, 1995). In a recent study of 2799 suicides in Queensland between 1990 and 1995, paracetamol and trycyclic antidepressants represented more than 30% of overdose deaths by suicide, and 46% of the trycyclic antidepressant deaths were from Dothiepin, 23% from amitriptyline, 20% from doxepin and 8% imipramine overdoses. On the positive side, the newer antidepressants (Moclobemide, Fluoxetine, Paroxetine and Sertraline) accounted for less than 1% of those deaths when combined together. (Baume et al 1997).

In other methods, an alarming fourfold increase in hanging, and a doubling in carbon monoxide suicides in both genders has been observed. There has been speculation that the decline in firearms may have resulted in the substitution of other methods but this view does not adequately reflect the observation that the rise in suicide by hanging and carbon monoxide is much greater than the respective decline in suicide by firearms. The increase in hanging has been noted in both the Indigenous and non-Indigenous populations and therefore may be suggestive of broader influences than simply cultural differences. It has been argued that the media coverage of deaths in custody may have promoted a symbolic association of suicide with hanging (Baume & Clinton 1997).

Hence it can be concluded that the increased availability of a culturally accepted method of suicide tends to result in an increase in the suicide rate for that method; that restricting the availability of a particular method of suicide is associated with a decline in suicide by that method; and that restricting access to a particular method of suicide often, but not always, is associated with a decline in overall suicide rates. (Cantor et al, 1996).

8. ATTEMPTED SUICIDES (PARASUICIDES)

Information about attempted suicides is difficult to obtain in Australia because there are no generally accepted reporting procedures nor well accepted definitions. The Australian Bureau of Statistics report hospital separations for suicide attempts but there are reliability problems with hospital coding of suicide attempts and most suicide attempts do not present to hospital. As for other countries, a true picture of attempted suicide is not available at this time. Rates for females have always been estimated to be much higher than the rate of males and recently the male to female ratio of hospital presentations for attempted suicide in Australia has been reported to be approximately 1.6 to 1 (Australian Institute for Health and Welfare (AIHW) 1994) (see Figure 11).

It is believed, however that the prevalence of suicide attempts is grossly underestimated because most research reports only on hospital contact. Studies generally have esti-

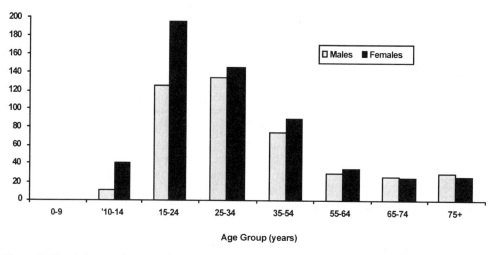

Figure 11. Hospital separation rates due to self-injury, by age group. Australia (excluding NT), 1992–1993. Source: AIHW.

mated that the ratio between non-lethal suicidal behaviour and suicide is between 20:1 and 100:1 (Sayer, Stewart & Chipps 1996, Kosky, 1987). The selection of method differs by age cohort and this appears, in part, to predict a non fatal outcome, thus explaining partly the fact that attempted suicide appears to be higher in the younger age groups. (See Figure 12.)

9. CONCLUSIONS

Aside from the loss of life, the human cost of suicide in terms of bereavement is great. Suicide is now the leading cause of death in young adults, there having been a three

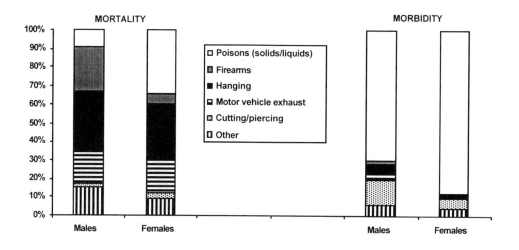

Figure 12. Death rates (1993) and hospital separation rates (1992–1993) for self injury, 15–24 years. Australia. Hospital inpatient data do not include NT. Source: AIHW.

to four fold rise in suicide in 15–24 year old males since 1960. While Australia has a relatively high rate of young (15–24) male suicide by international standards, the rate for older ages is more moderate. In many rural areas, youth suicide rates are higher and this may depend on the socioeconomic characteristics of the communities concerned. While there has been a significant decline in suicide by firearms and overdoses, this has been more than offset by an alarming rise in hanging and carbon monoxide poisoning. There is a need, therefore, for ongoing research towards understanding suicide in the Australian context.

A number of studies in Australia, as for other countries, have employed different terms and definitions which complicate the comparisons of research findings across studies. Furthermore, there appears to be a degree of confusion, especially in the area of attempted suicide, and how this may affect data collection. It is clear that careful attention must be paid to ensure validity and reliability of the instrumentation and methodology used to assess and classify suicidal behaviour in research studies. Hence the need to develop an acceptable nomemclature for Australia in conjunction with World Health Organisation.

Most information and knowledge of suicide in Australia continues to rely heavily on overseas data, indicating a need for more research to be undertaken on the epidemiology of suicide, the short and long term risk factors, and on protective factors in Australia compared to other countries. These efforts, however, need to be broad-based, culturally sensitive and use a multidisciplinary research approach.

In summary then, the collection of accurate data on suicide is essential to research, services and educational programs. Uniform and consistent standards for classifying suicidal behaviour should be developed and utilised, requiring that the current surveillance systems must be improved to identify and report attempted and completed suicide at the local, state and national levels. Collaborative efforts need to be established between mental health professionals and coronial offices to conduct systematic psychological autopsy studies on suicidal deaths. Finally, ongoing international comparisons are necessary to validate changes that may be taking place in this country.

REFERENCES

Australian Bureau of Statistics (1996). *Causes of Death, Australia 1995*. Catalogue number 3303.0. Canberra: Australian Government Publishing Service.

Australian Institute for Suicide Research and Prevention (1996). *Access to Means of Suicide by Young Australians*. A background report to the Commonwealth Department of Health and Family Services. Canberra, AGPS, 1996.

Australian Institute for Health and Welfare (1994). *Australia's health 1994*. Canberra: Australian Government Publishing Service.

Baume, PJM, Cantor, C & McTaggart, P. (1997*). Suicides in Queensland, a comprehensive study, 1990–1995*. Queensland Health Department.

Baume, PJM & Clinton, ME. (1997). Social and cultural patterns of suicide in young people in rural Australia. *Australian Journal of Rural Health*, 5, 115–120.

Buckley, N.A., Whyte, I.M., Dawson, A.H., McManus, P.R. & Ferguson, P.R. (1995a). Self-poisoning in Newcastle, 1987–1992. *Medical Journal of Australia*, 162, 190–193.

Buckley, N.A., Whyte, I.M., Dawson, A.H., McManus, P.R. & Ferguson, N.W. (1995b). Correlations between prescriptions and drugs taken in self-poisoning: implications for prescribers and drug regulation. *Medical Journal of Australia*, 162, 194–197.

Diekestra, R.S.W. (1985). Suicide and suicide attempts in the European Economic Community: An analysis of trends with special emphasis upon trends among young. *Suicide and Life-Threatening Behaviour*, 15, 27–42

Dudley M., Waters B., Kuk N. and Howard J. (1993). Youth suicide in New South Wales: Urban-rural trends, 1964–1988. *The Medical Journal of Australia*. 156(20); 83–88.

Dudley, M., Kelk, N., Florio, T., Howard, J., Waters, B., Haski, C., Alcock, M. (1996). Suicide among young rural Australians, 1964–1993: A comparison with metropolitan trends. *Social Psychiatry and Psychiatric Epidemiology*, 32, 1–10.

Hunter, E. (1993). *Aboriginal Health and History: Power and Privilege in Remote Australia*. Melbourne: Cambridge University Press.

Kosky, R. (1987). Is suicide behaviour increasing among Australian youth? *The Medical Journal of Australia*. 147. 164–166.

Sayer, G., Stewart, G. & Chipps, J. (1996). Suicide attempts in NSW: Associated mortality and morbidity. Public Health Bulletin, 7(6), 55–66.

UNICEF. *The Progress of nations*. New York, UNICEF, 1996.

Vale, J.A. & Proudfoot, A.T. (1995). Paracetamol (acetaminophen) poisoning. *Lancet*, 346, 547–552.

11

SUICIDE IN THE 18 YEARS AFTER DELIBERATE SELF-HARM

A Prospective Study

Gregory M. de Moore[1] and Andrew R. Robertson[2]

[1]Department of Consultation-Liaison Psychiatry
[2]Department of Psychiatry
Westmead Hospital
Westmead
Australia

The prediction of eventual suicide in those who harm themselves is notoriously difficult. The sensitivity and specificity of the risk factors are low (Pokorny, 1982; Nordentoft *et al,* 1993). Long-term follow-up studies of deliberate self-harm (DSH) are one method of improving our predictive ability and hence our clinical management.

Follow-up studies in the past few decades have usually been of 5–10 years duration at the most. Two notable earlier studies of much longer duration date from the 1940s and 1950s (Schneider, 1954; Dahlgren, 1977), since when there have been major changes in the epidemiology of both DSH and suicide (Hawton & Catalan, 1987). Australia has experienced a disturbing increase in youth suicide in the past 20 years, and now has one of the world's highest youth suicide rates (Kosky, 1987; Hassan & Carr, 1989).

1. BACKGROUND

Blacktown lies on the western outskirts of Sydney. In 1975 the population was almost 160 000 and was still increasing. Over one-third of the population was under 15 years of age. The population was predominantly of the lower socio-economic classes (Australian Bureau of Statistics, 1976 census).

Data came predominantly from patients taken to hospital as a result of DSH. Other sources were patients seen in their homes by community staff, and patients seen in hospital out-patient clinics or psychiatrists' private rooms as a result of DSH which had not led to hospital assessment.

Suicide Prevention, edited by Kosky *et al.*
Plenum Press, New York, 1998

1.1. Data Collection

A data collection sheet was completed by the assessor each time a patient with DSH was assessed. The assessment period occurred from October 1975 for twelve months. Data obtained included the following.

   a. Demographic information: name, address sex, age, country of birth, marital and parental status, with whom the subject was living, employment status, and date of DSH episode and of assessment.
   b. Clinical and social details of the episode: method and agent used; lethality and suicidal intent, each scored on a three-point scale as low, intermediate or uncertain, or high; whether significantly affected by alcohol; whether pregnant; presence or absence of environmental precipitants; and previous DSH.
   c. Presence of mental and physical illness: mental illness was defined as presence of schizophrenia, major depression, alcohol or drug dependence, dementia or clinically significant brain injury. Because of an error in the preparation of later data sheets, we had data for the presence and nature of physical and mental illness for only 162 of the 223 patients.
   d. Sequelae of the episode, for example whether admitted to hospital, whether still suicidal, and proposed management.

Any action of self-harm which might, however remotely, threaten life, led to inclusion. Patients who lived outside Blacktown were excluded.

Through the Office of Births, Deaths, and Marriages we identified those of the 223 patients who had died in NSW since 1975 to 1993. Through coroners' records, those who may have died in unnatural ways were identified. We studied the records, and decided whether to deem a death as suicide, using the criteria of 'probable suicide' (Adelstein & Mardon, 1975).

The possible predictors of suicide in the DSH population were those variables recorded at the time of DSH. Data were analysed using the x^2 test, and by logistic regression analysis using the SPIDA statistical package. Both univariate analysis for each variable and a best-fitting multivariate model were ascertained.

2 CHARACTERISTICS OF SAMPLE

There were 237 episodes of DSH, involving 223 patients (150 females and 73 males). Nine females and three males harmed themselves twice and one female did so three times. The age range for females was 14–73 years, mean 28.5, and for males 13–64 years, mean 32.2. Of all subjects, 42% were married, 35% were single, 9% were living in a *de facto* (common law) marriage, 10% were separated, 3% were widowed, and 1% were divorced; male-female differences were not statistically significant. Three per cent of both males and females lived alone. Thirteen per cent of the females and 19% of the males classed themselves as unemployed.

A medication overdose was taken by 93% of females and 82% of males. 'Cutting' was used by 6% of females and 7% of males. There were nine narcotic overdoses (eight males and one female). Most episodes were impulsive (86% in females 85% in males). The majority of episodes were of low lethality (69% of females, 61 % of males). With regard to intent, the numbers were fairly evenly divided between the three categories in both females and males. Of the episodes of both high lethality and high intent, 4 (2%) occurred in females and 8 (11%) in males (x^2=6.6, P=0.01).

Twenty-eight of the females (17%) and 34 of the males (45%) were considered to have been significantly affected by alcohol at the time of the episode ($x^2=19.1$, P<0.001).

A social precipitant, usually interpersonal conflict, was present in 90% of females and 82% of males.

There was a history of DSH in 27% of females and 28% of males.

Nine women (6%) were pregnant, or believed they were pregnant, at the time of the episode.

Eleven per cent of the females and 22% of the males were assessed as being physically ill, and 11% of the females and 26% of the males were mentally ill, as narrowly defined.

3 CHARACTERISTICS OF SUICIDES

Fifteen suicides (nine females and six males) occurred. Nine of these were unquestionable suicides. In five others, death was from overdose where evidence of clear and unambivalent suicidal intent was lacking. The remaining one case was included after considerable discussion; accidental death was recorded by the coroner, but review of the circumstances suggested that suicide was more likely. thus, 60% of suicides were unequivocal and 40% were equivocal.

The interval from the index episode to suicide ranged from 12 days to 16.9 years (Fig. 1). Four of the 15 suicides occurred within a year of the index episode.

The method of suicide was drug overdose in nine cases, shooting in two, hanging in two, and jumping or falling in two.

A striking finding was that four of the six male suicides had been aged 16–17 years at the index episode, and three of these four episodes had been narcotic overdoses.

Demographic variables at the time of the index episode of DSH were analysed, using univariate and multivariate logistic regression methods, to determine a best-fit picture for those who completed suicide. Statistical analysis was carried out for the DSH group as a whole, and for males and females separately. Results are presented in Table 1.

In view of the trend to significance for age of males in the univariate analysis, the data were re-examined by dividing age into two groups, teenagers and those aged 20 years

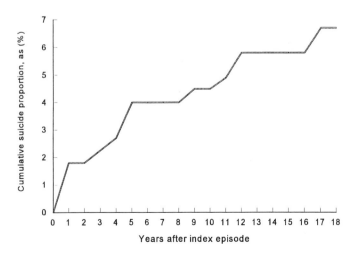

Figure 1. Cumulative proportion of suicide, as % of DSH population, with time.

Table 1. Univariate and multivariate analysis of risk factors in index DSH episodes associated with subsequent suicide

Risk factors	Suicide risk of all patients		Females only		Males only	
	Univariate P value	Best-fitting multi-variate model P value	Univariate P value	Best-fitting multi-variate model P value	Univariate P value	Best-fitting multi-variate model P value
Sex	0.05	—	—	—	—	—
Age	0.8	—	0.2	—	0.1	—
Any past DSH	0.3	—	0.08	—	0.5	—
More than one episode of DSH in year of study	**0.02**	**0.02**	0.08	—	0.08	**0.03**
High lethality	0.2	—	0.1	—	0.8	—
High intent	0.8	—	0.5	—	0.9	—
Planned attempt	**0.04**	**0.02**	**0.02**	**0.02**	0.8	—
Affected by alcohol	0.9	—	0.8	—	0.5	—
Narcotic overdose	**0.009**	**0.001**	0.9	—	**0.01**	**0.007**
Any drug overdose	0.8	—	0.3	—	—	—

and older. For males only, univariate analysis showed that being a teenager was a highly significant predictor of suicide (P= 0.01). It did not, however, alter the best-fit multivariate model for the males. However, narcotic overdose and being a teenaged male were highly confounded, and if the sample had been larger, both may have become independent predictors. There was no trend for being a female teenager predicting suicide; the trend if anything was for older females to complete suicide.

We had data on mental and physical illness for 162 DSH patients, and for 11 of the 15 suicides. We included mental and physical illness with the other variables and reanalysed the data. For this group of 162 patients, the best-fit multivariate model was planned attempt (P= 0.007) and being mentally ill (P= 0.03). For males, the best-fit multivariate model was being a teenage male (P=0.01). For females, the best-fit multivariate model was planned attempt (P = 0.02) and being mentally ill (P = 0.02).

Clinical evaluation of the case histories of the 15 suicides was undertaken. Three clinical subgroups, accounting for 13 of the 15 suicides, could be identified. (a) Four patients were suffering severe unresolved grief following a major interpersonal loss. These four were among the seven suicides in the first four years after the index episode. (This is the only apparent clinical difference between the early and late suicides.) (b) In seven patients, substance abuse appeared to be a way of life, or a means of dealing with or avoiding conflict. This group overlaps with (c), four females who repeatedly took overdoses as a result of chronic or episodic depression or as a habitual response to conflict.

4. DISCUSSION

There was a progressive increase in the cumulative proportion of suicide over the 18 years. Most recent studies have been of 8–10 years. The two earlier long-term studies of Schneider (1954) and Dahlgren (1977) gave somewhat similar results to ours, although Dahlgren's was an atypical sample, having an excess of males and of alcoholism. Our findings, like theirs, suggest that the risk of suicide after DSH, although diminishing over time, is probably a lifetime risk. The cumulative proportion of suicide with time in our study is compared with that in other studies in Table 2.

Table 2. Cumulative proportion of suicide (as a percentage of the DSH population) with time, in various studies

Study	Years of follow-up						
	5	8	10	12	18	28	35
de Moore & Robertson	4.0%	4.0%	4.5%	5.8%	6.7%		
Nordentoft *et al* (1993)			10.6%				
Suokas & Lonnqvist (1991)	3.2%						
Ekeberg *et al* (1991)	4.0%						
Nielsen *et al* (1990)	11.0%						
Beck & Steer (1989)			4.8%				
Hawton & Fagg (1988)		2.8%					
Cullberg *et al* (1988)			6.1%				
Dahlgren (1977)				6.0%			11.0%
Schneider (1954)			10.0%		11.8%	13.0%	

Four of the 15 suicides (27%) occurred in the first year after the index episode. This increased risk for early suicide is in accord with the findings of most other studies in recent times (Hawton & Fagg, 1988; Nielsen *et al,* 1990; Ekeberg *et al,* 1991; Suokas & Lonnqvist, 1991; Nordentoft *et al,* 1993).

Hawton & Fagg (1988) noted a low rate of suicide at eight years, 2.8%. Their data were collected in the early to mid-1970s, as was ours, and this period saw a large increase in self-poisoning. They speculated that their low rate of suicide may represent fewer 'genuine' suicide attempts, and hence fewer completed suicides. Our data showed a higher suicide rate.

Based on the expected, annual suicide rate for the sydney population in 1975–76, we would expect to have a suicide rate of 10 per 100,000 in our sample. Instead, the rate is around 360 per 100,000.

Table 3 presents the risk factors identified in the present study together with those from six other studies published in recent years. It is somewhat surprising that only two of the seven studies have shown that male sex is statistically significantly associated with completed suicide, in view of the much higher rate of male suicide in the general population. It may be that males tend to use more lethal methods, and so the DSH populations studied are skewed towards 'survivors' and females. If this is so, then preventive measures for males may need to be directed to risk factors additional to survival from DSH, such as gun law reform and alteration of social attitudes to teenage male alcohol excess (Cantor, 1994; Kosky & Goldney, 1994).

Although the studies in Table 3 vary considerably in design, some risk factors seem to be consistent, including the importance of multiple DSH episodes, psychiatric illness, abuse of alcohol and other sedatives, and planned attempts.

Other studies have noted the importance of increasing age as a risk factor, especially in males (Hawton & Fagg, 1988; Suokas & Lonnqvist, 1991; Nordentoft *et al,* 1993). Our study, in complete contrast to these, found male youth, associated with narcotic abuse, a major risk factor. This is not an isolated finding. Tenaged substance abusers seem to be at high risk for completed suicide (Tunving, 1988, Hawton *et al,* 1993). Most clinicians find such patients hard to engage in treatment (Kotila & Lonnqvist, 1988; Graham & Burvill, 1992) and so the preventive value of this finding may not be as useful as might be hoped (Kosky & Goldney, 1994).

Table 3. Risk factors in the index episode of DSH, statistically significant or showing a strong trend, associated with subsequent suicide, in various studies.

Risk factor	de Moore & Robertson	Nordentoft et al (1993)	Suokas & Lonnqvist (1991)	Nielsen et al (1990)	Beck & Steer (1989)	Hawton & Fagg (1988)	Cullberg et al (1988)
Male sex	No	No	Yes	No	No	Yes	No
Past or repeated DSH	Yes	Yes	Yes	No	No	Yes	Yes
Psychiatric illness	Yes	Yes	Yes	Yes	Yes[1]	Yes	Yes
Physical illness	No	—	—	Yes	—	Yes	—
Planned episode	Yes (F)	—	Yes	—	Yes	—	—
High lethality	No	—	Yes	—	—	—	—
High intent	No	—	Yes	—	Yes	—	—
Drug/alcohol abuse	Yes (M)	No	—	Yes	Yes	Yes	Yes
Increasing age	No (M)[2] Yes (F)	Yes	Yes	No	No	Yes (F)	No
Narcotic overdose	Yes (M)	—	—	—	—	—	—
Country of study	Australia	Denmark	Finland	Denmark	USA	England	Sweden

1. Alcoholism.
2. Opposite finding.
(F) females only, (M) males only

Like Hawton & Fagg (1988), we found that older female survivors of DSH are more likely to complete suicide than younger DSH suicide patients. We found that a planned episode was an important predictor of suicide in females, but not in males. We also found that severe mental illness, narrowly defined, was a significant predictor for females, although the smaller numbers and methodological difficulties must give rise to caution in interpreting this finding. We did not find that physical illness was a statistically significant predictor, this may reflect the relative youth of the population, the small number of patients who were physically ill, or the incompleteness of this part of the data collection. Certainly, other studies have found physical illness to be a significant predictor (Hawton & Fagg, 1988; Nielsen et al, 1993). The risk factor of repeated episodes of DSH has been demonstrated in this study, as in many others. Like Hawton & Fagg (1988), we found marital and employment status at the index episode to be non-predictive of subsequent suicide.

Five of the first eight suicides after DSH were suffering from unresolved grief. This is a potentially treatable group. Among the suicides were a group of women who habitually overdosed in response to conflict or crisis, and in whom substance abuse may also have been a problem. This is probably the same group identified by Cullberg et al (1988) as "depressed women with long- standing suicidal processes."

5. SUMMARY

I. teenage males who overdose on narcotics are at relatively high risk of subsequent suicide;
II. suicide risk after DSH gradually declines with time, but is a lifetime risk;
III. planned or frequently-repeated episodes of DSH, especially associated with substance abuse; chronic unresolved grief; and mental illness are relatively high-risk factors.

The limitations of the study include:

I. suicides which may have occurred outside NSW have not been included;

II. incomplete data on physical and mental illness limits conclusions on the predictive importance of these factor;

III. patient numbers are too small to determine whether the highly confounded variables of teenage male and narcotic overdose are independent risk factors for suicide.

ACKNOWLEDGMENTS

Thanks are due to Dr John Westerink, Ms Rosemary Pearson, Mr Colin Everingham, and Ms Kath Fyfe for helping to set up the original study, and Dr Willem Blignault for subsequent help and advice, Dr Karen Byth for statistical advice, Professor Russell Meares for helpful comments; and Ms Lena Melville for secretarial work.

REFERENCES

Adelstein, A. & Mardon, C. (1975) Suicides 1961–74. *Population Trends,* 2, 13–18.

Beck, A.T. & Steer, R.A. (1989) Clinical predictors of eventual suicide: a 5- to 10-year prospective study of suicide attempters. *Journal of Affective Disorders,* 17, 203–209.

Cantor, C.H. (1994) Clinical management of parasuicides: critical issues in the 1990s. *Australian and New Zealand Journal of Psychiatry,* 28, 212–221.

Cullberg, J., Wasserman, D. & Stefansson, C.G. (1988) Who commits suicide after a suicide attempt? *Acta Psychiatrica Scandinavica,* 77, 598–603.

Dahlgren, K.G. (1977) Attempted suicides - 35 years afterwards. *Suicide and Life Threatening Behaviour,* 7, 75-

Ekeberg, 0., Ellingsen, O. & Jacobsen, D. (1991) Suicide and other causes of death in a five-year follow-up of patients treated for self-poisoning in Oslo. *Acta Psychiatrica Scandinavica,* 83, 432–437.

Graham, C. & Burvill, P.W. (1992) A study of coroners' records of suicide in young people, 1986–1988, in Western Australia. *Australian and New Zealand Journal of Psychiatry,* 26, 30–39.

Hassan, R. & Carr, J. (1989) Changing pattens of suicide in Australia. *Australian and New Zealand Journal of Psychiatry,* 23, 225–234.

Hawton, K. & Catalan, J. (1987) *Attempted Suicide: A Practical Guide to its Nature and Management* (2nd edn). Oxford: Oxford University Press.

Hawton, K. & Fagg, J. (1988) Suicide, and other causes of death, following attempted suicide. *British Journal of Psychiatry,* 152, 359–366.

Hawton, K., Fagg, J., Platt, S., *et al* (1993) Factors associated with suicide after parasuicide in young people. *British Medical Journal,* 306, 1641–1644.

Kosky, R. (1987) Is suicidal behaviour increasing among Australian youth? *Medical Journal of Australia,* 147, 164–166.

Kosky, R., & Goldney, R.D. (1994) Youth suicide: a public health problem? *Australian and New Zealand Journal of Psychiatry,* 28, 186–187.

Kotila, L. & Lonnqvist, J. (1988) Adolescent suicide attempts: sex differences predicting suicide. *Acta Psychiatrica Scandinavica,* 77, 264–270.

Nielsen, B., Wang, A.G. & Bille-Brahe, U. (1990) Attempted suicide in Denmark. IV. A five-year follow-up. *Acta Psychiatrica Scandinavica,* 81, 250–254.

Nordentoft, M., Breum, L., Munck, L.K., *et al* (1993) High mortality by natural and unnatural causes: a 10 year follow up study of patients admitted to a poisoning treatment centre after suicide attempts. *British Medical Journal,* 306, 1637–1641.

Pokorny, A.D. (1982) Prediction of suicide in psychiatric patients. *Archives of General Psychiatry,* 30, 1089–1095.

Schneider, P.B. (1954) *La tentative de suicide. Etude statistique, clinigue psychologique et catamnestique.* Neuchatel, Paris: Delachauz et Niestle SA.

Suokas, J. & Lonnqvist J. (1991) Outcome of attempted suicide and psychiatric consultation: risk factors and suicide mortality during a five-year follow-up. *Acta Psychiatrica Scandinavica,* 84, 545–549,

Tunving, K. (1988) Fatal outcome in drug addiction. *Acta Psychiatrica Scandinavica,* 77, 551–566.

12

YOUTH SUICIDE

The Victorian Coroner's Study

J. W. G Tiller,[1] J. Krupinski,[2] G. D. Burrows,[3] A. Mackenzie,[4]
H. Hallenstein,[5] and G. Johnstone[6]

[1]Department of Psychiatry
 The University of Melbourne
[2]Mental Health Research Institute, & State Coroners Office, Victoria
[3]Department of Psychiatry
 The University of Melbourne
[4]Mental Health Research Institute, Victoria
[5]Magistrate & Former State Coroner
[6]State Coroner

1. INTRODUCTION

The suicide rate in Victoria has increased progressively, as it has nationally, particularly since the 1960s. The increased suicide rate in persons under 25 is predominantly in young adult males in the 20–24 year age group, but to a lessor degree affects all groups. A retrospective study of youth suicide identified these differences and was reported previously by this research group (Krupinski, Tiller, Burrows & Hallenstein, 1994). This increase has also been noted in other Australian states (Kosky, 1987). Rates of suicide amongst young people in Australia are higher than in many other western countries (Baume, 1996; Diekstra & Garnefski, 1985; World Health Organisation, 1996). The Victorian coroner, established a Working Party to study suicide. The Working Party decided on youth suicide as it's primary objective. In the early 1990s when the Working Party was established there was no contemporaneous Victorian data on the causes of youth suicide. It was determined to study all consecutive youth suicides in Victoria over an interval of time and compare those with people who attempted suicide who were first of all hospitalised for more than 24 hours, and those who presented to emergency departments but were not hospitalised. It was expected that the non-hospitalised group would be like those reported elsewhere as having made suicide attempts or para-suicides, and the hospitalised attempters would be intermediate with characteristics between those who made attempts and who committed suicide. Though it has been claimed that a prior suicide attempt is the

Suicide Prevention, edited by Kosky *et al.*
Plenum Press, New York, 1998

best indicator of suicide risk (Dudley & Waters, 1991), the majority of those who make attempts do not progress to suicide. A previous study by Krupinski, Stoller and Polke (1967) showed that suicide attempters consist of two different groups; there were those who wanted to but failed to die, and those who responded with a suicide gesture to family or relationship conflicts. It was determined to use data from this study to develop a predictive instrument to identify those persons making suicide attempts, who had characteristics like those who completed suicide.

2. AIMS AND METHODS

1. To compare a consecutive cohort of all persons under the age of 25 committing suicide in the state of Victoria with young persons presenting to hospital emergency departments, whether admitted or not, following a suicide attempt.
2. To delineate suicide attempters at high risk to commit suicide.
3. To develop a useful screen to enable early recognition of those attempters at risk of suicide.
4. To identify the demographic characteristics differentiating those making suicide attempts from those completing suicide.

The method was to match suicides with attempted suicides, hospitalised and non-hospitalised. Matching was by two age groups, 15–19 and 20–24 years, and where possible to match by sex. Data was obtained from coronial inquiry and hospitals using a youth suicide interview schedule developed by the investigators. The completed suicide schedules were filled in during the context of coronial inquiry, information being collected from family, significant others, doctors, other professional carers, teachers, police and from suicide notes, when available. Psychiatric registrars, psychiatrists and other health professionals collected hospital data from suicide attempters during clinical evaluation. The three samples were compared as a whole, and in two sex and two age groups by block design. In addition, three groups of 51 subjects each were compared matching by sex and age. Variables discriminating significantly between completed and attempted suicides, were included in a multiple logistic regression analysis (Lee, 1986) to determine relative odds to commit suicide. That data is reported in this book in "Predicting suicide risk among young suicide attempters (Krupinski, Tiller, Burrow & Mackenzie, 1997)."

3. RESULTS

148 consecutive suicides were studied over a 16 month period. In addition 105 hospitalised suicide attempters, and 101 non-hospitalised suicide attempters were studied. The highest suicide risk was amongst the young adult male with a ratio, male to female, of 6:1, while the highest attempted suicide risk was among young women with a ratio to men of 2:1. The suicide method was most commonly by hanging (37%), firearms (20%) and carbon monoxide (18%).

Typical Suicide

The profile of the typical young person committing suicide is that they are male, using a violent method, leaving a suicidal note, and having psychiatric problems or a worthless feeling. These people will have rarely asked for help before suicide.

Typical Suicide Attempter

In contrast to the suicide detailed above, the typical suicide attempter is a female, using drugs or poisons, giving reasons such as relationship and family conflicts, quarrels and family fights, and with a clear precipitant such as a broken relationship or a fight. These people characteristically have sought help prior to the attempt.

Why Do Fewer Women Commit Suicide?

The reason for fewer women committing suicide was not clear from our study, but possibilities included that young women have better networking skills, that they are more prepared to seek help, and that they have more adaptive communication skills. The example of notes left after suicide attempts clearly show young men can be aware of their feelings and have the capacity to communicate those feelings. However, it is clearly maladaptive to communicate after you are dead rather than while you are alive.

The implications of these differences mean that there one should look to trying to change attitudes and responses, especially among young men. It is important to improve men's communication skills, but also to change community attitudes and reduce stigma so that people will respond appropriately and constructively to young people's calls for help and assistance. In addition, there need to be available psychiatric resources for young adults and the ability to access those resources.

Assumptions Disproved

The data showed that in this sample there were no significant differences between the suicides and the community, in terms of country of birth, nor urban-rural differences. Threats or attempts did not discriminate between subsequent suicide attempts or suicide. Almost 90% who committed suicide had no identified help-seeking behaviour, in contrast to the common belief that the majority seek help before committing suicide. There was no specific event prior to suicide for the majority, with, for example, unemployment identified as a reason for under 5% of suicides. Those who committed suicide had fewer identified stressful life events than those who made attempts. Over half of those committing suicide were living at home and were not alone, homeless or in desperate solo situations. Past histories of physical or sexual abuse were related more to attempts than suicides and the majority of those who suicided were not using vast quantities of drugs or alcohol. Those who made attempts and were hospitalised were like the non-hospitalised attempters, not like those who committed suicide.

4. DISCUSSION

These data confirm the author's prior retrospective data that the group at greatest risk of youth suicide are young adult males. The typical suicide clearly contrasts with the suicide attempter. Women tend to use methods of self harm which do not overtly affect the appearance of their body (such as drugs or poisons), rather than violent methods such as hanging, shooting or carbon monoxide poisoning, of which the first to at least, can markedly disfigure the body.

An important background characteristic for suicides was psychiatric illness, especially depression and psychosis, with these being more marked in those who commit suicide. In contrast, relationship difficulties were more prominent for the suicide attempters. A quality of worthlessness, even in the absence of identified psychiatric illness was also typical of those who committed suicide.

Consideration of differences between suicides and suicide attempters raises the issue of why fewer women suicide. As noted above, networking skills, a preparedness to seek help and more adaptive communication carry with it implications for prevention.

Our initial hypothesis was that those presenting to hospital, and hospitalised after self harm, would be intermediate in characteristics between suicides and those making attempts and treated as outpatients. This hypothesis was not sustained. Those who attempted suicide and were hospitalised were in fact not significantly different from those who attempted suicide and not hospitalised, and quite different to those who committed suicide. Thus the hospitalised suicide attempters do not represent an intermediate group, but are like simply a different sample of the outpatient suicide attempters.

The common assumptions disproved also address a number of issues which may explain why some suicide prevention programs have been unsuccessful. While it is clear that amongst drug users a proportion will commit suicide, excessive drug and alcohol use did not show up as a major factor when considering the populations of suicides as a whole. Likewise with homelessness and unemployment, of those who are homeless and/or unemployed, some do commit suicide. However again, when looking at the population of suicides as a whole, these are small contributors to the total.

It is easy to become focused on means of suicide, without concentrating more on the underlying circumstances and mental state of the person planning suicide. There remains the prospect of individuals simply using available methods of suicide once the intent is clearly formed and action decided upon. Thus, firearm deaths are more common in the country where firearms are more generally available. Whereas jumping from high buildings or bridges, is rather easier in urban places than in the country.

It is also of importance to identify that a prior history of physical and sexual abuse relates more to suicide attempts than suicides, as again it is easy to divert resources given to a problem like physical and sexual abuse believing that attending to that may impact on suicide, when it may have a relatively minor influence on overall suicide rates.

5. RECOMMENDATIONS

As a result of the findings of this study, there is now a set of baseline data for the Victorian community. These are published in the report "A prospective study of completed and attempted youth suicides in Victoria (Tiller, Krupinski, Burrows, Mackenzie, Hallenstein & Johnstone, 1997).

It is clear that effective intervention needs a multi-layered prevention strategy with a range of interventions affecting the whole community and maintained over an extended period of time. There may be a role for some legislative changes at harm minimisation such as restricting access to firearms, and having carbon monoxide cut-offs when carbon monoxide levels are raised in the cabins of vehicles with internal combustion engines.

It is important to utilise a range of educational resources including the community as a whole, schools, education directed at professionals, politicians and opinion leaders, and the media generally.

There needs to be active education and skills development among young people to facilitate the recognition of feelings and to aid coping skills. Especially for young men, issues to do with mental health should accompany those to do with physical health starting from the earliest stages of school and continuing in an integrated way throughout the school years. This should hopefully help young men better identify their feelings, and be able to network, seek support and effective intervention on their own. This is especially important as the key for young men is to have this knowledge, and these skills and abilities when they leave school as their highest risk period is in young adulthood, after ceasing school.

It is important to have readily available and automatically available support and therapeutic services. There should not be bars to seeing health professionals like a local doctor, for example, not having the family Medicare card to get to medical help. Young people who may be reluctant to involve parents or other family members do need to know they can get medical and specialist help on their own initiative.

It is useful to have predictive screening especially for attempters and those with identified mental health problems, together with targeted prevention strategies for at-risk individuals. The prediction can be assisted with measures such as our predictive screening instrument, published elsewhere in this volume.

Finally, suicide interventions must be coordinated nationwide with effective evaluation so that those measures which prove successful and constructive can be further developed, and those which have marginal impact can be stopped. Some of these interventions will be expected to be years in progress before the value or not can be determined. In addition, it is essential that there is ongoing research in this area which results in the loss of so many young lives at the beginning of potentially productive adulthood.

REFERENCES

Baume, PJM. (1996). Suicide and young people. In B. McGrath, G. Groom & A. Wilde (Eds.).*General Practitioners and Adolescents: Dismantling the Barriers.* Canberra: Commonwealth Department of Human Services and Health.

Diekstra, RFW. & Garnefski, N. (1985). On the nature, magnitude, and causality of suicidal behaviours: An international perspective. *Suicide and Life-threatening behaviour, 25(1).* 36–57.

Dudley, M. & Waters, B. (1991). Adolescent suicide and suicidal behaviour. *Modern Medicine of Australia (September).* 90–95.

Kosky, R. (1987). Is suicidal behaviour increasing among Australian youth? *Medical Journal of Australia, 147.*164–166.

Krupinski, J., Stoller, A.. & Polke, P. (1967). Attempted suicides admitted to the Mental Health Department, Victoria, Australia: A socio-epidemiological study. *International Journal of Social Psychiatry, 13,* 5–13.

Krupinski, J., Tiller, JWG., Burrows, GD. & Hallenstein, H. (1994). Youth Suicide in Victoria: a retrospective study. *Medical Journal of Australia, 160.* 113–116.

Krupinski, J., Tiller, J., Burrows, G., Mackenzie, A., Hallenstein, H. & Johnstone, G. (1997). Predicting suicide risk among suicide attempters. In R. Kosky, R. Goldney and R. Hassan (Eds). *Suicide Prevention - The Global Context.* New York: Plenum Publishing Corporation.

Lee, J. (1986). An insight on the use of multiple logistic regression analysis to estimate association between risk factor and disease occurrence. *International Journal of Epidemiology, 15.* 22–29.

Tiller, J., Krupinski, J., Burrows, G., Mackenzie, A., Hallenstein, H. & Johnstone, G. (1997). A prospective study of completed and attempted youth suicides in Victoria. *A report from the Coroner's Working Party on Suicide.* Melbourne: Tiller, J., Burrows, G. and The University of Melbourne.

World Health Organisation. (1996). *World Health Statistics Annual.* Geneva: World Health Organisation.

13

PREDICTING SUICIDE RISK AMONG YOUNG SUICIDE ATTEMPTERS

J. Krupinski,[1] J. W. G. Tiller,[2] G. D. Burrows,[2] and A. Mackenzie[1]

[1]Mental Health Research Institute, Victoria
[2]Department of Psychiatry
 The University of Melbourne

1. INTRODUCTION

The rate of suicides among males, aged 15 to 24 years, has increased dramatically in most of the developed countries, including Australia, within the last 30–40 years, whilst the reasons for this increase is still unclear. General preventive measures are non-effective and difficult to apply because suicide is a rare phenomenon. Preventive measures should, therefore, concentrate on groups at risk. However as Shaffer, Phillips, Garland and Bacon (1990) stated, "the known risk factors are sensitive... but very non-specific." Dudley and Waters (1991) noted that a suicide attempt is the best indicator of suicide risk, as 30 to 50% of completed suicides have a history of previous attempts. Our previous study (Krupinski, Stoller & Polke, 1967) has shown that suicide attempters consist of two different groups, those who wanted, but failed to die, and those who responded with a suicidal gesture to family or relationship conflicts. It is, therefore, necessary to predict, who of the suicide attempters are at risk to complete a suicide.

2. AIMS AND METHOD

To determine the attempters who are high risk to complete suicide, we decided:

1. To compare completed suicides with severe and non-severe attempts in young people in the 15–24 years age group;
2. To delineate suicide attempters who are at high risk to commit suicide so that preventive actions can be focused on those most vulnerable; and
3. To develop a useful screen, which will enable recognition of those at risk.

The recently published prospective study of completed and attempted youth suicides in Victoria (Tiller, Krupinski, Burrows, Mackenzie, Hallenstein, & Johnstone, 1997a) en-

Suicide Prevention, edited by Kosky *et al.*
Plenum Press, New York, 1998

abled us to compare 148 completed suicides (all youth suicides completed within Victoria within 16 months) with 105 suicide attempters, hospitalised for at least 24 hours, and 101 non-hospitalised suicide attempters, seen in the emergency departments of the cooperating hospitals. A youth suicide schedule was developed and tested in a pilot study, covering the following areas: sex and age, method and circumstances of suicide or suicide attempt, previous suicide attempts and threats, family setting and relationships, study and work history, medical and psychiatric history, the use of therapeutic and non-therapeutic drugs, contacts with police and reasons for those, and life events in the last three months. The schedules for completed suicides were filled in within the framework of the coronial inquiry, information being collected from the family, significant others (including doctors and other professional carers), police and from suicide notes, when available. Psychiatric registrars and other health professionals collected the required information from suicide attempters during their clinical interviews. We compared the three samples as a whole, and in four sex and age groups (a block design). In addition, it was possible to compare three groups of 51 subjects each, matched by sex and age. Variables discriminating significantly between completed and attempted suicides, were included in a multiple logistic regressions analysis (Lee, 1986) to determine relative odds to commit suicide.

3. RESULTS

The variables, significantly discriminating between completed and attempted suicides are presented in Table 1. Those who completed suicide, used significantly more frequently violent than non-violent methods than both groups of suicide attempters ($p<0.0001$), even when controlled for sex and age. Both groups of suicide attempters

Table 1. Odds ratios to complete suicide—Univariate analysis

Variable	Percentage of attempted suicides N = 206	Percentage of completed suicides N = 148	Odds ratio	95% confidence interval
Violent method	10.7	93.2	115.42	53.94–251.63
No prior help sought	35.5	85.5	14.34	8.02–25.63
Male	37.4	85.8	10.13	5.90–17.41
Suicide note	5.3	36.5	10.18	5.09–20.37
Psychiatric problem as a reason	15.0	38.5	3.84	2.13–5.86
Feeling worthless as a reason	7.8	23.0	3.54	1.87–6.70
Close/warm family relations with family	24.3	52.7	3.48	2.21–5.47
Aged 20–24	54.9	75.7	2.56	1.61–4.08
Relationship problems as a reason	40.3	30.4	0.65	0.41–1.01
Aged 15–19	45.1	24.3	0.39	0.34–0.45
Family conflict as a reason	28.2	11.5	0.33	0.18–0.60
Quarrels/fights in family	40.3	16.2	0.29	0.23 -0.35
Laceration	8.3	2.0	0.23	0.06–0.80
Physical abuse	25.7	5.4	0.15	0.10–0.19
Help sought from family/friends	27.2	5.4	0.15	0.07–0.33
Female	62.6	14.2	0.10	0.08–0.12
Help sought from doctor	43.7	6.8	0.09	0.06–0.15
Use of drugs or poisons	79.6	4.7	0.06	0.04–0.08

Table 2. Multivariate analysis

Variable	Odds—including method of suicide	Odds—excluding method of suicide
Violent method	47.74	—
No prior help sought	6.18	12.71
Suicide not written	5.23	5.33
Psychiatric problems	2.40	3.40
Being male	2.37	9.49
Aged 20–24	1.78	2.00
Conflict in family	0.39	0.43
Physical abuse	0.32	0.31
Constant	−6.80	−6.17

sought more frequently help from doctors, family and others than those who completed suicide, whilst the latter left more often a suicide note, in which they expressed love to their family, blamed themselves, and asked for forgiveness for their suicidal behaviour. Family relationship was reported to be more often close and warm among those who completed suicide, whilst attempters reported it to be distant or cool and complained of quarrels and fights, including past physical abuse. Significantly discriminating reasons for suicide were psychiatric problems and feeling worthless in those who took their life, and family conflict and relationship problems among suicide attempters.

The univariate analysis of odds ratio has shown that a violent method, not seeking prior help, being a male, leaving a suicide note, having psychiatric problems, feeling worthless, having close and warm family relationship, and being in the 20–24 age group indicated high risk to complete suicide, whilst an overdose, seeking prior help, being a female, reporting a physical abuse, family conflict, fights and quarrels, and being in the 15–19 age group provided low risks odds in this regard.

As the methods of suicide had such an enormous bearing on the probability to commit suicide, multivariate analysis was carried out in two ways, with and without the inclusion of the method used (Table 2.)

The cumulative odds were afterwards expressed in percentage risks to commit suicide (Table 3). Using the arbitrary cut-off point of 40%, we would miss less than 7% of subjects, who killed themselves, if the method of suicide was included in the equation. On the other hand, almost 9% of attempters should be regarded at risk. The exclusion of the method of suicide would widen the net, what is acceptable from the preventive point of view.

Table 3. Prediction of suicide—probability of completing suicide

	Probability					% correctly predicted
	< 0.2	0.2 < 0.4	0.4 < 0.6	0.6 < 0.8	> 0.8	
Analysis included method of suicide						
Suicide completed	7	3	2	15	121	93.2
Suicide attempted	181	7	5	12	11	91.3
Analysis excluded method of suicide						
Suicide completed	4	16	14	54	60	86.5
Suicide attempted	142	26	12	18	8	81.2

4. DISCUSSION

There is no doubt about the representativeness of our sample, as all completed suicides in Victoria during a 16 month period were covered, and attempted suicides admitted to seven main Victorian hospitals were included. Regarding the reliability of the information collected, there is no doubt that such "hard" data as sex, age, or method of suicide reflect the true picture of the persons concerned. Some information, dealing with physical or sexual abuse, or utilisation of help, have to be regarded as minimum figures, with positive answers accepted at their face value. Questions can be raised, however, as to how reliable is the "soft" information on family relationships and on reasons for suicide. Did the picture presented in suicide notes on the close, loving relations with their families by those who completed suicide, reflect the true situation in the family, or did those who had already decided to take their life write especially positively about their families to lessen their pain? We are not able to answer this question, but have to accept that statements about the closeness of family relations in contrast to conflict, fights and quarrels are indicative of a serious wish to take one's life.

Another point of dispute could be whether the recognition of psychiatric problems in information collected by police on completed suicides during coronial inquiries is valid; police could have missed a proportion of them. However, the fact that psychiatric problems were recorded significantly more often in completed suicides indicates that this variable does discriminate between completed and attempted suicide.

We believe, therefore, that our study supports the notion that suicide attempts do not constitute a uniform group. The calculation of odds ratios allows us to select attempters most likely to commit suicide, and apply to them intensive, individually tailored preventive measures. It would be a great achievement in suicide prevention, if this approach will save from committing suicide the 30–50% of subjects with a previous attempt. We feel very strongly that this method should be used routinely in all admissions after a suicide attempt. This could be achieved by computing to allow automatic calculation of the percentage risk for each subject admitted after an attempted suicide, or by calculating the risk manually using the prediction instrument for suicide outlined in Appendix A.

However, one has to realise that the predicting variables, obtained from the Victorian Study, cannot be used in other countries with different socio-cultural values. But the method of this study can be used to determine predicting variables in each country. Following this, a simple screening method can be applied to detect those high at risk.

ACKNOWLEDGMENTS

The Rotary Australian Health Research Fund, the Victorian Department of Human Services and the Department of Psychiatry, The University of Melbourne helped with financing the study. The Victorian State Coroner, the Victorian Police and the staff of the cooperating hospitals assisted in collection of the data. Mr Norman Carson helped with the analysis of the odds ratios and with the development of the simplified method of their calculation.

REFERENCES

Dudley, M., & Waters, B. (1991). Adolescent suicide and suicidal behaviour. *Modern Medicine of Australia (September)*. 90–95.

Krupinski, J., Stoller, A.. & Polke, P. (1967). Attempted suicides admitted to the Mental Health Department, Victoria, Australia: A socio-epidemiological study. *International Journal of Social Psychiatry, 13,* 5–13.

Lee, J. (1986). An insight on the use of multiple logistic regression analysis to estimate association between risk factor and disease occurrence. *International Journal of Epidemiology, 15,* 22–29.

Shaffer, D., Phillips, I., Garland, A. & Bacon, K. (1990). Prevention issues in youth suicide. *In Prevention of Mental Disorders, Alcohol and Other Drug Use in Children and Adolescents.* DASP Prevention Monograph-2. Rockville, MD.

Tiller, J., Krupinski, J., Burrows, G., Mackenzie, A., Hallenstein, H. & Johnstone, G. (1997a). A prospective study of completed and attempted youth suicides in Victoria. *A report from the Coroner's Working Party on Suicide.* Melbourne: Tiller, J., Burrows, G. and The University of Melbourne.

Tiller, J., Krupinski, J., Burrows, G., Mackenzie, A., Hallenstein, H. & Johnstone, G. (1997b). A prospective study of completed and attempted youth suicides in Victoria. In R. Kosky, R. Goldney and R. Hassan (Eds). *Suicide Prevention—The Global Context.* New York: Plenum Publishing Corporation.

APPENDIX A. PREDICTION INSTRUMENT

Variables	Scores given to the selected variables	
	Including method of attempt	Excluding method of attempt
Violent method	4.0	—
No prior help sought	2.0	2.5
Leaving a suicide note	1.5	1.5
Psychiatric problems	1.0	1.0
Being a male	1.0	2.0
Aged 20–24	0.5	1.0
Reported conflict in family	−1.0	−1.0
Reported physical abuse	−1.0	−1.0
Constant	−4.0	−5.0

Summarise the total score and check in the table below for the percentage risk of suicide.

Score	% Probability to suicide
4	98
3	95
2	88
1	75
0	50
−1	25
−2	12

14

AN OVERVIEW OF INDIGENOUS SUICIDE

Ernest Hunter

University of Queensland
North Queensland Clinical School
Department of Social and Preventive Medicine
Cairns, Queensland

The public understanding of Aboriginal suicide has been shaped by specific events, in particular the Royal Commission into Aboriginal Deaths in Custody. The publicity surrounding the Commission contributed to a widespread view that Aboriginal suicide is common, most often occurring in custody, with indigenous prisoners being at much greater risk than non-indigenous inmates. While the Royal Commission demonstrated that these perceptions are incorrect, the images are tenacious and persistent. In fact, overall, indigenous Australians die by suicide at a rate very similar to that of the wider Australian population, the ratio of age-adjusted rates for deaths attributed to suicide for indigenous versus non-indigenous populations for the period 1990–1992 (excluding Queensland which did not, at that time, identify Aboriginality on death certificates) being 0.9 (Moller, 1996).

However, for the same populations and periods, when examined by age, it is clear that indigenous suicide clusters in a younger population, the rate being significantly higher for the age-group 25–34 years (Harrison & Moller, 1994). Furthermore, and looking at more recent figures (1993–1995) from South Australia, Western Australia and the Northern Territory, it is also clear the greatest burden of loss is suffered by young indigenous males, with the highest rate being for those aged 15 to 19 (Harrison, Moller & Bordeaux, 1997).

These findings need to be contextualised, both in terms of an increased risk experienced by indigenous youth for injuries and deaths from non-natural causes generally (with elevated risk again clustering in the same age-groups), and in terms of changes over time. In terms of the latter, there has been considerable attention given to the increase in suicide rates for young males in the wider population which have trebled over the last three decades (Harrison, Moller & Bordeaux, 1997). Unfortunately, comparable figures for indigenous populations are not available. However, it is clear that not only are young Aboriginal and Torres Strait Islander males at greater risk than their non-indigenous peers, their elevated suicide rate has increased from a base rate that three decades ago was, almost certainly, extremely low (Hunter, 1993).

Suicide Prevention, edited by Kosky *et al.*
Plenum Press, New York, 1998

Thus, at a time when suicide rates are increasing significantly for young adult males in the wider population, male sex and youth have also emerged as vulnerability factors for indigenous suicide. Indeed, given that this has been a relatively recent contributor to premature indigenous mortality, that is probably all that can be said; the pace of change is such that it would be foolhardy to presume that this will be the case two decades hence. In particular, it is far from clear whether suicide will remain contained within the youth and young adult populations, or whether the increased vulnerability of Aboriginal youth and young adults will be carried with them as they pass into and through their middle adult years, thus shifting to parallel the distribution found in the general Australian population.

Regardless of whether this turns out to be the case (and I believe that it will) we can at least say with certainty that increased vulnerability was first experienced by young Aboriginal males passing into and through adolescence in the late 1980s. As suicide is an endpoint (as are also, for example, increasing rates of alcohol abuse, self-mutilation, child abuse and domestic violence) I suggest that most is to be learnt by exploring the background and precursor factors rather than seeking a 'cause' in the immediate circumstances (although those circumstances may well have informed the expression as suicide per se). This demands exploring the social ambience of Aboriginal development for those reaching maturity in the 1980s, thus the world experienced and shaped by those young adults who were having children through the 1970s.

As I have argued previously (Hunter, 1993), this was a period of tumultuous change with significant consequences for social roles within Aboriginal Australia, particularly for men. The generation who were young adults at that time were buffeted by social forces that included, among many others, dislocation from traditional and transitional lands, entry into the cash economy with unemployment and welfare dependence, and increasing access to alcohol. The direct consequences born by that group included increasing rates of morbidity and mortality from accidents and injuries, and social disruption in communities that were already disadvantaged. The indirect consequences have included the impact of that social upheaval on family life, in particular, on paternal availability which, in turn, is consequential for the construction of male identity.

I suggest that indigenous young adult males of the 1980s were already increasingly emotionally vulnerable and that the circumstances of continuing social disadvantage and binge drinking provided a context in which the impulsive, aggressive expression of those conflicts and tensions resulted in escalating interpersonal violence and, subsequently and perhaps influenced by deaths in custody and deliberate self-harm. In this construction suicide must be considered within the wider spectrum of violent behaviour, a proposition supported by a much higher proportion of indigenous suicides by violent means. From the 1990–92 data noted earlier (Harrison & Moller, 1994), 93% of Aboriginal suicides resulted from hanging or firearms, compared to 43% of non-Aboriginal deaths. While it may be stating the obvious, these are also the most lethal (Australian Institute for Suicide Research and Prevention, 1996).

Given the availability of means (with guns being readily available in remote and rural settings and hanging being a matter of opportunity rather than means) and the simplicity of execution, the connection with alcohol intoxication and impulsivity is particularly salient. Indeed, research from the Kimberley revealed that impulses to self-harm and suicide were widely experienced by indigenous informants, with a moderate association to drinking status and pattern. However, acting on those impulses was strongly associated with alcohol and, furthermore, among those who were drinkers, it was the quantity consumed per drinking occasion rather than the frequency of consumption that predicted past self-harmful or suicidal acts (Hunter, Hall & Spargo, 1991). Thus, rather than being causal in an absolute sense, alcohol appears to function by enabling the acting out of simmering impulses that may be externalised or internalised. Regardless, for young adult males the objects of this violence are most frequently that individual's most important relational objects - partners, family and friends, and the self - core referents in the construction of identity.

There is not sufficient space to consider those underlying issues in more detail. Suffice it to say that they exist in an intercultural context and that, thirty years after the Commonwealth Referendum, the tensions experienced by young adult Aborigines in relation to the wider society are probably greater than were experienced by their parents at a similar age. The failure of our society to deliver on the opportunities that were so optimistically anticipated has resulted in frustration, hopelessness and anger, particularly for those whose roles and status are most obviously compromised, young males. Winston Seaton of Palm Island touches on many of the issues - drugs, alcohol, unemployment, family conflict, fatalism and emotional despair - in his poem "Questions that were never answered." I conclude with his words.

What is tormenting the Youth of Palm?
A question that's been asked from Butler Bay to Farm.
Is it society or is it alcohol and dope, maybe no job?
That's when they think there's no hope.

Could it be so much pressure building up inside...
The young mind thinking perhaps there's nowhere to hide.
Maybe a drink will solve the pain, and a smoke to calm the brain.

One thing leads on to another, arguing with family,
your Father and Mother. Run and hide and let out the tears,
the pain is there but not the fears.

Is it some force that's taking them away,
or pressure of society from living day to day?
No one knows what's in another's mind,
when a psychiatrist will try to seek and find.

Nothing works and nothing ever will,
its over...its gone over the hill.
It's slowly tearing the mind apart,
from head to toe then finally the heart.

Talking to someone but they just won't listen,
life is full of hits and misses.
Finally it's back to the drink and smoke
where it all ends at the end of a rope.

Winston Seaton (by permission of the author).

ACKNOWLEDGMENTS

This article appeared in Australasian Psychiatry, October 1997, p. 231, and appears courtesy of Blackwell Science Asia Pty Ltd.

REFERENCES

Australian Institute for Suicide Research and Prevention. (1996). Access to means of suicide by young Australians. Report for the Commonwealth Department of Health and Family Services, Youth Suicide Prevention Advisory Group. Australian Institute for Suicide Research and Prevention, Brisbane.

Harrison J & Moller J. (1994). Injury mortality amongst Aboriginal Australians. Australian Injury Prevention Bulletin, 7 (September).

Harrison J, Moller J & Bordeaux S. (1997). Youth suicide and self-injury Australia. Australian Injury Prevention Bulletin, 15 (March, Supplement).

Hunter E. (1993). Aboriginal health and history: Power and prejudice in remote Australia. Melbourne: Cambridge.

Hunter E, Hall W & Spargo R. (1991). The distribution and correlates of alcohol consumption in a remote Aboriginal population. Monograph No 12. National Drug and Alcohol Research Centre, Sydney.

Moller J. (1996). Understanding national injury data regarding Aboriginal and Torres Strait Islander peoples. Australian Injury Prevention Bulletin, 14 (December).

15

SUICIDE IN EARLY PSYCHOSIS

Could Early Intervention Work?

Patrick McGorry, Lisa Henry, and Paddy Power

Centre for Young People's Mental Health
Parkville, Melbourne
Department of Psychiatry
University of Melbourne
Parkville, Melbourne

1. INTRODUCTION

In Australia suicide rates among young males aged between 15–24 years have tripled over the last 30 years (Australian Bureau of Statistics, 1994 (ABS)). In 1994, Australia recorded the highest rate of youth suicide among all industrialised nations with an annual incidence of 16.4 suicides per 100,000 for Australian 15–24 year olds, with rates being especially high for males aged 20–24 years ("News: Suicide," 1994). Major psychiatric disorders are extremely common among these young people who commit suicide and it is at this particular age (below 25 years) that major psychiatric disorders such as affective disorders and psychosis have their peak age of onset (Hafner, Maurer, Loffler, *et al* 1995; Lewinsohn, Clarke and Rhode, 1994). Surprisingly, only a small percentage of these young people who commit suicide are actually being treated for mental illness at the time of their suicide (Isometsa, Henriksson, Aro, Heikkinen *et al.*, 1994; Shafii, Carrigan, Whittinghill and Derrick, 1985).

2. SUICIDE IN THOSE WITH SERIOUS MENTAL ILLNESS

People who have been diagnosed with a psychiatric disorder, face a higher risk of suicide than the general population. The risk of suicide among the mentally ill in the Australian state of Victoria is estimated at 15 times higher than for the general population (Victorian Suicide Prevention Task Force Report, 1997). Suicide is a consequence of a complex interaction of various determinants whereby mental illness holds a front-line position in the matrix of causation (Tanney, 1992). Retrospectively conducted psychological

Suicide Prevention, edited by Kosky *et al.*
Plenum Press, New York, 1998

autopsies consistently report that between 90% to 98% of adolescent suicide victims had suffered from a psychiatric disorder either before or at the time of their suicide (Brent, Kupfer, Bromet, *et al.*, 1988; Marttunen, Aro, Henricksson and Lonnqvist, 1991; Rich, Sherman, and Fowler, 1990; Runeson, 1988;). Shafii *et al.* (1985) concluded that 95% had a diagnosable major psychiatric disorder and 81% had two or more co-morbid mental disorders, compared with 29% of the controls. The research by Shafii *et al.* suggested that 76% of those adolescents who suicided, suffered a major affective disorder or dysthymia, 70% had an associated substance abuse disorder, 70% had a history of antisocial behaviours, 65% had 'inhibited' personality traits, and 50% had made a previous suicide attempt.

2.1. Suicide in Affective Disorder

Psychotic depression appears to carry a five times greater risk of suicide compared to non-psychotic depressive disorders (Roose, Glassman, Walsh, *et al.*, 1983). Similarly, bipolar disorders have a particularly high risk of suicide, especially around the time of switch of mood (Jamison, 1986). Mixed states of mania and depression also appear to constitute high risk periods, this possibly being due to the combination of dysphoria and impulsivity. However, suicide rarely occurs during a pure manic episode (Robins, Murphy, Wilkinson, Gasner and Kayes, 1959). Rates of suicide appear to be similar in both unipolar and bipolar disorders but are possibly higher in bipolar type II disorder (Goodwin and Jamison, 1990). Overall, suicide rates are similar in males and females with mood disorders, though female suicides tend to occur in the first 15 years of illness, while male suicides appear to be bimodally distributed between the early and late phases of illness (Goodwin and Jamison, 1990). Comorbidity with substance abuse disorders (Fawcett, Schefter, Fogg, Clarke, Young, Dedeker and Gibbons, 1990) appears to enhance the risk of suicide in affective disorders.

2.2. Suicide in Schizophrenia

Schizophrenia occurs in 1 per cent of the population. The onset of schizophrenia occurs in late adolescence and early adulthood. This stage of life involves the crucial step of developing one's identity and ability to individuate as a person. The development of the disorder at this time in the individuals life can disrupt the person's developmental trajectory. Their work or academic life may be impaired, along with their social relationships. Suicide is the major cause of premature death in persons with schizophrenia with 10 per cent of persons diagnosed with schizophrenia committing suicide. Among patients with schizophrenia who die by suicide, males outweigh females by a ratio of 4:1, with males usually committing suicide before 30 years of age and females before 40 years of age (Black and Winokur, 1988). The profile of those who suicide are usually young, single, unemployed, males in the first 10 years of onset of a severe chronic form of the illness (Roy, 1982). Fifty percent of suicide patients with schizophrenia have made previous suicide attempts (Caldwell and Gottesman, 1990; Roy, 1986). Other studies confirm some of these risk factors and identify additional risk factors for patients, such as having: the paranoid subtype of the disorder (Fenton and McGlashan, 1991); relatively higher intelligence (Westermeyer, Harrow and Marengo 1991); relatively better psychosocial functioning premorbidly and higher self expectations of performance (Drake and Cotton, 1986) complicated by more severe morbidity following the illness onset; early disturbed psychosocial adjustment (Modestin, Zarro and Waldvogel, 1992); greater levels of depression (Roy,

1982); greater awareness of their pathology (Drake and Cotton, 1986); and complicating substance abuse (Runeson, 1989). Suicide is less likely in deficit subtypes of psychosis (Fenton and McGlashan, 1997).

Drake, Gates, Cotton and Whitaker, (1984) reported that suicide rarely occurs in the acute psychotic phase of schizophrenia. Many patients show improvement in functioning and have periods of remission before the suicide. The suicide tends to have been planned and agitation appears to be the predominant feature at the time of suicide. 'Self-reported subjective distress,' 'awareness of illness and disintegration,' and 'hopelessness' all appear to be associated features. The period during the onset of the development of the symptoms of schizophrenia, prior to detection and treatment, can be a high risk time for suicide as individuals attempt to deal with the complexity and confusion which accompanies this period. Prescription and illicit drugs and/or alcohol may often be used to self-medicate in an effort to cope with the disturbed mental state. The peri-discharge period from hospital is also a vulnerable time for completed suicide, particularly among males (Roy, 1982) there is speculation about contributing factors such as shorter lengths of hospitalisation, loss of support, reduced supervision, noncompliance with treatment, treatment resistance, and renewed exposure to stressors in the post discharge period. Common associated stresses include family conflict and rejection by the family (Brier and Astrachan, 1984).

According to the Victorian Suicide Prevention Task Force Report (1997), suicide rates were higher where no community follow-up care had been organised after discharge from hospital for patients with schizophrenia.

2.3. Suicide Risk in Early Psychosis

In our clinical experience at the Early Psychosis Prevention and Intervention Centre (EPPIC), which is a component of the Centre for Young People's Mental Health (CYPMH), suicide ideation and behaviours are common, but transient phenomena. Suicidality in early psychosis appears to be influenced by multiple interacting factors (both aggravating and protective) that wax and wane during the course of illness. Important interactive influences appear to be that of subjective distress caused by acute psychotic or persistent negative symptoms, emerging insight into the illness, and pessimism about one's prognosis. Among the patients attending EPPIC, suicidal behaviours appear to occur most frequently during the phases of emerging psychosis, early recovery and early relapse/failed recovery, with suicide behaviours occurring most frequently during the early recovery phase. Refer to Figure 1, which depicts these phases of risk.

Suicide ideation in the early phase appears particularly common during the transition from prodrome to psychosis, and usually before contact has been made with health services. From our clinical experience, it appears to be dependent on factors such as the degree of subjective awareness of prodrome deterioration, the speed of onset and fluctuating nature of the process, the degree of instability of mood (mixed affective features), levels of anxiety, command hallucinations, positive symptoms that represent prominent depressogenic themes, positive symptoms that are associated with particularly severe subjective distress, the patient's subjective impression of entrapment and hopelessness induced by psychotic experiences, the patient's impressions of significant other's responses and the associated subjective impression of rejection or shame (Birchwood, 1996).

Suicide ideation during the early recovery phase appears to be more common as insight emerges during the resolution of the symptoms of psychosis. From our clinical experience, it appears to occur earlier if the patient's understanding of psychosis is coloured by expectations of poor prognosis or distress with treatment, or later, when the patient's in-

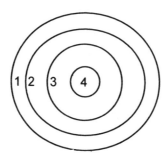

Phase 1: Pre-detection and entry to treatment.
Phase 2: First Episode Psychosis.
Phase 3: The Critical Period.
Phase 4: Prolonged Psychosis.

Figure 1. Phases of risk.

itial relief (gained by resolving psychotic symptoms, discharge from hospital, and escape from the intense level of clinical involvement) is superseded by distress due to the experience of persistent negative symptoms, post-psychotic depression, enduring psychosocial stressors, stagnation of life goals and loss of peer group. The period 1 - 3 months post-discharge from hospital is when suicide ideation and intent appears to peak in first episode psychosis patients. This is often a time when follow-up services are gradually reducing their involvement as the psychosis resolves, or the patient is experiencing difficulties remaining engaged.

During the last phase, suicidal ideation appears to occur when distressing psychotic symptoms fail to resolve, or re-emerge in the context of maintained insight, or when negative symptoms persist in the context of high personal, family, or staff, expectations.

3. SUICIDE RATES IN THE FIRST-EPISODE PSYCHOTIC POPULATION

Prior to the Early Psychosis Prevention and Intervention Centre's (EPPIC) inception, in 1992, treatment of first-episode psychotic patients in the Western region of Melbourne, was provided by an inpatient unit with outpatient treatment occurring by the regional community mental health centres. The number of new cases of psychosis treated by EPPIC has been approximately 250 per year. Since 1992, ten patients have committed suicided, despite the intensive level of interventions provided during this first-episode and 18-month follow-up phase. Nonetheless, this appears to be a reduction, in comparison to the rates of suicide among the pre-EPPIC population (5 suicides amongst 250 patients). Overall, between 1989–1997, approximately 1,350 people who were treated for first-episode psychosis and 15 people committed suicide. The method of suicide is in Table 1 below.

Table 1. Suicide methods used

Suicide method	Number
Hanging	6
Train/truck	3
Overdose	2
Electrocution	1
Asphyxia	1
Jumped from bridge	1
Unknown	1

The average age at death was 23 years old. The proportion of male to female was 11:4, respectively. Seventy-one percent of the suicides occurred within the first year of treatment, with the range being from 1 day through to 37 months. Therefore the length of follow-up appears not to be the problem as most of the suicides occured within the first 1–2 years of onset of symptoms. The time since the suicide victims were last in contact with a psychiatric service ranged from 1 to 11 days. Therefore all were in close contact with psychiatric services i.e., none had "dropped-out" from the service. The 15 suicides all occurred out of hospital, although 3 patients were 'on leave' from an inpatient hospital admission.

A substantial proportion of patients presented with or developed serious suicide ideation or behaviours at some stage during the course of their first episode of psychosis and recovery. A small number of patients from the service have died from either ambiguous or unexplained methods. Therefore, deciphering the intent behind these types of deaths can often blur the boundaries between suicide ideation or accidental death.

4. SUICIDE PREVENTION AT THE CENTRE FOR YOUNG PEOPLE'S MENTAL HEALTH

Service models that effectively reduce the suicide rates in those with early psychosis might be those that develop strategies to enhance: the early detection of psychosis; improved mechanisms for access to psychiatric services; 'user friendly' non-stigmatising mental health services for young people; adequate supports for carers of those with psychosis; effective treatments for those either already suffering from, or at risk of, developing early psychosis; and specific suicide prevention forums or structures within health services.

For those with early psychosis and identified as carrying a high risk of suicide, specific treatment interventions that might be effective in reducing the high risk of suicide may mediate their effect via mechanisms that: (a) ensure effective treatment, e.g. for depressive features, for side effects (akathisia), for those whose psychopathology is undetected, under-treated, or resistant to standard treatments; (b) ensure that secondary morbidity factors are being addressed, e.g. adjustment difficulties and hopelessness in the context of losses sustained (loss of relationships, employment, accommodation and importantly — loss of self esteem); and (c) address comorbid factors, e.g. substance abuse disorders, and premorbid factors, e.g., personality disorders or impaired social supports. Co-morbid conditions may be quite long-standing or entrenched, and may respond poorly to interventions. Commonly however they are simply overlooked.

The CYPMH Youth Access Team (YAT) provides early detection, assessment and crisis intervention. The team continues to develop links with various aspects of the community to ensure early detection. Such community links include: general practitioners, accident and emergency departments, teachers and youth support services. Co-ordination of these services is vital in the detection of early signs of suicidal behaviour and ideation.

The case management program at the CYPMH aims to offer continuity of care regardless of the phase of illness of the patient, i.e. whether as an inpatient or outpatient, the patient will have the same case manager. This model is operational within EPPIC and is currently being developed within OAS. This model is multidiscipline and multifaceted with the programs including: psychological, day program, family work and an accommodation service.

Individual cognitive-behavioural psychological interventions have demonstrated efficacy in psychosis (Jackson, McGorry, Edwards and Hulbert, 1996;) and have been trialed at EPPIC. These have shown probable indirect effects on reducing suicide risk in early psychosis through their effects on the primary/secondary symptoms of psychosis, adaptation issues, insight, treatment compliance, and by maximising protective influences against suicide through the instillation of hope in recovery.

Three suicide prevention projects have commenced at the CYPMH and are described below.

4.1. Individual Intervention for Young People Who Have Severe Mental Health Problems and Are at Risk of Suicide

A specific individual cognitive behaviour therapy intervention to address suicidality in psychosis is currently being developed and trialed at CYPMH as part of a Federally-funded national mental health initiative to introduce suicide prevention strategies for young people with serious mental illnesses (National Mental Health Strategy, 1995). This suicide prevention cognitive-behaviour therapy (CBT) based intervention is applied within the context of a crisis intervention model (given the urgent and transient nature of suicidality) and supplements standard case management. The therapy aims not only to address state-related risk factors, but also to provide: psychoeducation about the mechanisms of suicidality; coping strategies for suicide ideation; coping strategies to assist with the desensitisation of the impact of triggers; strategies to access assistance, augment protective factors such as 'hope' in recovery, self-esteem; education about psychosis; and assist with adjustment to losses. For those with active psychotic symptoms, a greater number of sessions may prove necessary due to the more complicated nature of suicidality in acute psychosis and the not infrequent impaired information-processing problems that may accompany active psychosis.

4.2. An Intervention Approach to Suicide and Self-Harm with Adolescents

The second research study aims to enhance access and early intervention and reduce suicidal behaviour by developing, implementing and evaluating a treatment program with a sample of adolescents, aged 14–18, with non-psychotic forms of serious mental illness and who present with suicidal or self-harming behaviour in the previous three months. They will be recruited from General Practitioners and two Accident and Emergency Departments in the Western suburbs of Melbourne. The treatment program, based on the work of Linehan and Lewinsohn, consists of an intensive group treatment over twelve weeks which will directly address health damaging behaviours, provide skills and enhance positive self-esteem.

4.3. An Analysis of Health Damaging Behaviours in Young People at High Risk Of Suicide

The third study is a prospective study of the incidence of suicide ideation and behaviours among a group of young people who are identified to be at high risk of later developing psychosis. This involves a comparison with a 'normal' control group and with a first episode psychosis group, to investigate which factors are associated with a high risk of developing suicide thoughts and behaviours at this early phase of illness development.

5. CONCLUSION

It is characteristic of all serious mental illnesses that they are associated with a substantial increase of suicide risk. The determinants of suicide risk may be different in each case but some common pathways may exist, such as demoralisation and acute stress. These pathways need to be avoided in an attempt to offer relevant and appropriate treatment to those at risk of suicide. Clinicians need a better understanding of the suicide matrix, that is, the complex sequence of components which may lead to suicide, and need to be able to target the intervening variables such as suicidal ideation and depression.

REFERENCES

Australian Bureau of Statistics.(1994). *Causes of Death* (Cat. No. 4102.0). Canberra: AGPS.

Birchwood, M. (1996). Keynote lecture at Verging on Reality, First International Early Psychosis Conference, June.

Black, D., Winokur, G. & Nasrallah, A. (1988). Effect of psychosis on suicide risk in 1593 patients with unipolar and bipolar affective disorders. *American Journal of Psychiatry,* 145, 849–52.

Brent, D., Kupfer, D., Bromet, E., et al. (1988). The assessment and treatment of patients at risk of suicide. In *American Psychiatric Review of Psychiatry, Vol 7.* eds: A. Frances & R. Hales, pp 353–385. Washington, D.C.: American Psychiatric Press.

Brier, A. & Astrachan B. (1984). Characterisation of schizophrenic patients who commit suicide *American Journal of Psychiatry*, 141, 206–9.

Caldwell, C. & Gottesman, I. (1990). Schizophrenics kill themselves too: A review of risk factors for suicide. *Schizophrenia Bulletin*, 16, 571–59

Drake, R.E., Gates, C., Cotton, P.G. & Whitaker, A. (1984). Suicide among schizophrenics: Who is at risk? *Journal of Nervous and Mental disease*, 172, 613–7.

Drake, R. & Cotton, P. (1986). Depression, hopelessness and suicide in chronic schizophrenia. *British Journal of Psychiatry*, 146, 554–59.

Hafner, H., Maurer, K., Loffler, W., *et al* (1995). Onset and early course of schizophrenia. In *Search for the Causes of Schizophrenia, Vol III.* Eds. H. Hafner & W.F. Gattaz, pp 43–46. New York. Springer.

Fawcett, J., Schefter, W., Fogg, I., Clarke, D., Young, M., Hedeker, D. & Gibbons, R. (1990). Time related predictors of suicide in major affective disorder. *American Journal of Psychiatry,* 147, 1189–94.

Fenton, W. & McGlashan, T. (1991). Natural history of schizophrenia subtypes. *Archives of General Psychiatry*, 48, 969–77

Goodwin, F. & Jamison, K. (1990). *Manic Depressive Illness.* New York: Oxford University Press.

Isometsa, E.T., Henriksson, M.M., Aro, H.M., Heikkinen, M.E., *et al.* (1994). Suicide and major depression. *American Journal of Psychiatry,* 151, 530–6.

Jamison, K. (1986). Suicide and bipolar disorders. *Annals of the New York Academy of Science*, 487, 301–15.

Jackson, H., McGorry, P., Edwards, J. & Hulbert, C. (1996). Cognitively Oriented Psychotherapy For early Psychosis (COPE). Ed. P. Cotton & H. Jackson. In *Early Intervention and Prevention in Mental Health,* pp 131–154. Melbourne, Australia. Australian Psychological Society.

Lewisohn, P.M., Clarke, G.N., & Rhode, P. (1994) Major depression in community adolescents: Age at onset, episode duration, and time to recurrence. *Journal of the American Academy of Child and Adolescent Psychiatry*, 33, 809–818.

Lewisohn, P.M., Rohde, P., & Seeley, J.R. (1996) Adolescent Suicidal Ideation and Attempts: Prevalence, Risk Factors, and Clinical Implications. *Clinical Psychology: Science and Practise* (3) 25–46.

Marttunen, M. J., Aro, H. M., Henricksson, M.M. & Lonnqvist, J.K. (1991) Mental disorders in adolescent suicide: DSM-III-R axes I and II diagnoses in suicides among 13 to 19 hear olds in Finland. *Archives of General Psychiatry*, 48, 834–839

Modestin, J., Zarro, I., Waldvogel, D. (1992). A study of suicide in schizophrenic inpatients. *British Journal of Psychiatry,* 160, 398–401

News: Suicide. (1994). *British Medical Journal*, 308, 7–11.

Rich, C.L., Sherman, M., & Fowler, T.C. (1990). San Diego suicide study: The adolescents. *Adolescence*, 25, 855–865.

Robins, E., Murphy, G., Wilkinson, R., Gasner S., & Kayes J. (1959). Some clinical considerations in the prevention of suicide based on a study of 134 successful suicides. *American Journal of Public Health*, 49, 888–898.

Roose, S.P., Glassman, A.H., Walsh, T., *et al.* (1983). Depression, delusions, and suicide. *American Journal of Psychiatry*, 140, 1159–1162.

Roy, A. (1982). Suicide in chronic schizophrenia. *British Journal of Psychiatry,* 141, 171–177.

Roy, A. (1986). Suicide in schizophrenia. In *Suicide* (ed: A. Roy) pp 97–112. Williams and Wilkins: Baltimore.

Runeson, B. (1989). Mental disorder in youth suicide: DSM-III-R Axes I and II. *Acta Psychiatric Scandinavia*, 79, 490–497

Shafii, M., Carrigan, S., Whittinghill, J.R., & Derrick, A. (1985). Psychological autopsy of completed suicide in children and adolescents. *American Journal of Psychiatry*. 142, 1061–1064.

Tanny, B. (1992). Mental disorders, psychiatric patients, and siucide. In R. Maris, A. Borman, J. Maltsberger and R. Yufit (Eds.), Assessment and Prediction of Suicide, The Guilford Press, New York, U.S.A..

Victorian Suicide Prevention Task Force Report, July 1997.

Westermeyer, J., Harrow, M., Marengo, J. (1991). Risk for suicide in schizophrenia and other psychotic and non-psychotic disorders. *Journal of Nervous and Mental Disease,* 179, 259–266.

16

SUICIDE AMONG THE CANADIAN INUIT

Antoon A. Leenaars,[1,2] Jack Anawak,[3] and Lucien Taparti[3]

[1]University of Leiden
The Netherlands
[2]Windsor, Ontaria, Canada
[3]Rankin Inlet, NorthWest Territories, Canada

Across the Arctic, Aboriginal people, the Inuit, have rates of suicide that are three to four times the Canadian average (Royal Commission of Aboriginal People, 1995). This is equally true for Aboriginal people in Alaska and Greenland (Kirmayer, 1994). There are very few people across the world with such staggering suicide rates. Our intent here, utilizing both nomothetic and idiographic approaches, is to share some epidemiology, history, stories of the land, and words on healing from the Inuit.

EPIDEMIOLOGY AND THE ARCTIC SCENE

Weyer (1932/1962) first suggested that suicide was a cultural trait of the Inuit (although he called them "Eskimos," a white man's word that means eater of blubber). Boas (1964) concurred that suicide was not uncommon. These early observers discussed suicide as a way of life. Documenting "altruistic" suicide, they noted that suicide, in the elderly, disabled, or sick, was undertaken to preserve the group. However, although suicide in the elderly occurred, later observers noted that both Weyer and Boas may have exaggerated the reports from specific cases in specific communities. Even more so, youth suicide was very scarce in the old ways (Kirmayer, 1994; Kirmayer, Fletcher, & Boothroyd, 1997). This, unfortunately, is not the case today. Suicide rates among Inuit in Canada, Alaska, and Greenland have increased dramatically in the last 30 years (Kirmayer, 1994). As an illustration, most Canadian Inuit live in the Northwest Territories (NWT) and that region of Canada has the highest rate of suicide in Canada. In 1991, *Statistics Canada* reported a rate of 40.3 per 100,000 (67.1 male; 11.4 female) in the NWT, compared to a total of 13.3 per 100,000 (21.6 male; 5:2 female) in Canada. Table 1 presents the rates of suicide for North West Territories and Canada from 1980 to 1992. However, these data present only a snapshot of the actual rates. Abbey, Hood, Young, and Malcolmson (1993) have reported rates of 54.5 to 74.3 per 100,000 in some communities. The highest risk group is young

Suicide Prevention, edited by Kosky *et al.*
Plenum Press, New York, 1998

Table 1. Suicide rates in Northwest Territories
and Canada

	Canada	Northwest Territories
1980	14.0	20.9
1981	14.0	21.9
1982	14.3	17.0
1983	15.1	43.4
1984	13.7	34.4
1985	12.9	25.5
1986	13.4	28.7
1987	14.0	29.0
1988	13.5	40.2
1989	13.3	58.1
1990	12.7	33/3
1991	13.3	40.3
1992	13.5	28.5

Rates are incidence per 100,000 population.
Source: 'Statistics Canada'

males (Kirmayer, 1994). There has been in fact an increasing rate for young males, but not females. Wotton (1985) in one northern community, reported rates as high as 295 per 100,000 for 15–25 year old males.

With regard to suicide attempts, there are few studies. Boyer and his colleagues (Boyer, Dufour, Preville & Beyold-Brown, 1994) reported life time prevalence of 14%. However in the young people (15–24 years) the lifetime prevalence is 27.6% for males to 25.3% for females. These events are much higher than for the general population of Canada. Domino and Leenaars (1994), for example, found 3% of the population reporting a lifetime prevalence of suicide attempts. Thus, it is an easy conclusion that suicide and suicide attempts are a serious problem in the Canadian Arctic.

A HISTORICAL BACKGROUND

The Inuit people of Canada live primarily in the eastern Arctic, as well as in northern Quebec and Labrador. Approximately 80 percent of the people of the eastern Arctic are Inuit. The present-day Inuit people stem from the Thule whale-hunting culture that dates back to about A.D. 900, who overlapped with the Dorset people (approx. 1700 B.C. - A.D. 1100), who in turn overlapped with the pre-Dorset and Denbigh people (approx. 3000 B.C. - 500 B.C.) (Houston, 1995; Kral, Arnakaq, Ekho, Kunuk, Ootoova, Popatsie, & Taparti, 1997). Archaeologists have found evidence that people resided in what is now Igloolik four thousand years ago (Purich, 1992). Canadian Aboriginal people, including the Inuit and Dene of the North have lived in northern Canada well before the Vikings arrived on the shores of Canada around 1008AD.

The Inuit had foreign visitors or Qallunat (Inuktitut for non-Inuit) long ago, but notably occurring after 1400AD with the arrival of British and other European fishing ships, along with steady colonisation, predominately by the English and French. The Qallunat did not begin to have a major impact in the Arctic, however, until the whaling expeditions and fur trade during the nineteenth century. Hostilities were common then. Great diseases were introduced by the Europeans and took tens of thousands of lives. By 1900, only about one third of the Inuit population was left alive (Leenaars & Kral, 1996). These epidemics continued during the first half of the twentieth century, and it has been estimated that by 1950 one-fifth of the Inuit population had tuberculosis (Kral et al, 1997). The pain and hostilities increased as the fur trade declined and ultimately collapsed in the 1930s. The Canadian welfare state was introduced in the Arctic and created a human disaster as the significant involvement of the federal government in the lives of the Inuit increased. The presence of missionaries, the government, and large-scale community relocations during the 1940s and 1950s of the Inuit, in the context of attempts at assimilation into Canadian society, changed northern life enormously (Kral et al, 1997; Tester & Kulchyski, 1994). The way of life in the Arctic continued to change. Food and other important resources changed, such that even caribou was lost from the diet in some communities. Lifestyles changed from extended family kinship and nomadic hunting practices to a modern economy. The establishment of new settlements resulted in traumatic experiences and aftershocks (Crisjohn & Young, 1996; Royal Commission of Aboriginal Peoples, 1995).

Oil exploration and wells began on Melville Island in 1959, further increasing the pain in the north. Significant increases in social problems and especially suicide occurred after 1960, primarily among young males (Durst, 1991; Kral et al, 1997; Travis, 1984). Suicide, in fact, increased dramatically with colonialism among Aboriginal peoples in Canada (Anawak, 1994). In the Arctic, from Alaska through the NWT and Greenland during the 1970s and 80s epidemic levels of suicide were reported (Kirmayer, Fletcher, & Boothroyd, 1997). The loss of traditional lifestyle has been linked to anomie, powerlessness, and youth suicide in Aboriginal cultures throughout North America, Australia, and the world (Berlin, 1987; Kahn, 1982; May, 1987).

The Inuit continue to experience social disintegration (Durkheim, 1897). They have one of the highest birth rates globally, double that of Canada. Fifty-nine percent of the Inuit population is under 25 years old, compared with 35 percent of all of Canada (The Globe and Mail, 1997). Infant mortality is 3.5 times higher than it is nationally, and life expectancy is up to fifteen years lower. The Inuit unemployment rate is almost in the 30 percent range (The Globe and Mail, 1997). There is also a significant housing shortage (Purich, 1992). Colonial hostilities have impacted upon each generation in different ways (O'Neil, 1986).

It is now well documented that the Canadian government, beginning in the late nineteenth century, systematically suppressed traditional Aboriginal beliefs and lifestyles through treaties, the Indian Act, residential schools and reservations, and the outlawing of spiritual ceremonies and persecution of those who were caught practicing traditional ways (Dickason, 1992; Kral et al, 1994; York, 1989). Residential schools were especially endemic (Crisjohn & Young, 1996). These attempts at supression are, hopefully, no longer in effect and Canada's Inuit are in a healing phase.

A healing has, in fact, recently been started in the Arctic by the Inuit themselves. The lifestyles of Inuit are being restored. A new Inuit territory called Nunavut, first proposed in 1976, will come into existence in the eastern Arctic in 1999, promising hope and deliverance to the people, with Jack Anawak being its first leader.

STORIES FROM THE LAND

Understanding suicide in the Arctic is complex, more complex than Weyer and Boas suggested. These Qallunat merely interpreted suicide as a cultural trait in the Inuit. Yet, it has increasingly been understood that the event is multifarious. Of course, as in all suicides, there is pain, mental constriction, frustration of needs, and so on (Shneidman,

1985). However, it is not simply these factors that explain the tragedy in the Arctic. As our account of the history shows, the Inuit have experienced profound cultural changes in their lives. This rapid change has had a major impact on the Inuit and all Aboriginal people (Royal Commission on Aboriginal People, 1995).

To understand suicide, we believe that giving voice to the people is a sound avenue to knowledge (Kral, Arnakaq, Ekho, Kunuk, Ootoova, Papatsie, & Taparti, 1997; Leenaars, 1995; Leenaars & Kral, 1996). Narrative accounts are, in fact, becoming increasingly common in the human sciences. Allport in 1942, in fact, had already argued for such idiographic documentation, showing the importance of personal documents in human science. He argued that letters, logs, memories, diaries, autobiographies, personal accounts - and we would add suicide notes - have a place in understanding people. The tabular, statistical, demographic approach has a place in understanding suicide among the Inuit. Yet, the idiographic involves the intense study of people themselves, allowing us to "do justice to the fascinating individuality" of these people.

Narrative knowing or story telling is the tradition of the Inuit. No statistics, in fact, can capture the pain of the people. We will, thus, report two types of personal documents in order to understand. However, we do not imply that the nomothetic approach has no place, only that both avenues are needed to comprehend suicide among the Inuit. The first type of document will be some stories about travel by the author (AL) to the Arctic; and the second will be the actual words of healing from an Elder from the land.

Here are the stories:

My plane was to pick me up at 5:00 p.m. from Pangirtung (population 1,000), a small hamlet near the Arctic Circle on Baffin Island. However, there was a snow storm. There are few tourist places in Pangnirtung. Fortunately, I was able to stay with Rev. Roy Bowkett and his family. Let me tell three little stories about the land:

1. I decided to cook supper; so, I went to the "Northern" (previously the Hudson Bay stores) and bought 2 cans of spaghetti, 1 1/2 lbs of hamburg, noodles, bread and peanut butter. The cost was $44.95. The cost of living is unbelievably high. Indeed, one carver I met said, "Groceries are more expensive than carvings."
2. As we were eating, a couple of Inuit children came in to join us. One said, "That smells good." I offered to share, provided they asked their parents. The oldest girl looked at me in a perplexed way and said, "I'm Inuk" (singular for Inuit). From my travels, I knew what this meant, Inuit children make their own decisions and parents respect the decisions, something maybe we should all learn.
3. One of the children - she was 11 - asked me "Where are you from?" I mentioned Windsor and noted the trees outside my home. She said, "I've never seen a tree."

To get an idea about the numbers of suicide, let me share with you my favourite trip on the land. I went out for a Kamotiq (sled) ride with two Inuit guides from Apex (pop. 200), a tiny hamlet near Iqaluit (pop. 3,000) on Baffin Island. We went over the ice of Frobisher Bay and went inland over the small lakes and land, while it was snowing. We travelled and travelled. The caribou were passing us. The land is not only beautiful but I found it healing. On the trip, we stopped at a camp for tea - after all it was 2:00 p.m. - and as we sat, one Inuk told about his sister and brother who had killed themselves. Everywhere there is pain. Regardless of where you go, one becomes aware of the vast number of suicides. All of the community is experiencing aftershock. The official statistics of NWT are likely unreliable. Research by Joshie Teemotee, an Inuk from Iqaluit, supports this perception; the statistics underreport the actual numbers.

Rankin Inlet is a beautiful community on the very north shore of Hudson Bay (pop. 1000). One of the most important sites in Rankin is their Inukshuk. Inukshuk are like stone figures; they are guideposts for the caribou hunts and for the travellers. They are found across the Arctic.

Once when I was in "Rankin," the first Keewatin Arts & Crafts Festival was being held. Keewatin artists are carrying on the tradition of fine art. There was a Northern Feast where traditional foods such as arctic char & caribou were served. It was a feast of feasts. It ended with a concert by Susan Aglukark who performed in the native language, Inuktitut. One of her songs, "Arctic Rose" is about a young Keewatin who goes south, leaving the land. She sings about how this man, who comes from a place where it is six months night, did not know darkness until he saw the city lights. He lost himself, turning to alcohol and drugs. The pain grew and in the end, he killed himself, being returned to the land by the spirits after his death. The song is prototypical of the pain of the people.

I was fortunate to meet with young people in the schools on Baffin Island. We talked about suicide. They told me about their friends who had killed themselves. They told me about suicidal people. These young people were quite knowledgeable about the facts about suicide (as much as the young people whom I have meet in the schools in the south). We talked about helping, the place for peer counsellors ... I could have been speaking in any school in Canada.

The students raised many issues that I have heard before: is suicide for attention? confidentiality, the lack of services, the need to know what to do. Some concerns were different, however. The magnitude of the problem is an obvious difference. Most of these young people have many suicides among their family members and friends. The pain is expansive.

During a visit to Rankin Inlet, I met with Jack Anawak, M.P. and Senator Willie Adams. Both men are federal leaders from the Arctic and deeply concerned about the rate of suicide. I asked what they had learned.

They told about abuse by white men. They shared with me tales of sexual abuse. Although they told tales about the rewards of the churches, it was clear that there is an anger towards the Western churches because of this....and equally, towards the Canadian government.

On one of my trips above the Arctic Circle, I met a young Inuk woman, Sandra Inutiq. She was the 1993 valedictorian at Iqaluit's Inuksuk High School. She also had been on the front page of the *Globe and Mail* (Canada's national newspaper) on August 2, 1993. The article had focused on the story that drugs, suicide, and abuse mean that most Inuit teens never finish high school. Sandra was featured in the article, highlighting that Northern leaders are in short supply to guide the young. This article had caused, understandably, a lot of upset in the north. "Was it the way the southern press reports the facts?," I asked Sandra. Indeed, she was very upset at the southern press, although she also stated that there are deep problems in the Arctic. She said, "We have witnessed and been deeply touched by so many of the social problems around us." She said that suicide is a major problem "that must be addressed by teachers and parents." Sandra said, "People have to stop saying "my child doesn't do that."" Yet, she believes people are working to make a successful future for young people. "Elders are available. We do have leaders." Sandra and many others are interested in helping and she said, "I think education is the number one priority if Inuit are going to heal."

Young people have been involved in suicide prevention; yet, the pain continues. One adolescent on a revisit to his class a year later shared with me the pain in his class. Many had left school during the year; school drop-out was a major problem. One girl was pregnant. There had been substance abuse. There had been suicide. As he told me, one senses that the pain had gotten deeper for this youth.

Yet young people in the Arctic offer hope. Here are a few of their words: "I have lost because of suicide... I want to learn. I want to do something about it." "Listen to us, children. Don't deny the problems." "Lets stop the pain."

Jack Anawak, has spoken to me many times. He tells me that the pain of the people is "deep in the psyche." He notes how traditional ways had been forgotten. Acculturation is the norm. People don't know who they are, where they came from, and where they are going. Jack Anawak says "How we think... how we talk... has been affected deep in our psyche." The best analogy I can offer is the iceberg. What people are beginning to struggle with in the north is likely the tip of the iceberg, and Arctic icebergs are large.

Jack Anawak noted that "only by re-learning the traditional ways with the new is healing possible." Jack Anawak does not believe that people can only heal by going back to the old; he and many leaders in the north see a need for growth and development. To go back to only the old ways, he says, is much too simplistic of a solution.

Jack Anawak admits that there are problems. Substance abuse is a major worry. Of course, there are those people in the south who also abuse drugs. Yet there are many efforts in the Arctic to fight substance abuse and "it is helping." The same is true for suicide.

Jack Anawak said how Inuit ways differ. These ways are complex. As an example, he said punishment was less known before the Qallunat. People were rarely punished. They were not told "you're stupid." "When the white people came we were punished and told we were stupid." "We believed that we were stupid." Such cognitions are obviously important in the suicidal mind. Traditionally, people talked to their children. They would not say one was bad; rather, "elders would guide us." "They would tell us what they had learned."

Elders, such as Jack Anawak, are again being respected in the north. In Pangirtung, I had heard an Elder speak. She told about the old ways and when the whalers came. People hunted. People cleaned the whale... "and then the Qallunat would take the catch, leaving only blubber for us." "In our way," she said, "we share the labour and the catch."

Jack Anawak believes healing is possible. Many people in the north believe healing is possible. People need to speak about the sexual abuse, the alcohol use... and more. Suicide must be discussed. Jack Anawak, at the end of one of our conversations said, "I have no questions about who I am. I'm an Inuk, but I can adapt to other ways."

Many Inuit have noted that there has been a lot of changes. They spoke to me about the assimilation, the acculturation, being "totally lost." Accepting the acculturation is hard; yet, they encouraged progress and "waking up." Elders are obvious experts about life and suicide. People have even spoken to me about subintentional suicides such as about the lone hunter who goes out to the land, asking "Was it an accident or a suicide?" During my travel, I have learned that the Inuit are beginning to talk. Yet, they will need to understand much. Healing will take a long time because these people have not only lost their way of life, but some of their soul. They were stripped of their dignity and respect by people. Their children were taken away from them. They were imprisoned for speaking Inuktitut. They were raped. They were abused.

Yet, there is hope. Lucien Taparti, an Elder and friend from Rankin Inlet, stated that "people have been crying inside for a long time"; however, there is direction. He stated: "It is up to each individual to help... It is up to us to preserve our culture... our people."

The honorable Taparti believes that people need to communicate. If not, he suggested with psychoanalytic wisdom, that "the pain builds up." As he says, "if you smile, I smile back." That is the heart of the people. He believes "love can overcome all."

STORIES OF HEALING

We should listen closely to the people of the Arctic in order to understand. The words of an Inuit Elder, Lucien Taparti, reproduced from a Foreword to a forthcoming book, *Suicide in Canada*, edited by Leenaars, Wenckstern, Sakinofsky, Dyck, Kral and Bland, published by University of Toronto Press, are quoted here, to allow some understanding of suicide in the north from him:

"In the past we hardly used to hear of suicides in our communities and would hear of them every so often only, because there were less people. Once in a blue moon you'd hear of suicides in one of the communities. But nowadays, in one year there would be quite a few suicides. It's hard to grasp the problem. I feel we should look for solutions and start giving this matter more consideration/attention....."

"So how could we rectify this, working together in our communities, not only in the harsh land, but all of us in Canada? We have to start helping, because we all feel the same way and we live the same way. We all have the same lives. So we need to look for resources that would help in our communities. I wonder how we could start working together on this."

I want people to consider more in their communities on how we could work together. We need to teach our young people of their own culture, whether it be Inuit culture, Qallunat culture or Dene culture. Some of us who are using modern ways and people who knew the old ways then, would be able to say that we are using a new way.

I think we have to start asking ourselves, "Where can we get help with suicidal people?" It is essential that we each have to ask outselves this. The Inuit must ask themselves. We Canadians will have to ask how we could start to initiate things and how we could rectify problems more so and promote the issue more, so that suicide could decline. It's obvious now, that we'll have to really work together on this issue.......

We really have to start thinking of ways to rectify things. I'm sure this can be achieved some-how, but I don't know the answer to it. If it came from a larger community it could be a start-ing point and even if they think they couldn't, they would be able to do so. Just as long as they have appropriate laws (rules) that they'd use. As long as the rules are capable of being fol-lowed. I'll use snow as an example: it is worked on by different people, some are very good with snow and some are capable to work with it but not as well. That's why we use different types of snow to work with. Snow was our means of survival, even when we were young and even when we became adults. I wasn't worried at all, knowing that we'll get an iglu, even when there was going to be a blizzard. That was one of the laws and I followed it, so that was our life and the iglus were where our lives were. That's how we used to live in the winter time.

If we started tackling different things that we were capable of doing on our own, we couldn't really think of other things to get into. Soon as we were capable to do things that we had to follow, we didn't have much to be concerned of, not like our young people I see today. That's how it is with our culture from the harsh region, our cultures are all different and we need to keep it visible. If we ignore the issue, it is obvious that it wouldn't get rectified.

We all have different lives, different cultures and we can't say that the Qallunat have a strong culture. All of us came from our ancestors and if we could grasp that back then there were less suicides, perhaps we could start utilizing our culture for prevention. We'll have to know more about our cultures of our ancestors, and try to follow them and try to help each other more. We can use many people's cultures, whether they may be Qallunat's, Dene's or even the Inuit's culture. If we can be more aware of people's cultures, I'm sure that we would be able to come up with something that would be of benefit......

Jack Anawak (1994) has said the same, healing is probable. At an Iqualit conference in 1994 of the Canadian Association for Suicide Prevention (CASP), he stated:

"As Inuit and Dene people we have survived in what is considered to be the most challenging climate in the world. We have coped for hundreds, even thousands of years and developed at-titudes, behaviours, values and beliefs that allowed us to face whatever had to be dealt with and to overcome great difficulties. We must call upon those same values that brought us to this day. We need to own this problem. We cannot give it over to the governments, authorities, specialists, professionals, scholars, organizations or consultants. We own this problem. Say it... Believe it! We are part of the problem if we do not acknowledge this fact and take both in-dividual and collective action to address it."

We have finally come to realize that:

- WE are the experts of our stories.
- WE know the strengths and weaknesses of our own communities.
- WE have a pretty good idea about how things got this way.
- We have a value system that is worth honouring... and WE do have the brains to figure out what to do about it

The Inuit is now confronting the genocide towards indigenous people in the Arctic (Chrisjohn & Young, 1996).

AN AFTERTHOUGHT

We hope that the epidemiology, the history, memoirs of our travels and the words of healing of an Elder allow you to understand somewhat the unbearable pain among the

Inuit. We would like to add one final story from an Elder: The Elder stated that all the change in the Arctic has not been negative. He tells how in the 1940's there was a famine on the land. Many people died. In search of caribou, he and his older brother had been lost on the land during a snow storm. When his brother became very sick, the Elder had attempted to drag him, to carry him, anything. However, in the end, he had to leave his brother to die. The Elder still now feels the pain, the painful guilt. The man stated, "There are no more famines." The Qallunat, he stated, "have helped in some ways." Yet, the Inuit have also helped themselves for centuries and must again help themselves. A healing is needed in the Arctic: Respect for all.

NOTE

With thanks to M. Kral. Parts of this presentation were presented elsewhere:

Leenaars, A. (1995). Suicide in the Arctic. A few stories. *Archives of Suicide Research, 1*, 131–140.
Leenaars, A. & Kral, M. (1996). Suizidalität unter kanadishen Inuit - nomethetishe und idiograpische Perspektivin. *Suizidprophlaxe, 5*, 60–66.

REFERENCES

Abbey, S., Hood, E., Young, L., & Malcolmson, S. (1993). Psychiatric consultation in the Eastern Canadian Arctic: III. Mental health issues in Inuit women in the Eastern Arctic. *Canadian Journal of Psychiatry, 38*, 32–35.

Allport, G. (1942). *The use of personal documents in psychological science.* New York: Social Science Research Court.

Anawak, J. (1994). Suicide and the community. Keynote addresses presented at the conference of the Canadian Association for Suicide Prevention, Iqaluit, NT (Nunavat).

Boas, F. (1964). *The central Eskimo.* Lincoln: University of Nebraska Press.

Berlin, I.M. (1987). Suicide among American Indian adolescents: An overview. *Suicide and Life-Threatening Behavior, 17*, 218–232.

Boyer, R., Dufour, R., Préville, M., & Beyold-Brown, L. (1994). State of mental health. In M. Jetté (Ed.), *A health profile of the Inuit: Report of Santé Québec health survey among the Inuit of Nunavich, 1992,* Vol. 2, pp. 117–144. Montreal: Ministère de la Santé et des Services Socieux.

Chrisjohn, R. & Young, S. (1996). *The Circle Game: Shadows and Substance in the Indian Residential School Experience in Canada.* A report to the Royal Commission on Aboriginal Peoples, submitted Oct. 1, 1994.

Dickason, O.P. (1992). *Canada's First Nations: A history of founding peoples from earliest times.* Toronto: McClelland & Stewart.

Domino, G., & Leenaars, A. (1994). Attitudes toward suicide among English-speaking urban Canadians. *Death Studies, 19*, 489–450.

Durkheim, E. (1951). *Suicide* (J. Spaulding & G. Simpson, Trans.). Glencoe, iL: The Free Press (Original published in 1897).

Durst, D. (1991). Conjugal violence: Changing attitudes in two northern native communities. *Community Mental Health Journal, 27*, 359–373.

Houston, J. (1995). *Confessions of an igloo dweller.* Toronto: McClelland & Stewart.

Inuit endorse gender-equal legislature. *The Globe and Mail,* Jan. 27, 1997, p. A6.

Kirmayer, L.J. (1994). Suicide among Canadian Aboriginal peoples. *Transcultural Psychiatric Research Review, 31*, 3–58.

Kirmayer, L., Fletcher, C., & Boothroyd, L. (1997). Suicide among the Inuit of Canada. In A. Leenaars, S. Wenckstern, I. Sakinofsky, R. Dyck, M. Kral & R. Bland (Eds)., *Suicide in Canada.* Toronto: University of Toronto Press.

Kral, M., Arnakaq, M., Ekho, N., Kunuk, O., Ootoova, E., Papatsie, M., & Taparti, L. (1997). Stories of distress and healing: Inuit elders on suicide. In A. Leenaars, S. Wenckstern, I. Sakinofsky, R. Dyck, M. Kral, R. Bland (Eds.), *Suicide in Canada.* Toronto: University of Toronto Press.

Leenaars, A. (1995). Suicide in the Arctic: A few stories. *Archives of Suicide Research, 1*, 131–140.

Leenaars, A. & Kral, M. (1996). Suizidalität unter Kanadishen Inuit - nomethetishe und idiograpische Perspektivin. *Suizidprophlaxe*, 5, 60–66.

Purich, D. (1992). *The Inuit and their land: The story of Nunavut.* Toronto: James Lorimer & Company.

Royal Commission on Aboriginal Peoples (1995). *Choosing life: Special report on suicide among Aboriginal people.* Ottawa: Minister of Supply and Services Canada.

Shneidman, E. (1985). *Definition of suicide.* New York: Wiley.

Taparti, L. (1997). Foreword. In A. Leenaars, S. Wenckstern, I. Sakinofsky, R. Dyck, M. Kral, & R. Bland (Eds)., *Suicide in Canada.* Toronto: University of Toronto Press.

Tester, F.J., & Kulchyski, P. (1994). *Tammarniit (mistakes): Inuit relocation in the eastern Arctic, 1939–1963.* Vancouver: University of British Columbia Press.

Travis, R. (1984). Suicide and economic development among the Inupiat Eskimo. *White Cloud Journal, 3(3)*, 14–21.

Weyer, E. (1962). *The Eskimos: Their environment and folkways.* Hamden, CT: Archan Books (Original published in 1932).

Wotton, K. (1985). Labrador mortality. In R. Fortuine (Ed.), *Circumpolar Health 1984*, pp. 139–142. Seattle: University of Washington Press.

York, G. (1989). *The dispossessed: Life and death in Native Canada.* Toronto: Lester & Orpen Dennys.

17

SUICIDE IN JAPAN

What Are the Problems?

Yoshitomo Takahashi

Tokyo Institute of Psychiatry
Tokyo, Japan

1. SUMMARY

Although Japan had a high suicide rate in the 1950s, the rate has stabilized since then. This is despite continuing social problems such as an increasing divorce rate, the collapse of pre-existing family systems, changes in traditional values, increases in the incidence of drug abuse and crime, intensified competition in society, and widening of the gap between rich and poor. There are now about 21,000–22,000 suicides every year in Japan, making the suicide rate about 17 per 100,000. This paper discusses current state of suicide and future strategies for prevention in Japan.

1.1. Change in Suicide Rate

The National Police Agency (NPA) provides annual statistics of suicide in Japan (NPA, 1995; Takahashi, 1992, 1994b). Figure 1 shows annual changes in the number of suicides in Japan. A peak occurred in the late-1950s, followed by stabilization, and then a second peak was observed in the mid-1980s. After 1986, when the number of suicides was the highest in the post World War II period, there was a downward trend. In 1986 there was a transient increase of suicides among the youth, because there were two major suicide clusters. In January a 14 year-old junior high school student killed himself, with a suicide note left describing the bullying he received from class mates. The mass media reported this sensationally, which triggered other students' suicide all over the country. In April, a famous pop singer, Yukiko Okada, jumped to her death. More than 30 youngsters took their own lives within two weeks after her death, and her influence lasted about a year. The suicide rate among young people showed a high tendency only in this year, and since then has been decreasing. In 1994, there were 21,679 suicides in Japan and the suicide rate was 17.3 per 100,000. (Figure 2)

Suicide Prevention, edited by Kosky et al.
Plenum Press, New York, 1998

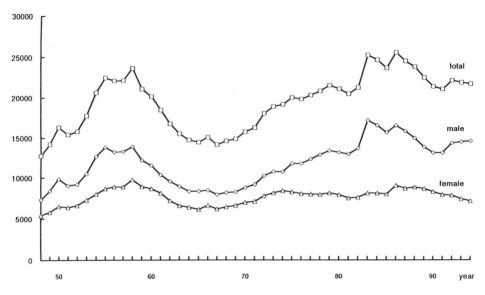

Figure 1. Annual changes in number of suicides in Japan.

Figure 3 shows changes in the suicide rate according to age group. A decrease in the rate among youth is evident from the 1950s to the 1990s for both males and females. In the 1950s and 1960s there were two peaks in the suicide curve, the young people and the elderly people. But the suicide rate of the young people has decreased since then. Contrary to the perception of the wider world, Japanese youth do not show a very high suicide rate. The recent trend is that the older the Japanese becomes, the higher the suicide rate is.

Needless to say, suicidal Japanese people have as many risk factors for suicide as those in other countries. These include prior suicide attempts, physical diseases, psychiat-

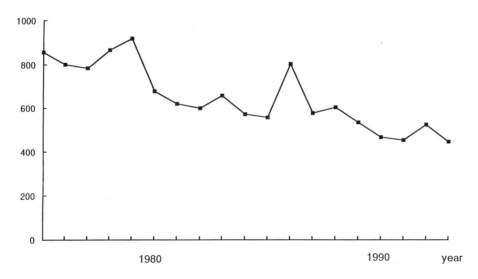

Figure 2. Annual changes in number of minor's suicide.

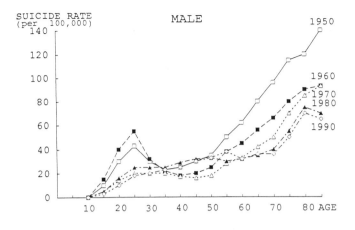

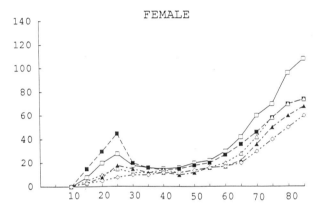

Figure 3. Changes in suicide rate according to age.

ric disorders (including mood disorders, schizophrenia, alcohol or substance abuse and personality disorders), lack of social support system, older age, male gender, various types of loss, physical or sexual abuse in childhood, accident proneness, a family history of suicide, and exposure to other people's tragic deaths (Takahashi, 1992, 1993a, 1993b).

1.2. Reasons

Figure 4 indicates reasons for suicide in Japan. The most common motive for suicide was suffering from physical illnesses (39.3% of all suicides) followed by suffering from psychiatric disorders (18.5%), financial problems (11.2%), family problems (9.0%), work-related problems (5.5%), love-related problems (2.6%), school-related problems (1.2%). There is a tendency for more males to commit suicide because of financial problems and work-related problems. According to the National Police Agency's report, the most frequent cause for suicide was suffering from physical illness, but other reports with a limited number of subjects conducted by mental health professionals including the author's researches (Takahashi, 1992), show that psychiatric disorders play a more important role.

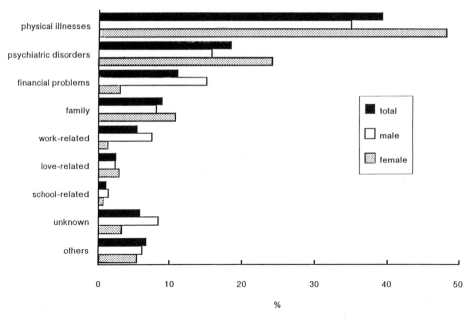

Figure 4. Reasons for suicide in Japan (1994).

1.3. Methods

Figure 5 summarizes the methods of suicide in 1994. The most frequently used method of suicide was hanging, (55.6%), followed by jumping off a high building (10.4%), drowning (8.5%), taking poison or drug overdose (5.6%), being run over by a train (5.2%) and so on. More males tend to use hanging as a suicide method while more females tend to use drowning. Suicide by gun is almost negligible, consisting of 0.2% of all suicides. There are strict gun control laws in Japan.

1.4. Comparison with Other Countries

Figure 6 shows a comparison between the suicide rates of some European countries and the United States of America and Japan. This indicates that Japan's suicide rate is not high compared with some European countries. Japan's recent suicide rate is about 17 per 100,000, which is almost similar to that of Sweden and Norway (Takahashi, 1995b).

1.5. Suicide of the Elderly

The suicide rate among young Japanese has generally shown a decreasing tendency over the past three decades. In contrast, suicide committed by senior citizens was and is an increasing problem in Japan. Individuals aged 65 and older accounted for 15% of the total population of Japan in 1994, yet there were 5,511 suicides in this age group, constituting 25% of all suicides. According to estimates made by the Ministry of Health and Welfare, the elderly population will grow to 24% of the total population by the year 2020. Therefore, suicide by the elderly has been and will be a big social problem (Takahashi, 1995a,

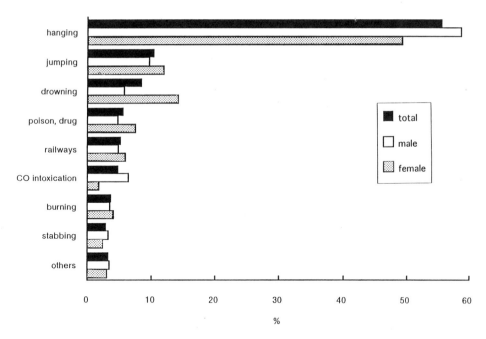

Figure 5. Methods of suicide in Japan (1994).

1995b, 1996b, 1996c; Takahashi, Hirasawa, Koyama, Asakawa, Kido, Onose, Udagawa, Ishikawa, & Uno, 1995).

Although the number is not yet high, suicide pacts between elderly couples could become a serious problem in the near future. One example is when an old spouse suffers from an incurable and chronically disabling disease such as senile dementia, and his/her partner also suffers from some form of illness due to advanced age. Because of the recent breakdown of the extended family system in Japan, such couples may not get enough support from their children or relatives. Neither do they want to be dependent on others. Such circumstances are made more difficult in that no adequate social system for supporting these lonely couples has yet been established. When a failing spouse with whom a partner has lived and shared his/her life can no longer function because of dementia, the other partner, usually the husband, might not be able to find any solution for this defeating struggle, and becoming depressed, decides to kill his wife and himself.

2. STRATEGIES FOR SUICIDE PREVENTION IN JAPAN

Compared with other nations, the author should admit that adequate social systems have not been established for suicide prevention in Japan and that there is still strong stigma against suicide.

Domino and Takahashi (1991) did a comparative study on people's attitude toward suicide in the United States of America and Japan. Japanese subjects tended to consider that suicide can be permissible in some situations and can be a behavior of normal conduct. In sharp contrast, Americans tended to think that suicide is a behavior based on aggression expressed toward oneself arising from some psychiatric problems and suicide

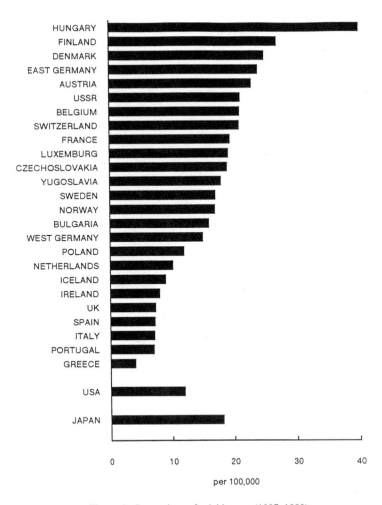

Figure 6. Comparison of suicide rates (1987–1989).

should be prevented. Strong stigma against suicide exists in Japan and against many kinds of activities for suicide prevention, which are being conducted in Europe and America, and are not available in Japan. The author would like to propose some areas to be improved in the future for suicide prevention in Japan as follows:

2.1. Decreasing Resistance toward Consulting a Mental Health Professional

Although the tendency has been changing gradually, there is still strong resistance among the general public to consulting a mental health professional. Japanese families are unwilling to accept the fact that their member may suffer from mental illness. They try to take care of the afflicted individual by themselves for as long as possible, and do not seek professional help until the condition has deteriorated (Takahashi, 1989, 1994b).

People do not talk about mental illness openly and tend to conceal the fact that someone may suffer from a psychiatric disorder in the workplace. If such a fact is known, it may become an obstacle to promotion or sometimes a reason for dismissal, either overtly or covertly. Because of this social stigma in general, people often miss a chance to seek professional help at an earlier stage. Therefore, more concerted efforts should be made to educate the public about mental health and the effectiveness of treatment in order to counter the stigma.

2.2. Educational Programs for Medical Students and General Practitioners

Although a curriculum for treating mental disorders is provided at medical schools, specific education focusing on suicide risk or its prevention is inadequate. Only a few medical schools offer special lectures on suicide prevention and the treatment of suicidal individual. Even these schools spare only a couple of hours for these topics in addition to other general subjects. It should be emphasized that medical students who will become core providers of accurate psychiatric knowledge in the future should be offered proper educational programs on suicide prevention.

In addition, Murphy (1986) has pointed out that the general practitioner can play an important role in detecting a patient's suicide risk at an earlier stage and initiating appropriate intervention for the suicidal crisis. This also applies to the present situation in Japan (Takahashi, 1991). According to an unpublished survey in Japan, nearly 80% of depressive patients first go to general practitioners complaining of various physical symptoms, but only about a quarter of them are properly diagnosed as suffering from depression and receive proper treatment. This shows how important it is to provide the general practitioner with up-to-date knowledge of psychiatric disorders and suicide risk. Furthermore, active interaction between psychiatrists and other medical specialists should be encouraged in order to exchange opinions on suicide prevention.

2.3. School (Community) Based Suicide Prevention Programs

When a suicide cluster of young people occurs, the mass media tend to sensationalise the tragedy, but no adequate countermeasures are discussed. School-based suicide prevention programs such as those conducted in the United States of America could be started in Japan, although some researchers have doubts about this (Shaffer, Vieland, Garland, Rojas, Underwood, & Busner, 1990).

Given that there is strong resistance against a suicide prevention program for high school students, the first step should be to educate parents, teachers or concerned people in community on suicide risk and how to make contact with mental health professionals. Parents and teachers especially can play an important role as responsible adults in detecting suicide risk among children and adolescents.

2.4. Suicide Prevention for the Elderly

As already touched upon briefly, suicide by the elderly is a big problem. The proportion of the elderly population in Japan will grow by about 200% within the next 30 years. Although the statistics show a high suicide rate among the elderly in Japan, clinicians have gained an impression that elderly patients rarely seek help from mental health professionals. The reasons for this are as follows (Takahashi, 1997; Takahashi, & Berger, 1996; Takahashi, et al., 1995):

    i. Elderly persons often experience various forms of loss, such as unemployment, retirement, death of a friend or spouse, or physical illness. Any given elderly individual may experience multiple losses within a short period, or at the same time. Because of this, people tend to regard their depressive state as "natural," especially considering the situation in which they are living. This erroneous psychological over-interpretation is made not only by persons associated with the elderly, but also the elderly themselves. Thus their depression is not considered a treatable condition, but rather something that the elderly must endure.

    ii. Elderly Japanese have a strong resistance to seeing a psychiatrist, and tend to put off asking for an appropriate psychiatric consultation. Depressed aged patients complaining of various physical symptoms often consult doctors in disciplines other than psychiatry. However, these general physicians often lack knowledge about psychiatric disorders and tend to stick superficially to the patient's ill-defined physical symptoms. Depression, therefore, is underdiagnosed and not treated properly. These circumstances lead to the tragedy that depression is left untreated, resulting in unnecessary suicide.

The most important point that the author would like to emphasize here is that educational programs should be started for the elderly, the general public, and physicians providing up-to-date knowledge of psychiatric disorders and suicide risk. Education should be provided for all those involved, with details of warning signs of depression and suicide. We should also establish a system of identifying high-risk groups, and start treatment as soon as possible. This would lead to elimination of the stigma associated with psychiatric disorders in the long run.

2.5. Psychological Help for Those Affected by Suicide

Ruth Benedict (1946) has called Japan a culture of shame. In such a culture the attitude of candidly speaking about a relative's or a friend's suicide cannot be recognized. Even though neighbours know that someone has committed suicide and his/her family or friends have difficulty in mourning, people try to avoid touching upon the subject and leave the persons concerned alone. It has been pointed out that others are greatly influenced psychologically by someone's suicidal behavior. It is also reported that the suicide rate among those who have experienced the suicide of a family member or friend is much higher than that among the general public (Roy, 1983). Therefore, those affected by suicide should be offered appropriate psychological help. We should consider providing psychological help by specially-trained mental health professionals and the formation of self-help groups.

2.6. Cooperation with the Mass Media

Japanese mass media do not always deal cases of suicide exaggeratedly, but there are some exceptions. Notorious examples are cluster suicide of young people. The mass media report such cases, explaining methods and motives in great details. The way they report is characterized by oversimplification of cause and effect, glorification, overgeneralization, and detailed explanation of suicide methods. Unfortunately, they themselves neither realize their role in developing suicide cluster nor have their own press code for reporting suicide.

However, efforts should be made to establish cooperative relationship with mass media since they could play an important role to educate the public accurate knowledge about psychiatric disorders, how to prevent suicide, and reduce stigma toward suicide in the public.

In the previous reports the author has made recommendations the media's reports on youth suicide (Takahashi, 1995c, 1996a). In summary, the mass media should: 1) avoid excessive reports on youth suicide; 2) refrain from over-simplified explanations for cause of suicide; 3) avoid glorification and exaggeration about suicide; 4) refrain from describing suicide methods in detail; 5) report youth suicide anonymously; 6) emphasize preventive measures; 7) put a concrete list of mental health professionals in community; 8) establish a closer relationship with mental health professionals before crisis actually occurs; and 9) prepare the press code by themselves in advance for prudent reporting.

3. CONCLUSION

Although the suicide rate in Japan has been stabilized recently, it is doubtful that this decreasing tendency will continue in the future, because Japan is now going through rapid and unprecedented social changes not experienced hitherto.

The extended family system has been gradually collapsing and the number of nuclear families has been increasing. As women have made advances into various fields of society, the social system has been changing. The divorce rate has also been increasing. Emphasis is now being placed on academic performance and the competition for entry to prestigious universities is so keen that even elementary school pupils go to supplementary schools and study until late at night. The gulf between the rich and the poor has been increasing, and the incidence of substance abuse, including alcohol, stimulants, solvents, and even cocaine, has been increasing among young Japanese recently. Furthermore, with the advent of an aging society, suicide by the elderly is already a big problem and will become more serious in the future.

Considering these social changes, there is a great likelihood that Japan will show an increase in the suicide rate again in the near future. The author believes that the time has come for Japanese to establish practical and effective systems in community to prevent suicide.

REFERENCES

Benedict, R. (1946). The Chrysanthemum and the Sword: Patterns of Japanese Culture. New York: New American Library.

Domino, J., & Takahashi, Y. (1991). Attitudes towards suicide in Japanese and American medical students. Suicide and Life-Threatening Behavior, 21, 345–359

Murphy, G. E. (1986). The physician's role in suicide prevention. In Roy, A. (Ed.) Suicide (pp.171–195). Baltimore: Williams & Wilkins.

National Police Agency (1995). National Police Agency's 1990 Annual Report, Tokyo: Printing Section of Ministry of Finance. (written in Japanese)

Roy, A. (1983). Family history of suicide. Arch Gen Psychiatry, 40, 971–974

Shaffer, D., Vieland, V., Garland, A., Rojas, M., Underwood, M., & Busner, C. (1990). Adolescent suicide attempters: response to suicide-prevention programs. JAMA, 264, 3151–3155

Takahashi, Y. (1989). Suicidal Asian patients: Recommendations for treatment. Suicide and Life-Threatening Behavior. 19, 305–313

Takahashi, Y. (1991). Risk factors for suicide. Journal of Japan Medical Association, 106, 1871–1876 (written in Japanese)

Takahashi, Y. (1992). Clinical evaluation of suicide risk and crisis intervention. Tokyo: Kongo-shuppan. (written in Japanese)

Takahashi, Y. (1993a). Suicide Prevention in Japan. In Leenaars, A.A. (Ed.) Suicidology: Essays in honor of Edwin S. Shneidman. (pp. 324–334) Northvale: Jason Aronson.

Takahashi, Y. (1993b). Depression and suicide. In Kariya, T. & Nakagawara, M. (Eds.) Affective Disorders: Perspectives on Basic Research and Clinical Practice. (pp. 85–98) New York: Brunner/Mazel

Takahashi, Y. (1994a). Characteristics of depression in Japan: Suicidal tendency. Japanese Journal of Clinical Psychiatry, 23, 55–63 (written in Japanese)

Takahashi, Y. (1994b). Suicide prevention. Japanese Journal of Clinical Psychiatry, 23, 809–815 (written in Japanese)

Takahashi, Y. (1995a). Suicide prevention for the elderly. Japanese Journal of Geriatric Psychiatry, 6, 178–183. (written in Japanese)

Takahashi, Y. (1995b). Recent trends in suicidal behavior in Japan. Psychiatry and Clinical Neurosciences, 49 (suppl. 1), S105–109.

Takahashi, Y. (1995c). Mass media and youth suicide. Kokoro to Shakai, 26, 90–97. (written in Japanese)

Takahashi, Y., Hirasawa, H., Koyama, K., Asakawa, O., Kido, M., Onose, H., Udagawa, M., Ishikawa, Y., & Uno, M. (1995). Suicide and aging in Japan: An examination of treated elderly attempters. International Psychogeriatrics, 7, 239–251.

Takahashi, Y. (1996a). Bullying and adolescent suicide. Gekkan Seito Shido, 14–19, March. (written in Japanese)

Takahashi, Y. (1996b). Suicide in the elderly. Japanese Bulletin of Social Psychiatry, 4, 197–200. (written in Japanese)

Takahashi, Y. (1996c). Epidemiology of depression in old age. Kokoro no Kagaku, No. 68, 118–122. (written in Japanese)

Takahashi, Y., Berger, D. (1996). Cultural dynamics and suicide in Japan. In Leenaars, A., & Lester, D. (Eds.) Suicide and the unconscious, pp.248–258, Northvale: Jason Aronson

Takahashi, Y. (Ed.) (1997). Life and Death from a Psychiatric Perspective. Tokyo: Kongo-shuppan (written in Japanese)

18

SUICIDES IN POLICE CUSTODY IN THE NETHERLANDS

The Identification of Potential Suicide Victims

Eric Blaauw[1,2] and Ad Kerkhof[2]

[1]Department of Clinical Psychology
Vrije Universiteit Amsterdam
The Netherlands
[2]Netherlands Institute for the Study of Criminality and Law Enforcement
(NISCALE)
Leiden, The Netherlands

1. INTRODUCTION

In many countries suicides in the criminal justice system are a matter of concern. It is consistently found that jail and prison suicide rates are higher than community suicide rates (cf. Hayes, 1983; Liebling, 1992). European and Australian prison system suicide rates are between three and eleven times the rate in the community (Liebling, 1992, p.4) and the United States prison system suicide rate is at least three times the national average (Tuskan & Thase, 1983). Criminal justice system suicides typically occur in the not yet sentenced jail population and usually within a few hours or a few days after the imprisonment (cf. Hayes, 1983). One conclusion that can be drawn from this is that the suicide risk is greater in the early stages of confinement than in the later stages.

The few existing studies on suicides in police custody show that police custody suicide rates are higher than prison system suicide rates. McDonald and Thomson (1993), who studied deaths occurring in police custody or prisons in Australia in the period 1980–1989, concluded that the suicide risk in custody, especially police custody, is much greater than the risk in the general population. Blaauw, Kerkhof and Vermunt (1997) studied police custody suicides in The Netherlands in the period of 1983–1993. They calculated that the 20 suicides in this eleven-year-period translated into a suicide rate of 210 per average daily population of 100,000 detainees, which suicide rate was twice as high as that in the Dutch prison system in the same time period, and sixteen times as high as that in a Dutch community with a corresponding sex and age distribution. The most extreme

Suicide Prevention, edited by Kosky *et al.*
Plenum Press, New York, 1998

result was reported by Memory (1984) who found that the suicide rate in South Carolina police department lock-ups was 250 times the rate in the state's general population. The conclusion that can be drawn from these studies is that suicides in custody give reasons for concern (see also Hardyman, 1983; Hayes, 1983).

A possible explanation for the excess of suicides in the criminal justice system is that the characteristics of lock-up situations induce stress and, as a consequence, heighten suicidal risk. Police stations, jails and prisons deprive people of their liberty, hetero-sexual relations, autonomy, personal safety, and goods and services (Sykes, 1966). Police custody detainees are usually provided with little more than food and drinks, limited time in the fresh air, some reading material, and occasional contact with others (Blaauw, Vermunt & Kerkhof, 1997). Police stations, jails and prisons disrupt people's employment and family ties, and leave people with uncertainty about their near future. It is thus possible that many people are not able to cope effectively with such extreme environments and that some react with suicidal behaviour patterns.

Another possible explanation for the suicides has to do with the characteristics of the police custody population. Before apprehension, many may have been experiencing an overwhelming crisis, perhaps having led to the desperate criminal act that resulted in their arrest (Felthous, 1994). Before the arrest (and during and after the arrest), some may be suffering from mental disorders. Furthermore, some people in custody may have character weaknesses marked by impulsiveness and low tolerance for frustration (Felthous, 1994).

In the following, we discuss whether factors that contribute to suicide risk in the community are also factors that contribute to suicide risk in police stations. We describe the characteristics of 20 detainees who committed suicide in police stations in The Netherlands in the period 1983–1993, and we compare these characteristics to those of the regular police custody population. For more information about the specifics of our study on suicides in police custody, we refer readers to our earlier article (Blaauw, Kerkhof and Vermunt, 1997).

2. RISK FACTORS

2.1. General Risk Factors for Suicide

The occurrence of suicidal behaviour can not be predicted with absolute certainty. It is usually possible, however, to identify a group with a heightened risk for suicide. Research showed that some identifiable factors are associated with heightened suicide risk in the community. Suicides are more prominent among men than among women, more prominent among older age groups than among younger age groups, more prominent among widowed or divorced people than among married people, and more prominent among the unemployed than among the employed (cf. Clark & Fawcett, 1992). Thus, sex, age, marital status, and employment status are demographic factors that are associated with suicide risk.

Psychiatric disorders also predispose people to taking their own lives. Suicides rarely occur in the absence of psychiatric pathology. It is reported that up to 93 percent, with a minimum of 88 percent, of suicide cases would have qualified for a psychiatric diagnosis (Clark & Fawcett, 1992; Clark & Horton-Deutsch, 1992). Depression is one of such psychiatric disorders that is well-known to be associated with heightened suicide risk. Eventually some 15% of severely depressed patients will commit suicide, and at least 50 percent of those who commit suicide suffer from a depressive disorder (see Sainsbury,

1986). Schizophrenia is another psychiatric disorder that is known to increase suicidal risk. At least ten percent of people suffering from schizophrenia will end up taking their own lives (Roy, 1986). Furthermore, the presence of personality disorder, especially borderline personality disorder or antisocial personality disorder, is known to be associated with heightened risk for suicide (cf. Modestin, 1989; Paris, 1990). Combinations of psychiatric disorders are even more indicative of suicide risk. Schizophrenia in combination with depression seems to be a hazardous combination (Roy, 1986).

There is also an association between suicidal behaviour and drug and alcohol abuse or dependence. About four percent of those who are alcohol dependent commit suicide, and between 25 percent and 41 percent of those who commit suicide are alcohol dependent (cf. Murphy, 1986, 1992; Roy, 1985, 1986). A San Diego study showed that drugs such as anxiolytics, hypnotics, antidepressants, and alcohol were detected in no less than 68% of suicides (Mendelson & Rich, 1993). Co-morbidity further increases suicide risk. For instance, in the presence of depression, acute overuse of alcohol is associated with short-term risk for suicide (Murphy, 1986, 1992).

Traumatic life events, social isolation, loss of status, and social deviance are often reported to be associated with heightened suicide risk (Clark & Fawcett, 1992). The same is true for violent or impulsive behaviour (cf. Plutchik, van Praag & Conte, 1985). Suicidal ideation, suicidal communication and previous suicidal behaviour may indicate imminent suicide (Clark & Fawcett, 1992). Most persons with high suicide risk are completely preoccupied with suicide and may send some direct or indirect signals to their environment, communicating their suicidal tendency. Nearly 40 percent of all persons completing suicide have made one or more previous non-fatal attempts (Clarke & Horton-Deutsch, 1992). Thus, overt expression of emotional turmoil, overt violent or impulsive behaviour, suicidal ideation and suicidal communication, and a history of suicidal behaviour are factors associated with risk of suicide.

2.2. Risk Factors among Police Custody Detainees

Three previous studies of 309 police custody detainees (see Blaauw, Kerkhof & Vermunt, in press) showed that 94 percent of the police custody population were male. Seventy eight percent, were single, not married, divorced, or widower. Sixty nine percent were mostly unemployed. The vast majority of police custody detainees were in their twenties or thirties, with a mean age of 29 years. Evidently, the regular police custody population is characterised by high prevalence rates of demographic risk factors for suicide.

It is not known how many of the regular police custody detainees suffer mental disorders. However, a study on psychopathology among Dutch jail detainees led to the conclusion that at least three percent of the Dutch jail population are considered unfit to be incarcerated because of a mental disorder and that at least seven percent are considered unfit to be incarcerated because of a serious personality disorder (Nota werkzame detentie, 1994). These percentages are of course minimum prevalence rates of mental disorders in Dutch jails because they only address the prevalence rates of those detainees that are considered to be unfit for incarceration. Studies in other countries also demonstrate that disproportionate numbers of individuals enter jails and prisons with current psychiatric problems such as psychosis, major depression, and schizophrenia (cf. Gibbs, 1987; Teplin, 1990). Prevalence rates of mental disorders in Dutch police stations may be even higher than are those in Dutch jails. Approximately 43 percent of people in Dutch police custody have had contact with Mental Health Care Services prior to their incarceration and about 21 percent have received some form of inpatient psychiatric treatment. Eighty nine percent of the detained persons in Dutch police stations had high scores on a depression scale in comparison to the male general population. Thus, the police custody population consists of many people with a history of psychiatric care, many people with high levels of depression, and some people with another mental disorder.

We also found that approximately 35 percent of police custody detainees used hard drugs (heroin, cocaine, etc.) on a daily basis, and approximately 22 percent of police custody detainees consumed a large quantity of alcohol every day. In total, approximately 53 percent could be regarded as alcohol dependent or drug dependent. Studies of Dutch forensic health services showed that approximately 15 percent of the police custody detainees abused alcohol and/or drugs shortly before their arrest (see Blaauw & Lulf, 1997). These high prevalence rates of substance abuse again demonstrate that the police custody population is characterised by high prevalence rates of risk factors for suicide.

Our studies among regular police custody detainees showed that many detainees considered their lock-up to be a traumatic event. A total of 63 percent felt unhappy to very unhappy, 52 percent felt anxious to very anxious, 30 percent felt confused to very confused, and 44 percent felt despaired to very despaired. Many detainees felt socially isolated because they were kept in isolation from their relatives and friends during their incarceration and they had minimal contact with their companions, because The Netherlands maintain a one-detainee-per-cell-policy. A total of 70 percent felt lonely to very lonely. Many detainees also experienced loss of status because they were dependent on police officers for the provision of goods and facilities. About 86 percent of the detained persons had above average to very high scores on the hostility scale (SCL-90) in comparison to the general population. Thus, the feeling of being confronted with a traumatic life event, social isolation, loss of status, deviance, and violent tendencies are probably common among police custody detainees.

Our studies also revealed that about 27 percent of the regular police custody population had a history of suicide attempts. About 12 percent tried to commit suicide at least once and 15 percent tried to commit suicide more than once. The majority of these attempters swallowed pills and/or cut themselves with a sharp object.

Many of the factors that are indicative for risk of suicide in the community are therefore present in the Dutch police custody population. The majority of detainees are male, single, widowed, unemployed, substance dependent, and with a history of psychiatric treatment. Many have a history of previous suicidal attempts. In addition, a relatively high percentage suffer from a mental disorder, experience the lock-up to be traumatic, and feel socially isolated, loss of status, deviant from others, and have violent impulses. Except for the fact that the majority of the Dutch police custody detainees are young, the characteristics of the detainees are almost in complete accordance with the characteristics that are often found among those who commit suicide. Because of this, the high suicidal rate while in police custody is understandable.

2.3. Suicidal Cases of Dutch Police Custody

Several characteristics of those who committed suicide in Dutch police custody in the period 1983–1993 were not available (see Blaauw, Kerkhof & Vermunt, 1997). Dutch police organisations do not routinely screen the apprehended persons for the presence of suicide risk factors. Psychiatrists are not always called in for unusual detainees. Furthermore, the reports of the Rijksrecherche that had been issued for the suicide cases were not always complete for the variables of interest. The Rijksrecherche, which is a special independent police force, investigates the circumstances of the deaths, the characteristics of the deceased, and the police investigation of suicide cases, in order to determine whether police officials or police organisations in some way contributed to the death. Of course, such an aim is entirely different from the aim of providing a suicide risk profile. As a consequence, there was little information about the prevalence of mental disorders among the suicide victims, little information about the backgrounds of the deceased, and missing data on other variables. Nevertheless, we were able to obtain valuable information about the characteristics of those who committed suicide in police custody in The Netherlands.

Nineteen of the twenty police custody suicidal cases occuring between 1983 and 1993 were males. The cases were predominantly in their twenties or thirties, with a mean age of 32 years. Seven out of ten suicide cases (remaining ten were unknown) were unmarried, divorced or widower and four out of nine cases (eleven unknown) were unemployed.

One of the police custody suicide cases had auditory hallucinations and appeared to be paranoid, which could indicate a psychiatric disorder. Another spoke in a depressed tone of voice and cried continuously, which could indicate the presence of some form of depression. A third suffered from hyperventilation and was very agitated, which could also indicate the presence of a psychiatric disorder. When we consider a history of recent psychiatric treatment to be an indication of the presence of a psychiatric disorder, we see that about 55 percent may have suffered from a psychiatric disorder (25 percent had received inpatient psychiatric treatment). Although the remaining suicide cases did not have a history of psychiatric treatment, or were unknown to have such a history, it is not certain that a psychiatric disorder was absent in these cases.

Five out of eighteen suicide cases (two unknown), (28%), regularly consumed a large quantity of alcohol. Eight out of eighteen cases (44%), regularly consumed hard drugs, and one out of eighteen cases (6%), regularly consumed hard drugs and large quantities of alcohol. According to the Rijksrecherche reports, these fourteen suicide cases (70%) were dependent on substances. At least seven suicide cases (35%), were intoxicated of alcohol or drugs at the time of arrival in the cellblocks.

The Rijksrecherche reports did not mention whether the police custody suicide cases were traumatised by their lock-up. Only limited information about the detainees reaction to lock-up was available. Seventeen of the suicide cases (85%), had a history of previous arrests and imprisonments. All suicides occurred in isolation, because of the Dutch one-person-per-cell policy. Twenty five percent of the suicide cases were arrested for very serious offenses and forty five percent for property offenses.

According to the reports of the Rijksrecherche, none of the suicide victims had behaved violently or impulsively during the lock-up, but two of the suicide cases had shown aggression during the arrest. In addition, four of those who committeed suicide while in custody had been arrested for aggravated assault.

Five of those who committed suicide (25%) had a history of previous suicide attempts and four did not, while this information was not available on eleven cases. Eight of the twenty persons (40%) who committed suicide, had threatened to kill themselves at some time during their incarceration. One of them requested a police officer to shoot him. Suicidal communication was thus frequently noticed among the cases in police custody who committed suicide.

3. SCREENING FOR SUICIDALITY

Almost all of the risk factors for suicide that have been identified in the general suicidology literature are common characteristics among suicide victims within police stations' cellblocks. However, almost all of these risk factors are also common characteristics among regular police custody detainees. As a consequence, several risk factors have limited discriminative power in a police custody population. Sex, age, and marital status were about equally distributed among those who committed suicide and those who did not. Although our data are incomplete, the same is probably true for such variables as depressive thoughts, loss of status, social isolation, and deviance. Therefore, predicting suicide risk on the basis of these factors will lead to many people being wrongfully depicted as suicidal.

Some other risk factors for suicide identified in the general suicidology literature seem to have at least some discriminative power in a police custody population. Unemployment was somewhat more common among the non-suicidal police custody population than among the suicide cases. Histories of psychiatric treatment were more prevalent among the suicide cases than among the non-suicidal detainees. Substance abuse and substance dependence were substantially higher among the suicide victims than among the non-suicidal police custody detainees. Although data are incomplete, suicide victims more often displayed suicidal ideation and suicidal communication, and more often had a history of previous suicide attempts. These factors will probably lead to better predictions than do the aforementioned factors. However, the police custody population is a far from normal population. Large numbers of detainees are characterised by several factors that are indicative of suicidal risk.

Further research on risk factors for suicide in police custody is needed. There are only a few studies that address suicides in police custody. Studies on suicide risk factors in a police custody population are extremely rare. Our conclusions are based on a study with missing data on some of the variables of interest and on a group of only 20 suicide victims. Because assessment and prediction of suicide risk is the first, and probably the most important, component of an effective prevention program, the high police custody suicide rates can only be decreased if more attention is given to this special area of research (Bonner, 1992).

REFERENCES

Blaauw, E., Kerkhof, A., & Vermunt, R. (1997). Suicides and other deaths in police custody. *Suicide and Life-threatening Behavior, 27,* 200–210.

Blaauw, E., Kerkhof, A., & Vermunt, R. (in press). Psychopathology in police custody. *International Journal of Law and Psychiatry.*

Blaauw, E., & Lulf, R.E. (1997). Arrestanten en de forensische geneeskunde [Police custody detainees and forensic medicine]. *Modus, 6(3),* 18–20.

Blaauw, E., Vermunt, R., & Kerkhof, A. (1997). Detention circumstances in police stations: Towards setting the standards. *Policing and Society, 7,* 45–69.

Bonner, R.L. (1992). Isolation, seclusion, and psychosocial vulnerability as risk factors for suicide behind bars. In R.W. Maris, A.L. Berman, J.T. Maltsberger and R.I. Yufit (Eds.), *Assessment and prediction of suicide* (pp. 398–419). New York: Guilford Press.

Clark, D.C., & Fawcett, J. (1992). Review of empirical risk factors for evaluation of the suicidal patient. In B. Bongar (Ed.), *Suicide. Guidelines for assessment, management and treatment* (pp. 16–48). New York/Oxford: Oxford University Press.

Clark, D.C., & Horton-Deutsch, S.L. (1992). Assessment in absentia: The value of the psychological autopsy method for studying antecedents of suicide and predicting future suicides. In R.W. Maris, A.L. Berman, J.T. Maltsberger and R.I. Yufit (Eds.), *Assessment and prediction of suicide* (pp. 144–182). New York: Guilford Press.

Felthous, A.R. (1994). Preventing jailhouse suicides. *Bulletin of the American Academy of Psychiatry and Law, 22,* 477–488.

Gibbs, J.J. (1987). Symptoms of psychopathology among jail prisoners: The effects of exposure to the jail environment. *Criminal Justice and Behavior, 14,* 288–310.

Hardyman, P.L. (1983). *The ultimate escape: Suicide in Ohio's jails and temporary detention facilities, 1980–1981.* Columbus, OH: Ohio Bureau of Adult Detention Facilities and Services.

Hayes, L.M. (1983). And darkness closes in ... A national study of jail suicides. *Criminal Justice and Behavior, 10,* 461–484.

Kaminer, Y. (1992). Psychoactive substance abuse and dependence as a risk factor in adolescent-attempted and - completed suicide: A review. *American Journal on Addictions, 1,* 21–29.

Liebling, A. (1992). *Suicides in prison.* London: Routledge.

McDonald, D., & Thomson, N.J. (1993). Australian deaths in custody, 1980–1989. *The Medical Journal of Australia, 159,* 581–585.

Memory, J.M. (1984). *Jail suicides in South Carolina, 1978–1984.* Unpublished paper. Columbia, SC: Office of the Governor, Division of Public Safety Programs.

Mendelson, W.B., & Rich, C.L. (1993). Sedatives and suicide: The San Diego study. *Acta Psychiatrica Scandinavica, 88,* 337–341;

Modestin, J. (1989). Completed suicide in personality disordered patients. *Journal of Personality Disorders, 3,* 113–121.

Murphy, G.E. (1986). Suicide in alcoholism. In A. Roy (Ed.), *Suicide* (pp. 89–96). Baltimore: Williams & Wilkins.

Murphy, G.E. (1992). *Suicide in alcoholism.* New York/Oxford: Oxford University Press.

Nota Werkzame Detentie [Note active detention] (1994). Den Haag, The Netherlands: Sdu.

O'Mahony, P. (1994). Prison suicide rates: What do they mean? In A. Liebling and T. Ward (Eds.), *Deaths in custody: International perspectives* (pp. 45–57). London: Whiting & Birch.

Paris, J. (1990). Completed suicide in borderline personality disorder. *Psychiatric Annals, 20,* 19–21.

Plutchik, R., van Praag, H.M., & Conte, H. (1985). Suicide and violence risk in psychiatric patients. *Biological Psychiatry, 20,* 761–763.

Roy, A. (1985). Suicide and psychiatric patients. *Psychiatric Clinics of North America, 8,* 227–241.

Roy, A. (1986). Depression, attempted suicide, and suicide in patients with chronic schizophrenia. *Psychiatric Clinics of North America, 9,* 193–206.

Sainsbury, P. (1986). Depression, suicide, and suicide prevention. In A. Roy (Ed.), *Suicide* (pp. 73–88). Baltimore: Williams & Wilkins.

Teplin, L.A. (1990). The prevalence of severe mental disorder among male urban jail detainees: Comparison with the epidemiologic catchment area program. *American Journal of Public Health, 80,* 663–669.

Sykes, G. (1966). *The society of captives: A study of a maximum security prison.* New York: Atheneum.

Tuskan, J.J., & Thase, M.E. (1983). Suicides in jails and prisons. *Journal of Psychosocial Nursing and Mental Health, 21,* 29–33.

19

SUICIDE IN SRI LANKA

Lakshmi Ratnayeke

Sumithrayo, Sri Lanka

It is a known fact that for well over a decade Sri Lanka has been faced with an ever increasing rate of suicide, and recently we have earned the dubious reputation of having the highest rate of suicide in the world, 47 per 100,000.

For those who may not already be aware, Sri Lanka is a tear drop shaped island in the Indian Ocean located at the southern tip of the sub-continent of India. It is a small island 270 miles long by 140 miles at its widest point with a multi-ethnic, multi-religious population of 18 million people, which I believe is as large a population as that of Australia.

Though 47 per 100,000 is a horrendously high figure, it is believed that it is an under-representation, as many of the suicides are recorded as accidental deaths. Reliable figures are not available for suicide attempts, as very often those too are recorded as accidental to save the victim and the family from further trauma, as suicide is still a criminal offence in Sri Lanka and also carries with it a social stigma (See Table 1).

If we take into consideration the five most recent years, between 1990 and 1995, a total of 38,517 people killed themselves during that period. The percentage increase in population over the same period of time is only 3.5% as against an increase of 15% in the number of suicides.

There is a further phenomenon hitherto unknown in Sri Lanka and that is the rapid increase in suicides of people aged 60 years and over. There has been a 50% increase in suicides in this group over these last five years, bringing the over 60's to the second most vulnerable age group, the first one being the 20–30 years age group. The suicides in this group has come down by 14.5% during the same period of time (See Table 2).

Table3 compares suicide figures in the island between 1991 and 1995, indicating the gender involved, the most vulnerable age groups, the most common methods and the most common motives for suicide. Three times as many men as women kill themselves in Sri Lanka. The most common method used was ingestion of poisons, and the second most common method used was hanging. Though Sri Lanka is a poor country the most common motive for suicide was not poverty, but disappointment in love, which contributes to the belief that suicide stems from ones inability to cope with negative feelings, emotions and urges coupled with poor coping and decision making skills. The second most common cause was mental illness (See Table 3).

Suicide Prevention, edited by Kosky *et al.*
Plenum Press, New York, 1998

Table 1. Suicides in Sri Lanka 1991–1995

	Year				
	1991	1992	1993	1994	1995
Total suicides	7411	7506	7364	7717	8519
Population (in millions)	17.2	17.4	17.6	17.8	18

Seventy five percent of the suicides in Sri Lanka occur in the rural areas. This is not surprising as in the countries of West Asia, though the cities are grossly over populated the greater part of the country's population is rural. For example, in Sri Lanka 78.5% is rural, including 6.5% on the tea plantations.

Many of the Asian countries are underdeveloped and even in the so-called developing countries, there are large areas of the country that are poverty stricken and have seen little or no development. Even in areas where rapid industrialisation has taken place, little or nothing has still been done to systematically uplift the quality of life of the people.

Over the last decade modern technology, in the form of TV and radio and other foreign influences, have penetrated remote village areas. Villagers in search of better employment have gone to the Middle East and affluent East Asian countries and returned bring with hem consumer items hitherto unheard of in their village environment. TV commercials and tele-dramas present a world of exotic consumerism and fantasy so different to anything that a villager would have seen or experienced before. For the first time they see another world so alien to their own and they become conscious of their own relative poverty and economic inadequacy. Comparisons tend to alter their perceptions of life and living standards, which leads to dissatisfaction with their lot in life and other kinds of complications leading to thoughts of suicide.

This gives you some idea of the epidemiology of suicide in the country. These figures refer to 1993 and 1994. You will note the highest rates of suicide are in the North Central Region—an unprecedented 101 and 118 per 100,000. This is an entirely farming area, where the villagers are dependent on paddy cultivation and cash crops. The Central Province, where the tea plantations are centered, comes next with figures of 56 and 63 per 100,000.

The rates of suicide in the states when compared with the Provincial rates and the over all rate of suicide for the country are very high. Statistics from 6 randomly chosen tea estates in the Central and Uva Provinces for 1993 and 1994 gave figures as high as 193 and 278 suicides per 100,000 workers respectively; whereas the overall suicide rates for the provinces where the estates are located were 56 and 24 per 100,000 for 1993 and 63 and 33 per 100,000 for 1994.

Agro-chemicals are widely used in the tea growing areas, not only by the tea industry but also by the small time market gardeners on the estates and surrounding villages. A large percentage of the suicides each year in these areas, 100% in many of the estates, are

Table 2. Characteristics of suicides

Total suicides 1991–1995	38,517
% increase in population from 1991–1995	3.5%
% increase in suicides from 1991–1995	15%
% increase in suicides of people over 60 years from 1991–1995	50%
% decrease in suicides of most vulnerable group (20–30years) from 1991–1995	14.5%

Table 3. Suicides in Sri Lanka 1991–1995 according to gender, vulnerability, methods and motives

	Year				
	1991	1992	1993	1994	1995
Total suicides	741	7506	7364	7717	8519
Males	5572	5689	5463	5638	6256
Females	1839	1817	1901	2079	2263
Most vulnerable group (20-30years)	2374	2238	2099	2212	2030
Second most vulnerable group (over 60years)	911	964	997	1095	1369
Most common method (poisons)	1801	1828	2109	1759	1801
Second most common method (hanging)	540	598	744	613	665
Most common motive (disappointment in love)	1083	1151	1134	1019	1084
Second most common motive (mental illness)	758	539	476	544	620

by the ingestion of insecticides or weedicides which are freely available and exists in the homes of nearly all the estate workers and villagers.

The high rates of suicide in the farming areas are also due to lethal agro-chemicals which are widely used by the farmers. Moreover, their potency is such that those who ingest them often die before admission to a hospital, usually situated in a town several miles away and transport is not always available. Another common method of attempting suicide is by eating the lethally poisonous seeds of the plant 'Kaneru,' the yellow Oleander which grows in abundance in all the villages in the dry zone.

As in most countries, the sale of dangerous drugs is carefully controlled by law in Sri Lanka, but not so the sale of agro-chemicals and other pesticides and weedicides. The high rate of suicide in the country could be directly linked to this lethal method used. In most de-

Table 4. Suicides in Sri Lanka—Provincial basis 1993–1994

Province (resources)	Population (million)	Total suicides		Per 100,000 population	
		1993	1994	1993	1994
Western (commerce, industry)	4.5	1817	2053	39	45
Central (estates—tea/rubber/industry)	2.3	1301	1437	56	63
Southern (estates—rubber/coconut, fishing, paddy cultivation)	2.3	855	777	36	33
North Western (fishing, farming, crop cultivation)	2.1	920	679	43	32
Sabaragamuwa (estates—tea/rubber, cash crops)	1.7	615	561	35	32
Eastern (commerce, fishing, farming)	1.3	480	560	37	43
Uva (estates—tea, cash crops)	1.1	265	369	24	33
North Central (paddy cultivation, cash crops)	1.0	1094	1282	101	118
Northern	not available	not available	not available	not available	not available

veloped countries only 3% to 5% of those who attempt suicide actually die but in Sri Lanka 20% to 25% of those who attempt suicide are successful in killing themselves. In the estate sector and very remote village areas, nearly 90% of the attempts are successful

In Sri Lanka, economically and emotionally crippled by a long, drawn out separatist war, the state is so pre-occupied with trying to maintain peace and provide the essential material needs of man, that little or nothing is done to improve the emotional well being of its people. Emotional and mental health is a neglected area, and perhaps not even recognised as an essential pre-requisite for human well being and is most often simply ignored. It is in this scenario that the Sumithrayo Befrienders in Sri Lanka and to the non government organisations in the field of mental health are working.

The Sumithrayo Befrienders are making a concerted effort to help in the field of prevention of suicide. Providing crisis intervention centres island wide, visiting national hospitals to befriend the survivors of suicide attempts, befriending in, and conducting awareness programmes in schools, and villages, training other non government organisation personnel, industrial factory personnel and officers from the armed forces to recognise and help those who may be depressed and/or suicidal are some of the many activities in the Sumithrayo Befrienders are currently involved in. Though the scope for Befriending activities is enormous in Sri Lanka, it is constrained by paucity of suitable man-power and finances.

The conventional Befriending approach that works in most parts of the world may not always be applicable in a developing country like Sri Lanka. Remote village areas seldom have access to social services that could offer support in times of crisis and village traditions discourage the villagers from revealing their personal difficulties to strangers.

The Sumithrayo Befrienders have been making efforts to address this situation and the volunteers attached to our rural centres have been trying to adapt traditional Befriending to suit the local situation. Research is in progress which would help in designing an outreach and prevention program located in the village and more in keeping with local norms. Such an outreach programme will have several benefits:

1. It can reach individuals and families before suicidal behaviour occurs.
2. It can reach individuals who would not come to a Sumithrayo Befriending Centre either because of the distance involved or because of other barriers, perceived or real.
3. It can produce greater public awareness of the Sumithrayo Befrienders and the befriending approach.

The work the Sumithrayo do with the suicidal in the rural areas is very slow and time consuming, but very rewarding. It may not have dramatic effects on the overall rate of suicide in the country, but our volunteers are doing good work, helping many people who would have otherwise given up on life.

20

THE METHODOLOGY, SYSTEM, AND SCOPE OF THE SUICIDE STATISTICS IN TURKEY[*]

M. Tomris Okman

Demographic Statistics Department
State Institute of Statistics
Ankara, Turkey

INTRODUCTION

The State Institute of Statistics (SIS) is responsible for compiling, evaluating and disseminating statistics used to characterise and monitor the changes and developments in the economic, social and cultural structure of Turkey. In summary, the SIS is the principal, organisation responsible for the Turkish Statistical Infrastructure. Compilation of data on suicide is one of the most important responsibilities of the Institute.

Suicide statistics have been compiled for the whole of Turkey since 1962. Initially these statistics were included in the "Yearbook of Justice Statistics' as summary information. Since 1974, 'Suicide Statistics' have been published as a separate publication each year. In order to offer wider and more comprehensive data to users, some new tables, figures and interpretation have been included since 1987.

The data on suicide statistics cover all inhabited places. For every single suicide occurring, a 'Suicide Statistics Form', which is prepared by our Institute, is filled out by the police or gendarme and is sent to the office of the governor in provinces and districts. At the end of every month, governors' offices send these forms to the State Institute of Statistics. The collected data is evaluated and published at the end of each year. The suicide statistics which have a close relation with many scientific branches have been presented to the use of researchers with diskettes and publications.

The suicide rate, which is one of the important indicators of the social and economic structures of the community, is motivated by various psychological, social, economic and cultural factors. For this reason, suicide can be seen in a broad population, by people who

---

[*] This paper was based on Suicide Statistics Publications, 1987–1995 which was originally published as 'The Methodology, System and Scope of the Suicide Statistics in Turkey'. The author is very grateful to the publisher for giving permission to use some materials from the above resource.

Table 1. Suicide rates in different countries

Country	Rate (%)
USA	12.2 (1989)
Japan	16.0 (1991)
Bulgaria	15.4 (1991)
Germany	15.8 (1990)
Italy	7.5 (1989)
Romania	9.3 (1991)
Australia	13.3 (1988)
France	20.1 (1990)
Turkey	2.4 (1995)

show no psychiatric symptomatology, but may also attempt suicide due to stressful life situations and by many who are seriously ill with psychiatric disorders like depression and schizophrenia.

Traditions, religious beliefs and social behaviours have an important influence on suicide in every country. It has been observed that Turkey has a very low suicide rate when compared to suicide rates of other countries (Table 1) . The reason may be that religious beliefs have a great influence on society in our country.

CRUDE SUICIDE RATE AND RATIO OF SUICIDES BY YEARS

Crude suicide rate has shown an increasing trend with some variations from 1987 (Figure 1). When male and female crude suicide rates are studied, it can be seen that there are the same changes for both sexes. For computing suicides rates for male and female population, it has been emphasised that the tendency to commit suicide is greater for males than females in general. According to the data in 1995, the crude suicide rate for males is 2.91 in 100,000 and for females 1.81 in 100,000.

As the data in Table 2 indicates males commit suicide more often than females and almost 60% of suicides occur in males per year in Turkey.

Table 2. Crude suicide rate and ratio of suicide per year

Year	Crude suicide rate 0/0000			Rate of suicide %	
	T	A	B	A	B
1987	2.09	2.49	1.68	60.38	39.62
1988	2.05	2.44	1.64	60.51	39.49
1989	2.14	2.58	1.68	61.18	38.82
1990	2.41	3.04	1.77	63.74	36.26
1991	2.14	2.68	1.59	63.35	36.65
1992	2.00	2.54	1.53	62.21	37.79
1993	2.07	2.43	1.69	59.56	40.44
1994	2.53	3.10	1.96	61.78	38.22
1995	2.37	2.91	1.81	62.12	37.88

T: Total
A: Male
B: Female

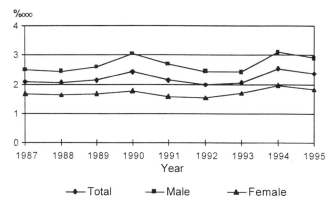

Figure 1. Crude suicide rate per year.

PERCENTAGE OF SUICIDES BY AGE GROUPS

When suicides are studied by age groups (Figure 2), it is seen that those who commit suicide are concentrated in the 15–34 age group for males and females. As age increases, the ratio of committing suicide decreases for both sexes.

Comparison between male and female suicide by age groups, shows that since 1987 females have commited suicide more as compared to males in young age groups (Table 3). About half of the suicides have occurred before age 35 for males and before age 25 for females. According to the data in 1995, 52.27% of females commit suicide before the age of 25 and 52.47% of males committed suicide before the age of 35.

PERCENTAGE OF SUICIDES BY CAUSES

When the suicide events are taken into consideration by physical or mental, or both, causes and years it is observed that the most important cause for suicides in Turkey is ill-

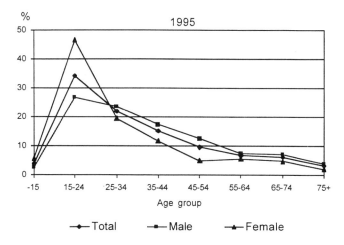

Figure 2. Percentage of suicides by age groups.

Table 3. Percentage of suicides per year, sex, and age groups

Year	Age group							
	−15	15–24	25–34	35–44	45–54	55–64	65–74	75+
1987								
T	3.69	30.97	20.83	12.59	11.65	10.89	5.21	4.17
A	3.45	23.55	21.82	14.29	13.50	13.03	6.44	3.92
B	4.06	42.24	19.33	10.02	8.83	7.64	3.34	4.54
1988								
T	4.13	29.67	21.97	13.05	12.21	9.77	5.54	3.66
A	4.66	22.52	23.60	14.91	13.66	10.40	7.45	2.80
B	3.32	40.62	19.48	10.21	9.98	8.79	2.61	4.99
1989								
T	4.23	28.96	20.33	12.59	12.06	11.09	5.11	5.63
A	3.72	24.36	19.63	14.33	12.75	12.32	5.73	7.16
B	5.02	36.30	21.46	9.82	10.96	9.13	4.11	3.20
1990								
T	3.54	31.17	21.81	15.40	10.91	8.25	4.20	4.72
A	3.47	26.01	21.96	18.73	10.98	9.60	4.28	4.97
B	3.66	40.24	21.55	9.55	10.77	5.89	4.07	4.27
1991								
T	3.42	29.72	21.83	15.56	10.91	9.28	5.21	4.07
A	3.21	25.07	23.14	16.20	11.95	10.15	6.04	4.24
B	3.78	37.78	19.55	14.44	9.11	7.78	3.78	3.78
1992								
T	4.63	33.16	20.65	13.88	10.11	10.11	4.63	2.83
A	4.41	25.20	22.04	17.77	11.43	11.57	4.41	3.17
B	4.99	46.26	18.37	7.48	7.93	7.71	4.99	2.27
1993								
T	5.70	32.63	20.67	15.46	9.19	6.51	5.04	4.80
A	4.10	25.96	21.99	18.17	10.66	6.97	5.87	6.28
B	8.05	42.45	18.71	11.47	7.04	5.84	3.82	2.62
1994								
T	3.65	32.23	21.16	15.37	10.02	8.85	5.01	3.71
A	2.21	26.66	21.50	18.12	11.59	10.12	6.22	3.58
B	5.96	41.23	20.61	10.90	7.50	6.81	3.07	3.92
1995								
T	3.56	34.25	21.92	15.07	9.52	6.44	6.16	3.08
A	2.31	26.68	23.48	17.20	12.35	7.17	7.06	3.75
B	5.61	46.66	19.35	11.57	4.88	5.24	4.70	1.99

T: Total
A: Male
B: Female

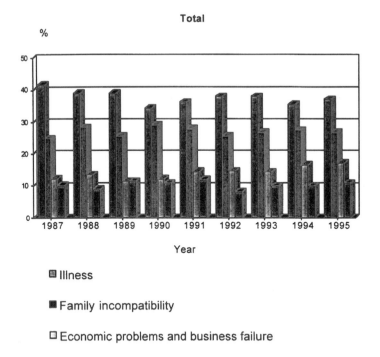

Figure 3. Percentage of suicides per year and main causes.

ness (Figure 3). The second and third important causes are family incompatibility and economic problems or business failure (Table 4). It becomes apparent that as the trend of illness increases, the trend of economic problems and business failure increase. According to the data in 1995, the rate of suicides for illness is 37.02%, for family incompatibility is 26.78% and for economic problems and business failure is17.23% (Figure 4).

As the data in Figures 3a and 3b shows that the main cause for committing suicide for males is illness. The second and third important causes are family incompatibility and economic problems and business failure respectively. The main cause for committing suicide for females is illness. The second and third important causes are family incompatibility and emotional relationships and not marrying the person wanted respectively.

In comparing male and female suicides with respect to causes of suicides, economic problems and business failure are observed as the main differences (Figure 4). It is assumed that work responsibilities and family continuity caused more suicides for males than females. Because of these, males are more likely to commit suicide for economic reasons than females. Family incompatibility has a high rate of suicide for females compared to males. At the same time, females with relationship problems who do not marry the person they wanted, have a higher rate than males.

PERCENTAGE OF SUICIDE BY DIFFERENT METHODS

It has been observed that the majority of suicides have occurred by hanging in Turkey (Figure 5). But, the rate of this method has shown decreasing trends per year. Taking

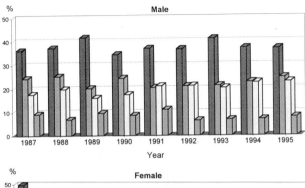

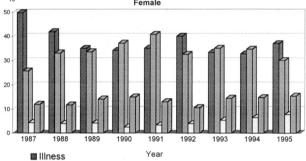

■ Illness

▨ Family incompatibility

☐ Economic problems and business failure

▨ Emotional relationship and not marrying the person wanted

Figure 3a&b. Percentage of suicides per year and main causes.

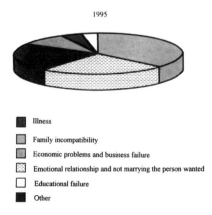

Figure 4. Percentage of suicides by causes.

Table 4. Percentage of suicides by year, sex, and causes

Year	Illness	Family incompatibility	Economic problems and business failure	Emotional relationship and not marrying the person wanted	Educational failure	Other
1987						
T	41.63	24.89	12.33	10.35	3.75	7.05
A	36.16	24.36	17.71	9.23	4.24	8.30
B	49.73	25.68	4.37	12.02	3.01	5.19
1988						
T	39.08	28.40	13.49	8.86	3.12	7.05
A	37.21	25.25	19.87	6.90	3.87	6.90
B	41.85	33.08	4.01	11.78	2.01	7.27
1989						
T	38.99	25.50	11.47	11.47	2.29	10.28
A	41.60	20.27	16.19	9.68	3.33	8.93
B	34.96	33.57	4.20	14.22	0.70	12.35
1990						
T	34.37	29.05	12.17	11.03	3.65	9.73
A	34.49	24.46	17.66	8.71	4.54	10.14
B	34.17	37.11	2.52	15.09	2.10	9.01
1991						
T	36.33	28.00	14.67	11.92	3.50	5.58
A	37.07	20.58	21.24	11.22	3.56	6.33
B	35.07	40.73	3.39	13.12	3.39	4.30
1992						
T	38.02	25.46	14.75	8.08	3.42	10.27
A	36.81	21.15	21.30	6.49	3.95	10.30
B	40.00	32.56	3.95	10.70	2.56	10.23
1993						
T	38.06	26.91	14.35	10.01	5.50	5.17
A	41.24	21.38	20.41	6.90	4.14	5.93
B	33.40	35.02	5.47	14.57	7.49	4.05
1994						
T	35.55	27.39	16.52	10.01	4.87	5.66
A	37.27	22.90	22.68	7.03	4.05	6.07
B	32.76	34.65	6.55	14.83	6.21	5.00
1995						
T	37.02	26.78	17.23	10.87	4.43	3.67
A	37.10	24.80	23.02	8.04	4.02	3.02
B	36.91	30.00	7.82	15.45	5.09	4.73

T: Total
A: Male
B: Female

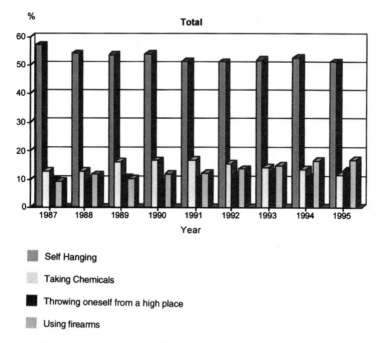

Figure 5. Percentage of suicides per year and main methods of suicide.

chemicals is the second method of suicide till 1993. After 1993, using firearms became the second, taking chemicals to the third most common method of suicide. As seen from Table 5, the rate of using firearms has shown to be an increasing trend. According to the data, in 1995 the rate of hanging is 51.3%, using firearms is16.92% and taking chemicals is11.51% (Figure 6).

When methods of suicide by sex are taken into consideration (Figures 5a and 5b), it is observed that the first common method of suicide for males is self hanging and the second most common method using firearms. Until 1992, the third most common method for males was taking chemicals. After this year, the method of taking chemicals has shown as decreasing, and the method of throwing oneself from a high place has shown an increasing pattern and became the third most common method. It is observed that the first most common method for females is hanging , the second is taking chemicals and the third most common method is throwing oneself from a high place.

PERCENTAGE OF SUICIDES BY LITERACY AND EDUCATIONAL LEVELS

Educational level is one of the most important factors that can affect the suicide events of a population. The data in Figure 7 shows that those who are literate commit sui-

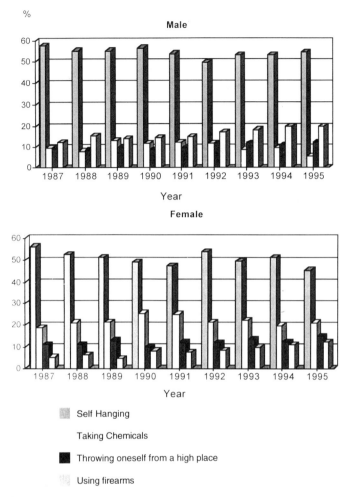

Figure 5a&b. Percentage of suicides per year and main methods of suicide.

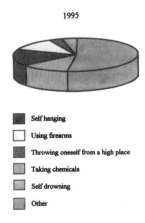

Figure 6. Percentage of suicides by different methods.

Table 5. Percentage of suicides per year, sex, and methods

Year	By hanging	Taking chemicals	Throwing oneself from a high place	By self drowning	Using firearms	By self burning	Using a sharp instrument	Using gas or ipg. etc.	Throwing oneself off a train or other motorized vehicle	Other
1987										
T	57.17	12.97	9.86	4.84	9.31	1.19	1.64	1.19	1.28	0.55
A	57.73	9.24	9.10	4.70	12.12	1.21	1.82	1.66	1.51	0.91
B	56.32	18.62	11.03	5.06	5.06	1.15	1.38	0.46	0.92	—
1988										
T	54.20	12.96	9.40	5.11	11.68	0.64	1.73	2.10	1.00	1.18
A	55.29	7.70	8.46	5.44	15.26	0.45	2.42	2.26	1.21	1.51
B	52.54	20.97	10.83	4.61	6.22	0.92	0.69	1.84	0.69	0.69
1989										
T	53.72	16.31	10.68	4.44	10.33	0.94	1.11	0.68	0.94	0.85
A	55.17	13.13	9.22	3.77	13.97	0.98	1.67	0.28	1.25	0.56
B	51.43	21.32	12.97	5.49	4.61	0.88	0.22	1.32	0.44	1.32
1990										
T	53.87	16.73	8.99	4.20	12.01	1.40	1.10	0.52	1.18	—
A	56.53	11.68	8.55	3.81	14.34	1.73	1.39	0.58	1.39	—
B	49.19	25.61	9.75	4.88	7.93	0.81	0.61	0.41	0.81	—
1991										
T	51.55	16.86	10.26	4.64	12.30	0.73	1.71	0.98	0.81	0.16
A	53.85	12.21	9.25	4.63	15.04	0.64	1.93	1.16	1.16	0.13
B	47.56	24.89	12.00	4.67	7.55	0.89	1.33	0.67	0.22	0.22
1992										
T	51.24	15.42	11.65	3.09	13.80	0.77	1.54	0.69	0.86	0.94
A	49.72	11.85	11.57	2.89	17.22	0.83	2.34	0.96	1.24	1.38
B	53.74	21.31	11.79	3.40	8.16	0.68	0.23	0.23	0.23	0.23
1993										
T	51.83	14.16	12.53	3.50	14.89	0.49	0.90	0.32	0.97	0.41
A	53.42	8.74	12.02	3.82	18.17	0.41	1.37	0.55	1.23	0.27
B	49.50	22.14	13.28	3.02	10.06	0.60	0.20	—	0.60	0.60
1994										
T	52.60	13.41	11.13	3.19	16.41	0.39	1.11	0.20	1.30	0.26
A	53.43	9.48	10.54	3.06	19.81	0.21	1.26	0.21	1.79	0.21
B	51.28	19.76	12.10	3.41	10.90	0.68	0.85	0.17	0.51	0.34
1995										
T	51.30	11.51	13.29	2.53	16.92	0.82	1.58	0.41	1.23	0.41
A	54.80	5.62	12.24	2.21	19.85	0.99	2.20	0.55	1.21	0.33
B	45.57	21.16	15.01	3.07	12.12	0.54	0.54	0.18	1.27	0.54

T: Total
A: Male
B: Female

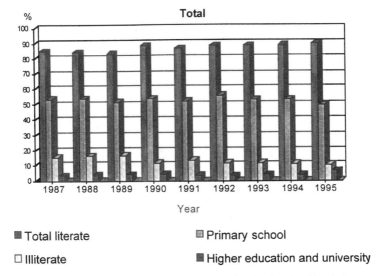

Figure 7. Percentage of suicides per year and main educational levels.

cide at a high rate. When literates commit suicide, and assessed for education level, it is observed that the rate of primary school and the rate of higher education have shown a steady pattern except in the year 1995. According to the data in 1995, the rate of illiterate people who committed suicide is 10%, the rate of primary school people who committed suicide is 49.31% and the rate of higher education and university people who committed suicide is 6.10% (Figure 8)

However, when male and female suicides are studied by literacy in Figures 7a and 7b, it can be seen that illiterate females commit suicide more than males. On the other hand, educated males commit suicide more than females in each education level. According to the data in 1995, (Table 6), the proportion of illiterate suicide is 6.5% for males and is15.73% for females. The proportion of the higher education and university suicides is 7.83% for males and 3.26% for females.

CONCLUSION

In conclusion, the crude suicide rate has shown an increasing trend in Turkey. Rapid social change, immigration from rural to urban, increasing unemployment and also easiness to get firearms may be the causes of the increasing trend.

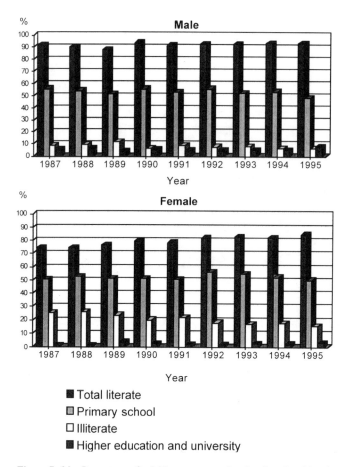

Figure 7a&b. Percentage of suicides per year and main educational levels.

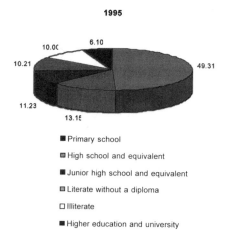

Figure 8. Percentage of suicides according to educational levels.

Table 6. Percentage of suicides per year, sex and educational levels

Year	Illiterate	Total literate	Educational level					
			Literate					
					Literate with a diploma			
			Literate without a diploma	Total	Primary school	Junior high school and equivalent	High school and equivalent	Higher education and university
1987								
T	15.22	84.78	12.84	71.94	53.36	8.40	6.82	3.36
A	8.51	91.49	13.75	77.74	55.16	9.33	8.18	5.07
B	25.44	74.56	11.47	63.09	50.62	6.98	4.74	0.75
1988								
T	15.89	84.11	10.53	73.58	53.80	6.43	9.65	3.70
A	9.39	90.61	11.00	79.61	54.53	8.25	11.17	5.66
B	25.74	74.26	9.80	64.46	52.70	3.68	7.35	0.73
1989								
T	16.56	83.44	12.91	70.53	51.65	8.19	6.95	3.74
A	12.02	87.98	12.76	75.22	51.90	10.56	8.80	3.96
B	23.58	76.42	13.15	63.27	51.25	4.54	4.08	3.40
1990								
T	11.40	88.60	12.77	75.83	53.72	9.50	8.59	4.02
A	6.41	93.59	11.27	82.32	55.28	11.50	10.44	5.10
B	20.30	79.70	15.43	64.27	50.95	5.92	5.29	2.11
1991								
T	13.52	86.48	12.05	74.43	52.04	9.93	8.96	3.50
A	8.61	91.39	12.08	79.31	52.96	11.18	10.67	4.50
B	22.00	78.00	12.00	66.00	50.44	7.78	6.00	1.78
1992								
T	11.57	88.43	11.74	76.69	55.87	7.63	9.85	3.34
A	7.58	92.42	11.29	81.13	55.65	9.37	11.57	4.54
B	18.14	81.86	12.47	69.39	56.24	4.76	7.03	1.36
1993								
T	11.55	88.45	11.80	76.65	53.21	10.09	9.52	3.83
A	7.92	92.08	11.07	81.01	52.19	12.43	11.47	4.92
B	16.90	83.10	12.88	70.22	54.73	6.64	6.64	2.21
1994								
T	11.07	88.93	9.76	79.17	53.26	9.24	12.96	3.71
A	6.74	93.26	8.54	84.72	53.84	10.54	15.49	4.85
B	18.06	81.94	11.75	70.19	52.30	7.16	8.86	1.87
1995								
T	10.00	90.00	10.21	79.79	49.31	11.23	13.15	6.10
A	6.50	93.50	8.71	84.79	48.73	12.57	15.66	7.83
B	15.73	84.27	12.66	71.61	50.27	9.04	9.04	3.26

T: Total
A: Male
B: Female

21

DEPRESSION AND ATTEMPTED SUICIDE

A Hospital Based Study of 437 Patients

Anthony T. Davis

University of Adelaide
Department of Psychiatry
Royal Adelaide Hospital
South Australia

1. INTRODUCTION

This is a report of one of several studies of attempted suicide conducted in Adelaide, South Australia, over a three-year period. These studies principally focused on the issue of depression in attempted suicide from 1986 to 1988 (inclusive).

Some of the principal concerns of clinicians working in the field of suicide prevention are the detection and management of depression in patients who have attempted suicide, and the identification of patients at risk for persistent depression and possible repeated attempted suicide or suicide.

Weissman (1974), in a comprehensive review of the epidemiology of suicide attempts between 1960 and 1971, found that depression was the most common psychiatric diagnosis made, accounting for 35–79% of all cases. However, the wide disparity in reports of the frequency of depression is striking, and warrants further consideration.

Researchers have offered conflicting views of the extent, nature and significance of depression in patients who have attempted suicide and have suggested a variety of therapeutic needs and interventions. A close analysis of the studies conducted prior to the advent of operational diagnostic criteria and structured interviews, reveals studies of non-similar patient samples, the use of diverse terminology and a multiplicity of study methods. Researchers have described various case-record reviews, clinical diagnoses based on diverse criteria, self-report questionnaires, observer rating scales and comparisons with other psychiatric patient groups. Some latter studies have utilised specific diagnostic criteria and/or structured clinical interviews, but these are surprisingly few in number. This approach certainly offers a chance of uniformity in study design and the opportunity to compare different findings.

Thus, the question of the nature and significance of depression in attempted suicide remains unresolved. What is more, there is very little information about the course of de-

Suicide Prevention, edited by Kosky *et al.*
Plenum Press, New York, 1998

pression following attempted suicide and the optimal short-term intervention for this large group of people. Clinical experience suggests that the majority of patients presenting to hospital following attempted suicide have a significant degree of depression, and that in some instances there is a significant reduction in the level of depression soon after hospitalisation, irrespective of the clinical diagnosis.

The major aim of this study was to provide a detailed analysis of aspects of depression in adults (aged 18–65) who have attempted suicide. The specific aims were to define the severity, type and symptomatic profile of depression in this group.

2. MATERIALS AND METHOD

2.1. The Setting

The Royal Adelaide Hospital (RAH) is the central adult teaching hospital for adults in the city of Adelaide, South Australia. It has 950 inpatient beds and an annual Accident and Emergency (A & E) attendance of approximately 60,000 patients during the 3 year study period. The RAH is responsible for approximately 25% of the A & E admissions in the Adelaide metropolitan area, and deals with approximately one third of the total number of attempted suicide admissions in Adelaide each year.

2.2. The Design

Stage 1: Survey of Attempted Suicide. A survey of the all "cases" of attempted suicide at the RAH was conducted over a 3-year period from 1986 to 1988. Patients were included in the survey if they had taken an overdose of medication or caused self-harm (e.g. wrist cutting, gunshot wound, hanging, CO poisoning, jumping from heights) with some degree of suicide intent as specified by the A & E medical officer. Patients with a primary drug or alcohol related disorder were not included in the survey.

For patients thus identified as possible "cases" of attempted suicide, all available demographic data, details of method of attempted suicide and day of admission were recorded.

Stage 2: Screening for Depression. A suicidal attempt was operationally defined according to Kreitman (1977) as a non fatal act in which an individual deliberately caused self-injury or ingested a substance in excess of any prescribed or generally recognised therapeutic dosage.

Patients who had attempted suicide were identified and asked to complete the Zung Self-Rating Depression Scale (SDS) (Zung 1965) and the Levine-Pilowsky Depression (LPD) Questionnaire (Pilowsky et al 1969). It was explained that these instruments were self-report measures of a variety of physical and psychological symptoms. Patients were asked to report on their thoughts, feelings and symptoms as they were over the 2 to 3 days prior to the suicidal attempt.

3. RESULTS

Stage 1

Over the 3-year period, a total of 2211 episodes of attempted suicide were identified by the survey (these episodes involved 1723 patients). The mean age of the patients was

Table 1. SDS Index of study group (n=437)

	Male	Female	Total
Below 50 (within normal range)	32 (17%)	24 (10%)	56 (13%)
50–59 (minimal to mild depression)	39 (20%)	32 (13%)	71 (16%)
60–69 (moderate to marked depression)	73 (38%)	79 (33%)	152 (35%)
70+ (severe to most extremely depressed)	50 (26%)	106 (44%)	156 (36%)

31.1 years, with a standard deviation (SD) of 13.1. The age range was 13 to 86 years. The female to male ratio was 1.3:1. Seven hundred and fifty five (79%) males and 974 (80%) females were aged less than 40 years. There was no significant difference in mean age between sexes. Following A & E assessment, 70% of the total were admitted to hospital.

Stage 2

A total of 504 days were defined as "study days." On those days, 784 patients aged between 18 and 65 were admitted to hospital. Four hundred and thirty seven (55.7%) of them consented to participate in the study and completed the Zung SDS and the LPD questionnaire. The mean age of this group was 31.5 years (with SD of 11.2). There were 194 (44.4%) males and 243 (55.6%) females.

3.1. Depression Ratings

Zung SDS. The mean SDS Index of the group was 64.9, with a SD of 12.7. The SDS Index was divided into 4 categories, as specified by Zung (1965). Table 1 shows the breakdown of scores.

For females, the mean SDS Index was 67.4 (SD =13.0). For males, the mean SDS Index was 61.7 (SD =11.7). This difference in mean SDS Index was highly significant (t = −4.67, df = 433, p < 0.001).

As well, there was significant difference in categories of depression between these groups with more females than males in the most severe category and less in the normal range and minimal to mild categories (X^2 = 17.3, df = 3, p < 0.001).

For the total group, age was not significantly correlated with mean SDS Index. For the sexes, statistically significant age and SDS Index correlations were found, although the r values were small and explained a minimal percentage of the variance (males: r = 0.81, p < 0.01; females: r = −0.19, p < 0.01).

LPD Questionnaire. The mean LPD score was 11.1, with a SD of 4.6. Males had a mean score of 10.6 (SD = 4.4) and females 11.6 (SD = 4.6). This difference was statistically significant (t = −2.39, df = 424, p < 0.05).

The LPD categories are shown in Table 2.

Table 2. LPD categories of study group (n=437*)

	Male	Female	Total
Non-endogenous depression	72 (38%)	65 (27%)	137 (31%)
Endogenous depression	67 (36%)	121 (51%)	188 (43%)
Not depressed	49 (26%)	51 (22%)	100 (23%)

*Missing values = 12 (3%)

There was a statistically significant difference in categories of depression between sexes, with more females than males in the endogenous depression category and less in the non-endogenous category ($X^2 = 10.40$, df = 2, p < 0.01).

For the total group, age was not significantly correlated with mean LPD score. For the sexes, statistically significant age and LPD score correlations were found, although the r values were small and once again explained a minimal percentage of the variance (males: r = 0.19, p < 0.01; females: r = −0.25, p < 0.01).

3.2. Non-Screened Group

A total of 352 hospitalised patients were not screened for depression. 185 were discharged from the medical and surgical wards out of study hours (generally at week-ends), 39 discharged themselves against medical advice, 57 refused to consent to participate in the study, 64 had cognitive impairment which precluded them from the study, 1 had language problems and 6 died following admission.

The patients screened for depression were compared on a number of variables with those not screened for depression. No significant differences were found between the groups in terms of mean age, sex, method of attempt, marital or occupational status. Not surprisingly, there was a significant difference in day of admission, with screened patients admitted less on Fridays and Saturdays than the non-screened group ($X^2 = 26.9$, df = 6, p < 0.001).

4. DISCUSSION

Before discussing the above findings, it is necessary to acknowledge an important limitation of the study. The use of only self-report measures of depression limits the extent to which conclusions can be drawn about the nature of depression in the suicidal subjects. A more rigorous appraisal of this could be achieved through combining self-report measures with observer ratings and a clinical assessment. For practical reasons, this approach was not possible during this screening for depression, although this combined approach was utilised in a further study of a subgroup of the screened subjects (Davis, 1995). Despite this limitation, the measures employed are considered to provide useful means of detecting symptoms of mood disorder and directing further enquiry into this important issue. Another limitation is that there was a low response rate, although the screened and non-screened groups were similar in many characteristics.

Both depression measures showed that the majority of patients hospitalised for attempted suicide have a depressive disorder, with the majority of these categorised as "moderate," "marked," or "severe" depression by the Zung SDS, or "endogenous" depression by the LPD questionnaire. Furthermore, a substantial number of suicidal subjects have a high frequency of symptoms usually associated with endogenous-type depression. The findings suggest that this may be particularly so for females. While this does not necessarily mean that each subject requires pharmacological treatment for depression, it certainly suggests that this possibility needs to be carefully considered, through a thorough clinical appraisal and close follow-up of each person.

The findings of the study are in keeping with several reports in the literature, which have also focused on the need for careful appraisal of depression in all suicidal individuals. (Morgan et al 1975, Weissman & Myers, 1978, Newson-Smith & Hirsch, 1979, Goldney & Pilowsky, 1980, Reeves et al 1985). Nonetheless, in making comparisons between studies, it is important to be mindful of important methological differences, including the type of research setting, the use of inclusion and exclusion criteria, the actual definition of attempted suicide, the rating instruments used and the representativeness of local populations.

In this study, 30% of the A & E subjects were not hospitalised, and could not be usefully compared with study subjects. Nonetheless, the study group did appear to be representative of the total hospitalised group, and therefore the findings may be generalised to reflect clinical issues in this important group.

In considering the significance of these findings, it is useful to review the findings of a previous study (Davis, 1989), when the LPD questionnaire was used to compare the characteristics of depression in 176 attempted suicide patients and 65 psychiatric inpatients with a diagnosis of major affective disorder. The study showed that despite significant age and sex differences, there was a striking similarity between the groups on all measures of depression, including severity and "endogenicity" of depression. This finding adds considerable weight to the argument that there is a clinically significant degree of depression in the majority of patients hospitalised for attempted suicide, and this needs to be carefully evaluated in every case.

It is important to continue to explore the issue of depression in attempted suicide, not the least because depression can usually be treated and clinicians can vigorously pursue this when it is detected. Furthermore, through treating depression, it is highly likely that clinicians can contribute to a significant reduction in the morbidity and mortality through suicide of this vulnerable group.

REFERENCES

Davis, A.T. (1989). Depression and attempted suicide : a comparative study. Australian & New Zealand Journal of Psychiatry, 23, 59–66.

Davis, A.T. (1995). Attempted suicide and depression : initial assessment and short-term follow-up. In "Impact of Suicide." B.L. Mishara (Ed).

Goldney, R.D. & Pilowsky, I. (1980). Depression in young women who have attempted suicide. Australian & New Zealand Journal of Psychiatry, 14, 203–211.

Kreitman, N. (1977) (Ed). "Parasuicide." London : John Wiley and Sons.

Morgan, H.G., Burns-Cox, C.J., Pocock, H., and Pottle, S., (1975). Deliberate self-harm : clinical and socio-economic characteristics of 368 patients. British Journal of Psychiatry, 127, 564–574.

Newson-Smith, J.G.B., and Hirsch, S.R. (1979). Psychiatric symptoms in self-poisoning patients. Psychological Medicine, 9, 493–500.

Pilowsky, I., Levine, S. and Boulton, D.M. (1969). The classification of depression by numerical taxonomy. British Journal of Psychiatry, 115, 937–945.

Reeves, J.C., Large, R.G. and Honeymoon, M. (1985). Parasuicide and depression : a comparison of clinical and questionnaire diagnoses. Australian and New Zealand Journal of Psychiatry, 19, 30–33.

Weissman, M.M. (1974) The epidemiology of suicide attempts, 1960–1971. Archives of General Psychiatry, 30, 737–746.

Weissman, M.M. and Myers, J.K. (1978). Rates and risks of depressive symptoms in a United States urban community. Acta Psychiatrica Scandinavica, 57, 219–231.

Zung, W.W.K. (1965). A self-rating depression scale. Archives of General Psychiatry, 12, 63–70.

22

LIFE EVENTS OVER THE LIFE CYCLE AND DEPRESSION IN LATE LIFE

V. Kraaij, I. Kremers, E. Arensman, and A. J. F. M. Kerkhof

Leiden University
Department of Clinical and Health Psychology
Leiden, The Netherlands
Vrije Universiteit
Department of Clinical Psychology
Amsterdam, The Netherlands

1. INTRODUCTION

Depression in late life is a severe problem. Depressive symptoms constitute a major risk factor for suicidal behavior for the elderly. Researchers have focused primarily on the effects of negative life events on adult depression, finding that loss-experiences (e.g., physical, social and psychological losses) and abuse are important risk factors for depression (Allers, Benjack, & Allers, 1992; Anderson, Yasenik, & Ross, 1993; Bifulco, Brown, & Adler, 1991; Moeller, Bachmann, & Moeller, 1993; Paykel, 1994; Weismann-Wind, & Silvern, 1994). However, looking at the available literature, elderly depression has received little attention.

In order to be able to prevent elderly depression and (attempted) suicide and to make effective prevention and intervention programs, it is important to identify risk factors for elderly depression. Studies concerning elderly depression primarily investigated the association between recent life events and depression in late life. Recent negative life events (e.g., bereavement, chronic social difficulties, personal physical illness and moving during the past year) appear to be correlated with depression in late life (for a review, see Katona, 1993). The influence of early negative life events and how they may pervade in old age has not yet been extensively studied.

The aim of the present study was to examine which life events occurring at different stages in life are related to depression in late life. This study is a pilot-study in preparation of a larger study. Therefore, the results presented here are to be considered preliminary.

Suicide Prevention, edited by Kosky *et al.*
Plenum Press, New York, 1998

2. METHOD

A total of 171 Dutch elderly people were asked to participate. Seventy-four (43%) agreed to be interviewed. The mean age of the sample was 82.3 years (SD 6.7, range 68–97) and 75% were female. All subjects were living in a nursing home or service flat. They were interviewed in their residences by trained psychology students.

Depressive symptoms were measured by the 30-item Geriatric Depression Scale (GDS; Yesavage, Brink, Rose, Lum, Huang, Adey, & Von Leirer, 1983). The GDS has a high reliability and validity (Kok, 1994). A cut-off score of 11 for depression was used.

Life events were measured by the Life Events Questionnaire (Kerkhof, Van Egmond, & Arensman, 1989). This instrument contains 96 items concerning stressful and traumatic life events. Information was recorded on the period in which an event occurred: childhood and early adolescence (0–14 year), late adolescence and adulthood (≥ 15 year) and the year prior to the interview.

3. RESULTS

The mean score on the GDS was 8.4 (SD 4.9). Eighteen elderly subjects (24%) met the GDS-diagnosis of depression.

First, the correlation between each life event and depressive symptoms was examined. Not all stressful and traumatic life events could be investigated; some were not reported (suicide[-attempt] by others or self, sexual and physical abuse).

Of all the life events that were reported, 15% occurred in childhood/early adolescence, 73% in late adolescence/adulthood and 12% in the year prior to the interview. Twelve life events correlated significantly with the severity of depressive symptomatology (see Table 1).

Three events in childhood/early adolescence were significantly correlated with depressive symptomatology. These events reflected a separation from parents and problems

Table 1. Significant Pearson product-moment correlations between life events in different periods and the GDS-scores

Stressful and traumatic life events	Throughout life	Childhood/ early adolescence	Late adolescence/ adulthood	Year prior to the interview
Problems with friends	0.24*	0.14	0.20*	0.05
Cheated by someone important	0.20*	—	0.20*	0.01
Mentally mistreated by brother(s) or sister(s) #	0.22*	0.05	0.22*	0.18
Problems in contact with brother(s) or sister(s) #	0.28**	—	0.28**	0.22*
Chronic, life-threatening disease child(ren)	0.25*		0.24*	0.10
Brought up by others than parents #	0.20*	0.20*		
Divorce/separation of parents #	0.20*	0.20*	—	—
Serious financial worries	0.28**		0.24*	0.21*
Loss of friends and relatives after relocation	0.21*	0.14	0.26**	0.05
Problems in making contact with other people	0.26**	0.14	0.14	0.32**
Problems in making friends	0.21*	0.21*	0.12	0.33**
Convicted or sentenced to jail #	0.20*	—	0.20*	—

*p<.05. ** p<.01.
#: fewer than 5 people answered with "yes"
—: the coefficient could not be computed

Table 2. Spearman correlations between sum variables of life events in different periods and the GDS-scores and variance accounted for

Life events	Correlation	Variance accounted for
Sum of childhood/early adolescence events	0.15	2.2%
Sum of late adolescence/adulthood events	0.25*	6.4%
Sum of recent events	0.30**	8.9%

*p<.05. ** p<.01.

in making friends. Significant correlations were mainly found for events occurring in late adolescence/adulthood. These events showed a large degree of heterogeneity. Four events represented problems with friends and family, the other events were illnesses of child(ren), financial worries, loss of contact after relocation and convicted or sentenced to jail. Life events in the year prior to the interview which were correlated with depressive symptomatology concerned problems with other people (brother[s], sister[s] and friends), problems in making contact and serious financial worries.

In order to examine the contribution of life events in different periods to depression, the sum of life events in each different life-phase were correlated with depressive symptomatology (see Table 2). The sum of events which occurred in late adolescence/adulthood and the sum of recent events were significantly correlated with depressive symptomatology, the sum of recent events accounting for most of the variance.

4. DISCUSSION

The study described in this paper examined the relationship between negative life events in different periods and depression in late life. Interpreting the results, one should take into consideration the fact that the study was conducted among a relatively small and selective (i.e., nursing home and service flat) sample. Therefore, one should be careful in generalizing the results.

A number of negative life events, which are related to adult depression, appeared to be correlated with depression in late life as well. These events included chronic social difficulties (problems in contact with others [friends and family]), financial worries, separation from parents, relocation, physical illnesses of child(ren) and sentenced or convicted to jail. In the present study, loss-experiences were not correlated with depression. However, all elderly people in the sample had experienced the loss of a loved one. The fact that a number of negative life events relating to depression were the same for adults and elderly people, provides support for the idea that depression in late life is not (only) age related. This may have further implications for treatment and prevention programs for depression in the elderly.

The majority of life events significantly correlating with depressive symptomatology occurred in late adolescence/adulthood. This may be explained by the length of the period. However, the available studies all focused on recent life events which could be related to depression. The findings of the present study indicate that negative life events occurring earlier in life may be important as well.

The correlation between a number of traumatic events and depression could not be investigated, because events as suicide, sexual abuse and physical abuse were not reported. A possible explanation for not reporting these traumatic events is that older people may be reluctant to talk about suicide and abuse, because these are "forbidden" topics. Another explanation is repression or amnesia of those painful memories.

In agreement with findings of other studies (for a review, see Katona, 1993), the negative life events experienced in the year prior to the interview showed the highest correlation with depressive symptomatology and accounted for most of the variance, even though the total number of reported life events were lowest in this period.

The population included in this study was a non-psychiatric population with relatively few depressive individuals. Therefore, in a clinical population, the correlations between different negative life events and depression may be stronger.

5. CONCLUSION

The results of the present study showed that not only recent events correlated with elderly depression, but life events that occurred throughout life also appeared to be related to depression in late life. Further research, in particular with psychiatric populations, is needed to investigate whether specific events in childhood and later life are related to depression in late life. The role of mediating factors such as coping and personality should also be investigated.

REFERENCES

Allers, C.T., Benjack, K.J., & Allers, N.T. (1992). Unresolved childhood sexual abuse: Are older adults affected? *Journal of Counseling & Development, 71,* 14–17.

Anderson, G., Yasenik, L., & Ross, C.A. (1993). Dissociative experiences and disorders among women who identify themselves as sexual abuse survivors. *Child Abuse & Neglect, 17,* 677–686.

Bifulco, A., Brown, G.W., & Adler, Z. (1991). Early sexual abuse and clinical depression in adult life. *British Journal of Psychiatry, 159,* 115–122.

Katona, C. (1993). The aetiology of depression in old age. *International Review of Psychiatry, 5,* 407–416.

Kerkhof, A.J.F.M., Van Egmond, M., & Arensman, E. (1989). Life Events Questionnaire. In A.J.F.M. Kerkhof, W. Bernasco, U. Bille-Brahe, S. Platt, & A. Schmidtke (Eds.). *WHO/EURO multicentre study on parasuicide, European parasuicide study interview schedule (EPSIS) (pp.37–49).* Leiden, The Netherlands: Leiden University, Department of Clinical and Health Psychology.

Kok, R.M. (1994). Zelfbeoordelingsschalen voor depressie bij ouderen. *Tijdschrift voor Gerontologie en Geriatrie, 25,* 150–156.

Moeller, T.P., Bachmann, G.A., & Moeller, J.R. (1993). The combined effects of physical, sexual, and emotional abuse during childhood: Long-term health consequences for women. *Child Abuse & Neglect, 17,* 623–640.

Paykel, E.S. (1994). Life events, social support and depression. *Acta Psychiatrica Scandinavica, Suppl 377,* 50–80.

Weissmann-Wind, T., & Silvern, L. (1994). Parenting and family stress as mediators of the long-term effects of child abuse. *Child Abuse & Neglect, 18*(5), 439–453.

Yesavage, J.A., Brink, T.L., Rose, T.L., Lum, O., Huang, V., Adey, M., & Von Leirer, O. (1983). Development and validation of a geriatric depression screening scale: A preliminary report. *Journal of Psychiatric Research, 17,* 37–49.

23

RISK FACTORS FOR SERIOUS SUICIDE ATTEMPTS AMONG YOUNG PEOPLE

A Case Control Study

Annette L. Beautrais

Canterbury Suicide Project
Christchurch School of Medicine
PO Box 4345, Christchurch, New Zealand

1. INTRODUCTION

In New Zealand, as in a number of countries, considerable concerns have developed in recent years about the issue of suicidal behaviour among young people. These concerns have been stimulated by several lines of evidence. Firstly, international comparisons suggest that New Zealand has one of the highest rates of youth suicide among developed countries with a suicide rate for young males aged 15 to 24 years of 40 deaths per 100 000 (World Health Organisation, 1993). Secondly, examination of historical time series data shows a marked recent increase in male youth suicide rates in New Zealand, which have quadrupled in the last two decades and are higher now than at any point in New Zealand's history (Deavoll, Mulder, Beautrais & Joyce, 1993). Finally, suicidal behaviour among young people is a significant source of morbidity and psychiatric emergency, with hospital admission rates for suicide attempts of approximately 220 per 100 000 annually for those aged 15 to 24 years (New Zealand Health Information Service, 1995).

This evidence have led to a growing realisation that suicidal behaviour is a serious problem in New Zealand. The present study was undertaken in an effort to contribute to knowledge about youthful suicidal behaviour and presents findings from a case control study in which a consecutive series of 129 young people who made medically serious suicide attempts were compared with 153 control subjects of similar age who were randomly selected from the community. This paper aims to provide an overview of the extent to which different domains of risk factors contribute to risk of serious suicide attempt among young people, using case-control methodology as the principal analytic process. The broad aims of this analysis were as follows:

a. To examine the extent to which a series of sociodemographic factors were associated with risk of serious suicide attempt;
b. To examine the contribution of a range of mental disorders to risk of serious suicide attempt;
c. To examine the association between a series of childhood experiences and family characteristics, and risk of serious suicide attempt;
d. To examine the association between a range of personality traits and cognitive styles, and risk of serious suicide attempt;
e. To examine the extent to which a series of stressful life events was associated with serious suicide attempts;
f. To examine joint linkages between sociodemographic factors, psychiatric morbidity, childhood experiences, personality factors, stressful life events and vulnerability to serious suicide attempt.

The overall goal of the study was to identify risk factors for suicidal behaviour and to relate these to points of intervention relevant to suicide prevention programmes.

2. METHOD

2.1. Overview

The findings in this study come from the Canterbury Suicide Project which is a case control study of completed suicide (202 cases), medically serious suicide attempts (302 cases) and 1028 randomly selected community control subjects. This paper describes risk factors for serious suicide attempts among young people from this study.

2.1.1. Cases. The cases consist of a consecutive series of 129 individuals aged under 25 years who made medically serious suicide attempts from 1/09/91 to 31/05/94 in Christchurch (New Zealand) which is a mixed urban/rural region with a population of 430 000.

Medically serious suicide attempts were defined as those for which hospital admission for more than 24 hours was required and which, during admission, required specialised treatment and/or care. A description of medically serious suicide attempts for this study has been published (Beautrais, Joyce & Mulder, 1996).

The response rate for cases was 97.7%. Almost equal numbers of males (45.7%) and females (54.3%) made serious suicide attempts. The mean age of cases was 19.4 years (SD = 3.0, range 13–24 years); (males: mean , 20.2 years, SD, 2.8 years; females: mean , 18.7 years, SD. 3.1 years).

2.1.2. Control Subjects. Control subjects were selected from local electoral rolls. An age and gender stratified sample was obtained in which the sample was stratified by gender and age with the number of subjects in the age by gender stratum selected at a rate proportional to the known age by gender distribution of the population aged 18–24 years. In total, 153 subjects selected for the control sample were aged under 25. The mean age of control subjects was 21.4 years (SD, 1.6) (males: mean, 21.5, SD, 1.5; females: mean, 21.3, SD, 1.6). The subjects in this age stratum were part of a larger sample of 1028 control subjects aged 18 and older and the estimated response rate for the total control sample was 85.7%. Official estimates from the national Electoral Roll Office suggested 95.5% of the eligible population were enrolled on Canterbury electoral rolls during the data collection period of the study.

The study was approved by the Ethics Committees of the Canterbury Area Health Board and the Southern Regional Health Authority. Written informed consent was obtained from all study participants after the aims and procedures of the study had been explained. For children aged 16 and under, the consent of both the child and the parent/guardian was obtained.

2.2. Data Collection

A semi-structured interview was conducted personally with each subject in the study by trained experienced interviewers to retrospectively reconstruct a life history and to obtain information about potential risk factors for serious suicide attempts. For each subject a parallel interview was conducted with a 'significant other' who knew the subject well and was nominated by the subject.

From the database of the study, the following measures were selected for analysis, based upon previous research from both the present study (Beautrais, 1996) and other studies (see, for example, reviews by Diekstra, Kienhorst & de Wilde, 1995; Shaffer & Piacentini, 1994) which suggested that these factors were associated with suicide attempt risk:

2.2.1. Social and Demographic Measures. Subject socio-economic status was measured using the occupational scale for socio-economic status in New Zealand (Elley & Irving, 1976).

Educational qualifications were assessed on a three point scale which classified subjects according to the highest educational qualification achieved: no formal educational qualification; secondary school qualification (usually obtained from 16 to 18 years); trade or technical qualification, university degree or diploma.

Religious affiliation was classified as: Church of England; Presbyterian; Roman Catholic; other Christian denomination; agnostic/atheist/other denomination.

Church attendance in the preceding year was classified as: at least once a month; two to three times a year; once a year or less often.

Ethnic/cultural identification was defined on subject self-identification and was dichotomised as Maori or non-Maori. Individuals who classified themselves as being part Maori were included in the Maori classification.

Personal income was defined as after tax annual income during the year prior to interview. For subjects living with partners (7.8% of cases; 24.2% of controls) personal income was defined as 50% of the joint family income.

Principal occupation was classified as: working in paid employment for >30 hours per week; secondary school or tertiary student; not a student and not in full-time employment.

2.2.2. Measures of Childhood and Family Risk Factors. Parental death was defined as the death of either or both parent figures during childhood. (Childhood was defined here, as for all family and childhood risk factors, as the period from birth to 16 years).

Parental separation or divorce was defined as the divorce or long term separation of the subject's parent figures during childhood.

Measures of maternal care, maternal control, parental care and parental control were obtained for each subject's principal parent figures, using the Parental Bonding Instrument (PBI) (Parker, 1989). PBI scores were dichotomised to produce measures of low care and high control, according to criteria recommended by Parker (1983) and MacKinnon, Henderson, Scott and Duncan-Jones (1989).

Childhood sexual abuse was assessed by asking each subject whether or not, during childhood, they had been "physically or psychologically forced by anyone to engage in any unwanted sexual activity, such as unwanted sexual touching of his/her body or sexual intercourse," a definition previously used by Murphy (1985). Subjects who responded positively to this question were then asked further questions relating to this activity. Subjects were classified as having a history of childhood sexual abuse if they responded positively to the initial question and subsequent questioning established a history of childhood sexual abuse.

Childhood physical abuse was assessed by asking each subject whether or not they believed they had, in their opinion, experienced physical abuse during childhood. Subjects who responded positively to this question were asked to provide specific examples of the abusive behaviour they had experienced. Subjects were classified as having a history of physical abuse if they responded positively to the initial question and responses to subsequent questions established a history of physical abuse.

Poor parental relationship was assessed by a global rating on a four point scale by each subject of their impression of the quality of the relationship of their major parent figures during childhood.

Parental imprisonment was defined as the imprisonment of either parent figure during the subject's childhood.

Poor economic circumstances was defined if the subject considered that "lack of money had caused difficulties for the subject or family" during childhood.

In care as a child was defined as institutional care during childhood (including foster care and Government Department of Social Welfare care).

Parental alcohol problems were defined if the subject specified parental alcohol problems as a family problem during childhood.

Parental violent behaviour was defined if the subject specified violent behaviour by either parent toward any other person as a family problem during childhood.

2.2.3. Measures of Current Psychiatric Morbidity. The interview for each subject included a modified version of the SCID interview (Spitzer, Williams, Gibbon & First, 1988) to generate DSM-III-R diagnoses of selected mental disorders (American Psychiatric Association, 1987). Data from both subject and significant other interviews was integrated in a diagnostic conference to produce, for each subject, best estimate diagnoses of mental disorders (according to DSM-III-R criteria). In the present analysis the following diagnostic groupings for disorders in the month prior to suicide attempt (or interview) were used: a) Affective disorders; b) Substance use disorders; c) Anxiety disorders; d) Eating disorders; e) Non-affective psychosis. For antisocial disorder (conduct disorder or antisocial personality disorder) a lifetime history was obtained. Multiple diagnoses were permitted on Axis I. The reliability of the best estimate diagnostic procedure was ascertained by a re-evaluation of a random sample of 20% of all cases (subjects and controls). The test-retest agreement was high with kappa coefficients (Fleiss, 1981) for the principal diagnostic categories ranging from 0.95 to 0.99.

2.2.4. Measures of Personality Traits and Cognitive Styles. For   some   personality traits, selected items from standardised questionnaires were used to form measures in an effort to curtail the length of the interview. The personality measures used in the analysis included:

Impulsiveness: The 30 item Barratt Impulsivity Scale (Barratt, 1985) was used to evaluate each subject's perception of impulsive aspects of his/her typical behaviours during recent years. Reliability was assessed using Cronbach's alpha (Cronbach, 1953), which showed the impulsiveness measure to be of good internal consistency ($\alpha = .78$).

Neuroticism and extraversion: The short form of the Eysenck Personality Questionnaire (MacKinnon, Jorm, Christensen, Scott, Henderson & Korten, 1995) was used to obtain measures of neuroticism, and introversion/ extraversion. The 10 items of each scale were summed to produce neuroticism and extraversion scores. The reliabilities of the resulting scales were good: extraversion ($\alpha = .88$); neuroticism ($\alpha = .86$).

Self-esteem: Seven items form the Coopersmith Self-Esteem Inventory (Coopersmith, 1981) were selected and summed to determine a measure of self-esteem. This measure was of good internal consistency ($\alpha = .89$).

Hopelessness: Ten items were selected from the Beck Hopelessness Scale (Beck, Weissman, Lester & Trexler, 1974) and summed to determine a measure of hopelessness. This measure was of high internal consistency ($\alpha = .89$)

Locus of control: Seven items were selected from the Locus of Control of Behaviour scale (Craig, Franklin & Andrews, 1984), and summed to determine a measure of the extent to which an individual perceives that events are a consequence of his/her own behaviour and therefore potentially under his/her control (Lefcourt, 1976). This measure was of moderate internal consistency ($\alpha = .65$).

2.2.5. Stressful Life Events. The short list of Threatening Life Experiences (Brugha, Bebbington, Tennant, Hurry et al, 1985) was used as a basis to evaluate each subject's perception of life events which had occurred during the preceding year, and was amended by the addition of several further items which prior research had indicated might also have significant threat.

For the present analysis, measures of life events were classified into seven related categories of life events which included: a) Interpersonal issues; b) Work issues; c) Financial issues; d) Serious problems with the law or police; e) Personal illness issues; f) Family illness or bereavement issues; g) Other life events (including rape, unwanted pregnancy, changes of residence and parental marital separation).

3. RESULTS

3.1. Bivariate Associations between Risk Factors and Risk of Serious Suicide Attempt

The contribution of particular risk factors to risk of serious suicide attempt was examined by comparing the 129 subjects who made serious suicide attempts with the control sample of 153 subjects. For each risk factor domain (sociodemographic factors, family and childhood factors, personality traits, mental disorders, life events), each table contrasts the percentages of cases and controls with each risk factor, tests the association between each risk factor and risk of serious suicide attempt using the chi squared test of independence, and gives odds ratios for risk of serious suicide attempt, relative to a specified reference category.

Table 1 examines the association between social and demographic factors and serious suicide attempt risk. Individuals who made serious suicide attempts had elevated odds of a range of social and demographic characteristics when compared with control subjects. In general these features were indicative of social disadvantage and included: Lack of formal educational qualifications (p<.0001), low socioeconomic status (p<.0001) and low an-

Table 1. Rates of social and demographic characteristics of young people who made serious suicide attempts, and control subjects

Characteristic	Serious suicide attempt		Controls		OR	p
	N	%	N	%		
Educational qualification						
University /tertiary qualifications	11	8.6	46	{30.0}	1	<.0001
Secondary school qualification	53	41.4	89	58.2	2.5	
No formal qualification	64	50.0	18	11.8	14.9	
Socio-economic status						
SES classes 1–2	1	0.8	21	14.1	1	<.0001
SES classes 3–4	19	15.0	56	37.6	7.1	
SES classes 5–6	107	84.3	72	48.3	31.2	
Personal income ($ per annum)						
≥20,000	12	9.6	52	34.4	1	<.0001
10,000–19,999	19	15.2	51	33.8	1.6	
<10,000	94	75.2	48	31.8	8.5	
Principal occupation						
Employed	36	27.9	78	51.0	1	<.0001
Student—school/tertiary	48	21.7	55	2.6	1.9	
Not employed–not student	45	34.9	20	13.1	4.9	
Religious affiliation						
Church of England	11	8.6	30	19.6	1	<.0001
Presbyterian	8	6.3	16	10.5	1.4	
Roman Catholic	12	9.4	15	9.8	2.2	
Other Christian	61	47.7	32	20.9	5.2	
Agnostic/atheist/other	36	28.1	60	39.2	1.6	
Frequency of church attendance						
Once a year or less	97	75.2	127	83.0	1	<.01
2–3 times a year	4	3.1	11	7.2	0.5	
At least once a month	28	21.7	15	9.8	2.5	
Ethnic/cultural identification						
Non-Maori	110	85.3	141	92.2	1	<.10
Maori	19	14.7	12	7.8	2.0	

nual income (p<.0001). Those who made serious suicide attempts were less likely to be working (p<.0001), more likely to hold Christian beliefs (p<.0001) and more likely to attend church regularly. There was a marginally significant tendency for ethnicity to be linked with suicide attempts with Maori having twice the odds of serious suicide attempt compared to non-Maori.

Table 2 compares cases and controls with respect to a series of measures of childhood and family functioning. Risks of serious suicide attempt were significantly related to a range of family and childhood factors including parental separation or divorce (p<.0001), poor parental relationship (p<.0001); childhood sexual abuse (p<.0001); childhood physical abuse (p<.0001), parental violent behaviour (p<.02) parental problems with alcohol (p<.0001), poor economic or material circumstances (p<.01), and being in care as a child (p<.0001). Those who made serious suicide attempts were more likely than control subjects to report lower parental care scores (p<.0001) and higher parental control scores (p<.01) on the PBI.

Table 3 contrasts cases and controls in terms of a series of measures of personality traits and cognitive styles. Risks of serious suicide attempt were significantly related to a range of personality traits including hopelessness (p<.0001), neuroticism (p<.0001), introversion (p<.0001), impulsiveness (p<.0001), low self-esteem (p<.0001)and external locus

Table 2. Rates of family characteristics of young people who made serious suicide attempts, and control subjects

Family characteristics	Serious suicide attempts		Controls		OR (95% CI)	p
	N	%	N	%		
Parental loss						
Parental death	8	6.3	6	3.9		>.30
Parental separation	47	36.7	25	16.3	3.0 (1.7,5.2)	<.0001
Parental care characteristics						
Low maternal care	23	18.0	7	4.6	4.6 (1.9,11.0)	<.0001
Low paternal care	44	34.4	12	7.8	6.2 (3.1,12.3)	<.0001
High maternal control	52	40.6	36	23.5	2.2 (1.3,3.7)	<.002
High paternal control	50	39.1	37	24.2	2.0 (1.2,3.4)	<.01
Abusive experiences						
Sexual abuse	43	33.6	11	7.2	6.5 (3.2,13.3)	<.0001
Physical abuse	27	21.1	3	2.0	13.4 (3.9,45.2)	<.0001
Family experiences						
Poor parental relationship	45	35.2	12	7.8	6.4 (3.2,12.7)	<.0001
Parental violent behaviour	11	8.6	3	2.0	4.7 (1.3,17.2)	<.02
Parental alcohol problems	17	13.3	3	2.0	7.7 (2.2,26.8)	<.0001
Parental imprisonment	4	3.1	1	0.7		>.10
Poor economic circumstances	30	23.4	17	11.1	2.5 (1.3,4.7)	<.01
In care as a child	21	16.4	3	2.0	9.8 (2.9,33.7)	<.0001

of control (p<.0001), with those individuals who scored in the highest quartile of each of these measures having elevated odds of serious suicide attempt.

Table 4 contrasts rates of current DSM-III-R disorders amongst cases and control subjects. Individuals who made serious suicide attempts had clearly elevated rates of a range of mental disorders at the time of the attempt including affective disorders (p<.0001), substance use disorders (p<.0001), anxiety disorders (p<.01), eating disorders (p<.001) and a lifetime history of antisocial behaviour (p<.0001). Overall, 89.2% of those who made serious suicide attempts met criteria for at least one mental disorder at the time of the attempt compared to 31.4% of controls (p<.0001).

Table 5 compares rates of a range of life events during the preceding year for cases and controls. Risks of serious suicide attempt were associated with a range of life events during the preceding year, with individuals who made serious suicide attempts having elevated rates of the following categories of life events: interpersonal losses or conflicts (p<.0001); work issues (p<.005); serious financial problems (p<.0001); serious problems with the law or police (p<.0001), personal illness issues (p<.02) and other life events (p<.0001).

Table 3. Rates of personality traits of young people who made
serious suicide attempts, and control subjects

Personality traits	Serious suicide attempts		Controls		OR	p
	N	%	N	%		
Hopelessness						
1 Low	13	10.2	65	42.5	1	<.0001
2	12	9.5	52	34.0	1.2	
3	31	24.4	30	19.6	5.2	
4 High	71	55.9	6	3.9	59.2	
Neuroticism						
1 Low	12	9.4	57	37.3	1	<.0001
2	15	11.7	45	29.4	1.6	
3	40	31.3	33	21.6	5.8	
4 High	61	47.7	18	11.8	16.1	
Extraversion						
1 High	21	16.4	43	28.1	1	<.0001
2	28	21.9	59	38.6	1	
3	30	23.4	32	20.9	1.9	
4 Low	49	38.3	19	12.4	5.3	
Impulsiveness						
1 Low	20	15.6	51	33.3	1	<.0001
2	29	22.7	47	30.7	1.6	
3	28	21.9	34	22.2	2.1	
4 High	51	39.8	21	13.7	6.2	
Self esteem						
1 High	10	7.8	51	33.3	1	<.0001
2	20	15.6	49	32.0	2.1	
3	31	24.2	40	26.1	4.0	
4 Low	67	52.3	13	8.5	26.3	
Locus of control						
1 Low (internal)	9	7.2	62	40.5	1	<.0001
2	31	24.6	44	28.8	4.9	
3	29	23.0	21	13.7	9.5	
4 High (external)	57	45.2	26	17.0	15.1	

In summary, the preceding analyses suggest that those young people most at risk of serious suicide attempt tended to be characterised by social disadvantage, childhood adversity, personality difficulties, current psychiatric disorder and recent stressful life events.

3.2. Multivariate Associations between Risk Factors and Risk of Serious Suicide Attempt

Since some of the risk factors shown to make significant contributions to risk of serious suicide attempt in the bivariate analyses above might be intercorrelated with: a) other risk factors within the particular risk factor domain, and/or: b) with risk factors from other domains, the net effects of each factor were examined by fitting logistic regression models to the data in a sequential process, taking account of: a) intercorrelations among risk factors of a particular category and, b) antecedent risk factors. The results of these analyses are summarised in Table 6 indicating those analyses which were adjusted for the

Table 4. Rates of DSM-III-R mental disorders (in month prior to suicide attempt) for young people who made serious suicide attempts, and for control subjects

Mental disorder	Serious suicide attempts		Controls		OR(95% CI)	p
	N	%	N	%		
Major depression	80	62.0	14	9.2	16.2 (8.4,31.2)	<.0001
Bipolar I or II disorder	11	8.5	—	—		<.0001
Any affective disorder	91	70.5	14	9.2	23.8 (12.2,46.3)	<.0001
Alcohol abuse/dependence	40	31.0	24	15.7	2.4 (1.4,4.3)	<.002
Cannabis abuse/dependence	15	11.6	4	2.6	4.9 (1.6,15.2)	<.005
Other drug abuse/dependence	12	9.3	2	1.3	7.7 (1.7,35.3)	<.002
Any substance use disorder	50	38.8	25	16.3	3.2 (1.9,5.7)	<.0001
Any eating disorder	11	8.5	1	0.7	14.2 (1.8,111.3)	<.001
Any anxiety disorder	19	14.7	8	5.2	3.1 (1.3,7.4)	<.01
Any non-affective psychosis	1	0.8	2	1.3	—	>.50
Any anti-social disorder	45	34.9	12	7.8	6.3 (3.2,12.6)	<.0001
Any mental disorder	115	89.2	48	31.4	18.0 (9.4,34.5)	<.0001

Table 5. Rates of life events during past year for those who made serious suicide attempts, and control subjects

Life event	Serious suicide attempts		Controls		OR (95% CI)	p
	N	%	N	%		
Interpersonal issues	102	79.1	52	34.0	7.3 (4.3,12.6)	<.0001
Work issues	71	55.0	46	30.1	2.9 (1.7,4.5)	<.001
Financial issues	41	31.8	16	10.4	4.0 (2.1,7.5)	<.0001
Legal issues	31	24.0	3	2.0	15.8 (4.7,53.2)	<.0001
Personal illness issues	56	43.4	40	26.1	2.2 (1.3,3.6)	<.0001
Family illness/bereavement Issues	72	55.5	84	54.9	—	>.10
Other life event	40	31.0	13	8.5	4.8 (2.5,9.6)	<.0001
Any life event	127	98.5	128	83.7	12.4 (2.9,53.5)	<.0001

Table 6. Summary of odds ratio estimates for key factors
for serious suicide attempts among young people

Risk factor	Odds ratio
1. Socio-demographic Factors	
No educational qualification	7.7
Low socio-economic status	2.3
2. Family and Childhood Factors (adjusted for 1)	
Poor parental relationship	3.3
Childhood sexual abuse	4.3
Parental alcohol problems	6.1
3. Personality Traits (adjusted for 1, 2)	
High hopelessness	13.2
High neuroticism	3.2
4. Psychiatric Disorder (adjusted for 1, 2, 3)	
Affective disorder	12.6
Substance use disorder	3.9
5. Life Events (adjusted for 1, 2, 3)	
Interpersonal issues	2.7
Problems with law/police	6.3

effects of antecedent factors, and showing, for each risk factor which was significant in the logistic regression, the odds ratio adjusted for intercorrelations between risk factors.

When account was taken of intercorrelations between sociodemographic factors, two key social and demographic factors were significantly related to risk of serious suicide attempt: educational qualifications and social class. The findings implied that those who lacked formal educational qualifications and those who in the lowest socio-economic classes were at increased risk of serious suicide attempt. Adjusted odds ratios for these factors ranged from 2.8 (for low socio-economic status) to 7.7 (for lack of educational qualifications).

The principal family factors associated with risk of serious suicide attempt included: exposure to childhood sexual abuse, poor parental marital relationship and parental problems with alcohol. Odds ratio estimates were adjusted for the effects of social and demographic factors and other family factors, and ranged from 3.3 (for poor parental relationship) to 4.3 (for childhood sexual abuse) to 6.1 (for parental alcohol problems).

Two personality traits were associated with suicide attempt risk: hopelessness and neuroticism. Odds ratio estimates were adjusted for socio-demographic factors, family factors and other personality traits and ranged from 3.2 (for those with scores in the highest quartile for neuroticism) to 13.2 (for those with scores in the highest quartile for hopelessness).

The principal mental disorders associated with suicide attempt risk were affective disorders and substance use disorders. Odds ratio estimates were adjusted for the effects of socio-demographic factors, family factors, personality traits and other mental disorder categories, and ranged from 3.9 (for substance use disorders) to 12.6 (for affective disorders).

The life events found to be significantly related to suicide attempt risk were exposure to interpersonal losses and conflicts, and to problems with the law and/or police. Odds ratio estimates were adjusted for the effects of sociodemographic, family and personality factors, and other life events, and ranged from 2.7 (for interpersonal life event exposure) to 6.3 (for legal problems).

The results of the present analysis suggest that these risk factors may act cumulatively to determine the extent of individual risk to serious suicide attempt. The next table

Table 7. Rates of risk factor occurrence for those who made
serious suicide attempts, and control subjects

No. of risk factors	Serious suicide attempts		Controls		OR (95% CI)
	N	%	N	%	
0	0	0	40	26.1)	1
1–2	11	8.5	81	52.9)	
3–4	37	28.7	29	19.0	10.1 (4.3,23.6)
≥5	81	62.8	3	2.0	127.4 (48.6,334.2)

shows the number of risk factors present for those making suicide attempts. This table was constructed by computing a simple points score for each subject: each subject received one point for each of the eleven risk factors shown to be significant in the previous logistic regression analyses. The score thus ranged from 0 for those subjects with no identifiable risk factors to 11 for those with all of the possible risk factors identified in this study. The table compares the distribution of the number of risk factors for cases and control subjects, and gives the odds of suicide attempt risk conditional upon the risk factor score. The following conclusions are evident from inspection of the table:

a. Young people who made serious suicide attempts were characterised by relatively high levels of risk factor exposure. The mean number of risk factors for those who made suicide attempts was 5.3 compared to the mean of 1.5 risk factors for the control series. Whilst almost two thirds (62.8%) of those who made serious suicide attempts scored in the highest category of risk factor exposure, only 2.0% of control subjects scored in the same highest risk factor category.
b. It is clear that with increasing risk factor exposure, odds of risk of serious suicide attempt rose dramatically: the odds of suicide attempt for those with five or more risk factors, relative to those with less than 3 risk factors, was 127.4.

4. DISCUSSION

The aims of this paper have been to provide an overview of the extent to which different domains of risk factors contribute to risk of serious suicide attempt among young people, using case-control methodology as the principal analytie process.

The key findings of this analysis suggested that the principal factors associated with serious suicide attempt risk included lack of formal educational qualifications; low socio-economic status; exposure to childhood sexual abuse, poor parental marital relationship and parental problems with alcohol; high levels of hopelessness and neuroticism; current psychiatric morbidity (including affective disorders and substance use disorders) and recent exposure to life events relating to interpersonal losses and conflicts and legal problems.

The results from this study may be viewed in two ways. The first way of conceptualising these findings is that they provide a means of constructing a profile of the range of characteristics which may contribute to suicide attempt risk among young people. The outcome of this analysis, suggests that the young person who is likely to be at greatest risk of serious suicide attempt is characterised by: a) a socially and educationally disadvantaged background; b) a history of exposure to adverse family circumstances during childhood; c) high levels of hopelessness and neuroticism; d) significant psychiatric morbidity including, in particular, affective disorders and substance use disorders and e) high levels of exposure to adverse life events, including interpersonal and legal difficulties.

These findings of this study strongly support an accumulative risk model in which the individual risk of serious suicide attempt rises dramatically with the risk factor burden to which an individual was exposed, with those who had five or more risk factors having elevated odds of serious suicide attempt which were over 120 times those who had fewer than three risk factors. This analysis clearly suggests that serious suicide attempts are not simply a consequence of current psychiatric disorder, nor of current stressful life events, but rather represent the culminations of adverse life course sequences which have been marked by accumulations of risk factors from the domains of social disadvantage, childhood adversity, personality factors, psychiatric disorder and adverse life events.

One possible criticism of these conclusions is that the association between these factors and risk of serious suicide attempt may reflect recall bias with those making suicide attempts more likely to report adverse life circumstances in an effort to better explain their suicide attempt. It was possible to address this issue in the current research design by collecting a series of parallel measures of risk factors from interviews with significant others for each subject. Analysis of these significant other data produced substantially similar results to those obtained from analyses of data derived from self report (Beautrais, 1996). To the extent that similar results were obtained for both significant other and self report data, the case for arguing that the results reflect a recall bias would appear to be diminished.

An alternative way of interpreting the findings from this study is suggested by the conceptual model shown in Figure 1. This model assumes that:

    a. Three correlated sets of factors (social background, childhood and family factors, personality factors) act as broad determinants of an individual's vulnerability to suicidal behaviour. Those most vulnerable tend to come from socially disadvantaged backgrounds, to be exposed to childhood adversity and to have high levels of hopelessness and neuroticism.

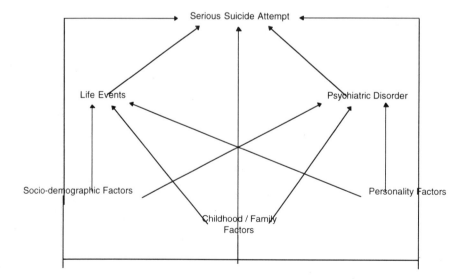

Figure 1. Conceptual model of risk factors domains for serious suicide attempt.

b. These vulnerability factors influence both an individual's susceptibility to psychiatric disorder and his/her level of life event exposure.

c. In combination, sociodemographic factors, childhood and family factors, personality factors, life events and psychiatric disorder make both direct and indirect contributions to an individual's risk of serious suicide attempt.

The major advantage of this model is that it provides a general overview and synthesis of the way in which various risk factor domains may combine to influence suicide attempt risk. The model suggests a life course process in which social background factors, childhood adversities, personality factors, psychiatric disorder and life events all combine to influence the likelihood of suicidal behaviour, with these factors being inter-related to each other. Whilst this model is clearly only approximate and should be subjected to further tests it serves the purpose of synthesising the large array of data collected over the course of this study into an orderly and interpretable framework that is generally consistent with prior research and theory in this area.

While the results of this analysis suggest that the aetiology of suicide attempt risk is multicausal and cannot be attributed to a single factor which clearly leads to suicide attempt, there does appear to be a theme that seems to unite all of the findings, and that suggests that, in one way or another, key predictors of serious suicide attempts in young people seem to be symptoms or consequences of life history courses marked by disadvantage, adversity and unhappiness. Moreover, the results suggest an accumulative model in which an individual's likelihood of making a suicide attempt rises almost exponentially with the number of adverse life course risk factors to which he is exposed.

The results of this study suggest that there are two major opportunities for prevention of serious suicide attempts among young people. The first approach involves the use of strategies which attempt to reduce the number of children exposed to unsatisfactory, disadvantaged or dysfunctional childhood environments which lead to suicide attempt risk. The types of interventions which are likely to be successful in addressing the role of family adversity in the development of suicidal behaviour are those strategies based on programmes which endeavour to improve parenting practices, to ameliorate adverse family circumstances and to increase individual life opportunities.

A second focus for intervention involves efforts to improve the recognition and management of psychiatric disorders among young people. A number of strategies for reducing the risk of psychiatric disorders and suicide attempt in the community have been proposed and include: improved organisation and structure of mental health care delivery systems to young people; improved identification, treatment and management of psychiatric illness, and particularly of affective disorders, by health professionals; improved training of primary mental health care providers to better recognise, refer and manage mental disorders; treatment protocols for those who have made suicide attempts who are at high risk of further suicide attempt behaviour and suicide.

An important recent finding from this study is that almost 80% of young people making serious suicide attempts have had previous contact with psychiatric and other health services for psychiatric reasons, with almost three quarters having been in contact with these services during the year prior to their serious suicide attempt. These findings clearly point to the need to embed suicide prevention programmes for young people into the context of mental health services.

In summary, the results of this study suggest a life course model of the development of suicidal behaviours that includes a combination of elements including social and demographic factors, family background factors, childhood experiences, personality traits, psychiatric morbidity and life events, which combine in various ways to increase the likelihood that serious suicide attempt will occur. The major themes that pervade this analysis are very similar to those which occur in other adolescent and young adult psychosocial disorders (including, for example, depressive disorders, substance use disorders, conduct disorders and youth offending behaviours) (see, for example, Rutter & Smith, 1995) and suggest that the major life pathways and processes which lead to serious suicide attempt overlap and correlate very substantially with those which lead to young adult psychosocial and mental health problems. These commonalities have two major implications for the understanding and prevention of serious suicide attempt behaviour among young people.

Firstly, they suggest that rising suicide rates among young people are part of a wider trend of substantial increases in rates of a range of psychosocial disorders among young people, and suggest that explanations for rises in youth suicide rates might more usefully be sought by considering changes in suicidal behaviours as part of broader social changes rather than considering suicide in isolation from other psychosocial disorders. Secondly, they imply that suicide prevention activities should be integrated into broader health promotion and health care delivery programs aimed at reducing the incidence of a range of psychosocial disorders amongst young people.

ACKNOWLEDGMENTS

This research was supported by the Canterbury Area Health Board, Healthlink South and the Health Research Council of New Zealand.

REFERENCES

American Psychiatric Association. (1987). *Diagnostic and Statistical Manual of Mental Disorders (3rd Edition—Revised) (DSM-III-R)*. Washington, DC: American Psychiatric Association.

Barratt, E.S. (1985). Impulsiveness defined within a systems model of personality. In C.D. Spielberger & J.D. Bulcher (Eds.), *Advances in Personality Assessment*. Vol 5. Hillsdale, NJ: Lawrence Earlbaum Associates.

Beautrais, A.L. (1996). Serious suicide attempts in young people: A case control study. Ph.D. Thesis, University of Otago.

Beautrais, A.L., Joyce, P.R, & Mulder, R.T. (1996). Risk factors for serious suicide attempts among youths aged 13 through 24 years. *Journal of the American Academy of Child and Adolescent Psychiatry, 35:* 1174–1182.

Beck, A.T., Weissman, A., Lester, D. & Trexler, L. (1974). The measurement of pessimism: The hopelessness scale. *Journal of Consulting and Clinical Psychology, 42:* 861–865.

Brugha, T., Bebbington, P., Tennant, C. & Hurry, J. (1985). The list of threatening life experiences: A subset of 12 life event categories with considerable long-term contextual threat. *Psychological Medicine, 15:* 189–194.

Coopersmith, S. (1981). *SEI—Self Esteem Inventories*. Palo Alto, CA: Consulting Psychologists Press *Data*. London: Methuen.

Craig, A.R., Franklin, J.A. & Andrews, G. (1984). A scale to measure locus of control behaviour. *British Journal of Medical Psychology, 57:* 173–180.

Cronbach, L.J. (1953). Coefficient alpha and the internal structure of tests. *Psychometrika, 16:* 297–334.

Deavoll, B.J., Mulder, R.T., Beautrais, A.L & Joyce, P.R. (1993). One hundred years of suicide in New Zealand. *Acta Psychiatrica Scandinavica, 87:* 81–85.

Diekstra, R.F.W., Kienhorst, C.W.M. & de Wilde, E.J. (1995). Suicide and suicidal behaviour among adolescents. In Rutter, M. & D.J. Smith (Eds). *Psychosocial disorders in young people: Time trends and their causes* (pp 686–761). Chichester: John Wiley & Sons.

Elley, W.B. & Irving, J.C. (1976). Revised socio-economic status for New Zealand. *New Zealand Journal of Educational Studies, 11:* 25–36.

Eysenck, H.J. & Eysenck, S.B.J. (1975). *Manual of the Eysenck Personality Questionnaire (Junior and Adult)*. Seven Oaks, Kent: Hodder & Stoughton

Fleiss, J.L. (1981). *Statistical Methods for Rates and Proportions. 2nd ed*. New York: John Wiley.

Lefcourt, H.M. (1976). *Locus of control current trends: Theory and research*. New York: Wiley.

MacKinnon, A.J., Henderson, A.S., Scott, R. & Duncan-Jones, P. (1989). The Parental Bonding Instrument (PBI): An epidemiological study in a general population sample. *Psychological Medicine, 19:* 1023–1034.

MacKinnon, A.J., Jorm, A.F., Christensen, H., Scott, L.R., Henderson, A.S. & Korten, A.E. (1995). A latent trait analysis of the Eysenck Personality Questionnaire in an elderly community sample. *Personality and Individual Differences, 18:* 739–747.

Murphy, J.E. Untitled news release. (Available from St Cloud State University, St Cloud, MN56301). June (1985)

New Zealand Health Information Service. (1995). *Selected Morbidity and Hospital Data—Vol.1 (1993)*. Wellington: Ministry of Health.

Parker, G. (1983). Parental 'Affectionless control' as an antecedent to adult depression. *Archives of General Psychiatry, 40:* 956–960.

Parker, G. (1989). The Parental Bonding Instrument: Psychometric properties reviewed. *Psychiatric Development, 4:* 317–335.

Rutter, M. & D.J. Smith. (1995). (Eds.). *Psychosocial disorders in young people: Time trends and their causes*. Chichester: John Wiley and Sons.

Shaffer, D., Piacentini, J. (1994). Suicide and Attempted Suicide. In M. Rutter, E. Taylor & L. Hersov (Eds). *Child and adolescent psychiatry: Modern approaches (*pp 407–424). Oxford: Blackwell Scientific Publications, 3rd ed.

Spitzer, R.L., Williams, J.B.W., Gibbon, M. & First, M.B. (1988). *Structured Clinical Interview for DSM-III-R—Patient version, (SCID-P, 6/1/88)*. New York State Psychiatric Institute, New York: Biometrics Research Department.

World Health Organisation (1993). *World Health Statistics Annual* Geneva: World Health Organisation

24

GENDER DIFFERENCES IN PSYCHIATRIC DISORDER FOR DELIBERATE SELF POISONING PATIENTS WITH MULTIPLE INPATIENT SERVICE UTILISATION

G. L. Carter, I. M. Whyte, N. T. Carter, and K. Ball

Newcastle Mater Misericordiae Hospital
Waratah, NSW, Australia

1. BACKGROUND

The Self Poisoning Patients: A Multiple Service Use (SPP:MSU) Project was conducted by the Self Poisoning Research Group at the Newcastle Mater Misericordiae Hospital (NMMH) to provide a quantitative account of multiple service use by self poisoning patients in the clinical service known as the Hunter Area Toxicology Service (HATS). This paper reports on a three year cohort (1992 to 1994) of deliberate (intentional) self poisoning patients (DSP), referred from a defined geographical area, and serviced by a single integrated clinical service. All analyses presented are for deliberate self poisonings, based on index DSP admissions or all DSP admissions as specified.

The SPP:MSU Project was funded under a 1994/95 NSW Health Outcomes Project Grant. The core clinical research group of the SPP:MSU Project comprises Dr G.L. Carter (Department of Consultation-Liaison Psychiatry and Primary Investigator), Dr I.M. Whyte and Dr A.H. Dawson (Department of Clinical Toxicology and Pharmacology). Additional positions were Ms K. Ball and Mrs N.T. Carter (part time Research Assistants).

The *NSW mental health goals and targets and strategies for health gain* (1995) has identified a number of targets to meet in order to achieve the goal of reducing suicide in NSW. These are *inter alia*:

Target 2.3.   reduce the suicide re-attempt rate by 25 percent over 10 years.

Target 2.4.   reduce the proportion of suicide re-attendances for self poisoning over 10 years.

This paper may provide relevant information concerning baseline rates of multiple service utilisation, psychiatric diagnoses and gender differences which may inform the development and implementation of these goals.

Suicide Prevention, edited by Kosky *et al.*
Plenum Press, New York, 1998

History of Hunter Area Toxicology Study

In 1987 the Clinical Pharmacology and Toxicology Department at the Royal New-castle Hospital took responsibility for the management of all self poisoning patients pre-senting to that hospital. By 1991 this had become an Area based service called the Hunter Area Toxicology Service (HATS) and was subsequently transferred to the NMMH. This expanded role required the provision of a primary and secondary referral service to a population of approximately 385,000 in the Greater Newcastle area and a tertiary referral service to the 100,000 population of the Lower and Upper Hunter.

Operationally it was decided that all self poisonings presenting to hospital were to be admitted under the Clinical Toxicologist on HATS. The service was multidisciplinary with an integrated Consultation-Liaison Psychiatry service so that all deliberate self poi-soning patients received joint medical and psychiatric assessment and care. Psychiatric as-sessment was provided for all self poisoning admissions and, on request, for other poisonings (accidental, recreational, iatrogenic and other). Staff education emphasised that self poisoning patients were entitled to a legitimate "sick role." Specific education in the medical and psychiatric aspects of patient care was instituted, which emphasised that treatment should be appropriate, rational and medically indicated rather than punitive.

A relational database for collecting prospectively recorded data on poisoned patients was in use from 1987. The complexity of this database has been progressively developed. Details of the service are available in a report to the NSW Department of Health (Carter, Whyte, Dawson and Buckley, unpublished). The clinical model of service delivery and the clinical outcomes of mortality, morbidity and length of stay for this model have also been reported (Whyte, Dawson, Buckley, Carter and Levey, in press).

2. OBJECTIVES

The objectives of this paper were to:

- describe the rates of multiple service use by describing the rates of repeat or re-peated deliberate self harm and multiple psychiatric hospital admission for a three ·year cohort of deliberate self poisoning (DSP) patients from a geographically de-fined area; and
- compare the DSM-IV psychiatric disorder rates for males and females in these categories.

3. DEFINITIONS

This project was interested in "multiple service use" in two settings:

- those deliberate self poisoning (DSP) patients who showed repetition of DSP be-haviour requiring further admission to the HATS in the general hospital; and
- those DSP patients who showed multiple admissions to the public psychiatric hos-pitals in the area.

Repeat Deliberate Self Poisoning (RDSP-1) was defined as a DSP admission in 1992 to 1994, plus at least two admissions for DSP occurring within an interval of one year, in the period 1992 to 1995. Non-Repeat Deliberate Self Poisoning (Non-RDSP-1) was then defined as a DSP admission in 1992 to 1994 but without any two DSP admissions occurring within an interval of one year, in the period of 1992 to 1995.

Multiple Psychiatric Hospital Admissions (MPHA-1) was defined as a DSP admission in 1992 to 1994 plus at least two admissions to a public psychiatric hospital within a one year interval, in the period 1992 to 1995. Non-Multiple Psychiatric Admission (Non-MPHA-1) was defined as a DSP admission in the period 1992 to 1994 but less than two admissions to a public psychiatric hospital within a one year interval, in the period 1992 to 1995.

Index DSP admission is the first DSP admission in the 1992–1994 period.

4. METHOD

The sample consisted of unselected, consecutive hospital referred self poisoning patients classified by the HATS staff as DSP. These patients were from a geographically defined area with a total population of approximately 485,000 persons of all ages.

Prospective data collection of clinical variables was undertaken. Psychiatric diagnosis was determined by clinical interview by a psychiatric registrar or psychiatrist according to DSM-IIIR and each diagnosis reviewed at a weekly meeting. DSM-IIIR diagnoses were "mapped" onto DSM-IV major diagnostic categories for the purposes of these analyses. Analyses for psychiatric diagnosis was done when an admission had at least one psychiatric diagnosis recorded from a DSM-IV major diagnostic category, with no consideration of comorbidity. The most common major diagnostic groups are reported.

The Hunter Area Mental Health Services medical records were searched for HATS patients with DSP admissions and data on presentations and admissions to the psychiatric hospitals were collected for the period of 1992 to 1995.

Statistical method for the comparison of groups was Fischer's exact test.

5. RESULTS

In 1992–94 HATS treated 1458 self poisoning patients, accounting for 1831 admissions. Of these, 1238 were classified as DSP patients and accounted for 1568 admissions.

Table 1 shows the distribution by gender of RDSP-1 and Non RDSP-1 patients and admissions for 1992 to 1994. 165 (13.3%) DSP patients for 1992–94 were classified as RDSP-1.

Table 1. Comparison of patients with repeated deliberate self poisoning (RDSP-1), multiple psychiatric hospital admissions (MPHA-1) and those who were admitted on one occasion only; by sex

Patients admissions					
Male	Female	Total	Male	Female	Total
RDSP-1			Non-RDSP-1		
57	108	165	449	624	1073
161	305	466	460	642	1102
MPHA-1			Non-MPHA-1		
90	116	206	416	616	1032
167	260	427	454	687	1141

Table 2. Psychiatric Diagnoses for repeated deliberate self poisoning

Diagnosis	At index admission		Across all admissions	
	Male n=57	Female n=108	Male n=57	Female n=108
Substance abuse disorders	19	22	28	34*
Psychotic disorders	13	12	15	17
Mood disorders	8	23	13	36
Adjustment disorders	13	22	17	42
Personality disorders	12	27	21	53
Other (v codes)	3	6	6	16

*Significant at $p<0.05$.

Table 1 also shows the gender distribution for MPHA-1 and Non MPHA-1 for patients and admissions for 1992 to 1994. Two hundred and six (16.6%) DSP patients for 1992–94 were classified as MPHA-1.

Eighty-four patients were recorded in both categories of multiple service use.

Table 2 shows the rates of psychiatric disorder at the index DSP admission for male and female RDSP-1 patients and the rates of psychiatric disorder for male and female RDSP-1 patients across all DSP admissions.

There were no statistically significant gender differences at index DSP admission. When considering all DSP admissions in the study period, substance related disorders were more common in male RDSP-1 patients.

The most common major diagnostic group at index DSP admission for male RDSP-1 patients was substance related disorders. The most common for female RDSP-1 patients was personality disorders.

Table 3 shows the rates of psychiatric disorder at the index DSP admission for male and female MPHA-1 patients and the rates of psychiatric disorder for male and female MPHA-1 patients across all DSP admissions.

There was a significant predominance of MPHA-1 males diagnosed at the index DSP admission with substance related, psychotic and personality disorders and MPHA-1 males with substance related disorders when analysing across all DSP admissions.

The most common psychiatric major diagnostic group at index DSP admission for male MPHA-1 patients was substance related disorders. The most common for female MPHA-1 patients was mood disorders. However, when considering diagnoses across all

Table 3. Diagnoses for patients with multiple psychiatric hospital admissions

Diagnosis	At index admissions		Across all admissions	
	Male n=90	Female n=116	Male n=90	Female n=116
Substance abuse disorder	34	16*	40	23*
Psychotic disorders	28	20*	29	24
Mood disorders	23	31	27	42
Adjustment disorders	12	18	15	30
Personality disorders	26	30*	32	50
Other (v codes)	1	6	4	12

*Significant at $p<0.05$.

DSP admissions, the most common diagnostic group for female MPHA-1 patients was personality disorder.

6. CONCLUSIONS

In this study there were modest gender differences in deliberate self poisoning patients who make multiple use of general hospital and psychiatric hospital inpatient services. It was also notable that deliberate self poisoning patients who show a pattern of multiple inpatient service use, show some separation in the services that they use, with at least half of the repeat deliberate self poisoning (RDSP)-1 group not showing multiple psychiatric hospitalisation whilst less than half of the multiple psychiatric hospital admissions (MPHA)-1 group showed repeat deliberate self poisoning sufficient to require multiple general hospital admission. These multiple service users showed a reasonable range of psychiatric disorder: the most common were substance related disorders and for females personality disorders.

This information could be used in the planning for services for deliberate self poisoning patients, taking into account the pattern of flows between services, the underlying diagnostic groups and the gender differences in diagnosis. It suggests that the treatment of substance related disorders for male deliberate self poisoning patients should be a prominent consideration in service planning. The extent of unmet need for these services in this population is unknown.

ACKNOWLEDGMENT

This project was supported in part by a NSW Health Outcomes Grant (94/95).

REFERENCES

Carter GL, Whyte IM, Dawson AH and Buckley NA. (1996) *Self poisoning patients: assessment, management, prevention and clinical outcomes 1989–1994.* Health Outcomes Report to the NSW Department of Health.

NSW Mental Health Expert Party. *NSW mental health goals and targets and strategies for health gain.* NSW Health Department. 1995.

Whyte IM, Dawson AH, Buckley NA, Carter GL, Levey CM. A model for the management of self poisoning. *Medical Journal of Australia* 1997 (in press).

25

SELF-INFLICTED INJURY AND COPING BEHAVIOURS IN PRISON

Greg E. Dear, Donald M. Thomson, Guy J. Hall, and Kevin Howells

Edith Cowan University
100 Joondalup Drive
Joondalup
Western Australia 6027

1. INTRODUCTION

Previous research (Bonner & Rich, 1990; Liebling, 1992; Liebling & Krarup, 1993) has suggested that self-harming prisoners are "poor copers," but has not provided detail as to how they differ from other prisoners in terms of their actual coping behaviour. Liebling (1992) found that self-harmers were more likely to have serious difficulties with other prisoners, less likely to have outside supports (either family or probation), spent more time in their cell (partly through being on restrictive regime and partly because they were hiding from teasing and intimidation), and were less able to articulate constructive ways of filling their time. Liebling concluded that "inmates with the fewest opportunities to occupy themselves (for whatever reason, some self-induced) were those who were least able to cope with the isolation and boredom of confinement to a cell for long periods of time" (p. 144). Essentially, however, poor coping ability was inferred from the greater levels of distress and disorder reported and there was no direct assessment of coping behaviour. It is yet to be determined whether prisoners who self-harm differ from other prisoners in terms of their coping behaviour. A more specific test of Liebling's assertion would be to examine whether prisoners who self-harm are less likely to employ effective coping strategies or are more likely to employ ineffective or counter-productive strategies.

It is not clear, however, what constitutes an effective coping strategy. Aldwin and Revenson (1987) remarked that "we are far from describing a "magic bullet" coping strategy that can instantly solve problems and restore emotional equilibrium" (p. 338). Nearly a decade later, Steed (1995) undertook an extensive review of the coping literature and concluded that "there are no strategies which can generally be regarded as more effective than others, rather, it depends on the nature of the stressor, particularly its controllability" (p. 100). On a more general level, however, studies have consistently found that problem-

Suicide Prevention, edited by Kosky *et al.*
Plenum Press, New York, 1998

focussed coping (strategies aimed at managing or changing the situation causing the distress) leads to a reduction in stress (Kohn and O'Brien, 1997; Steed, 1995). Steed (1995) reports that the results are more equivocal for emotion-focussed coping (strategies aimed at regulating the emotional response to the situation). Kohn and O'Brien (1997), however, reviewed research on avoidance-focussed coping (strategies aimed at removing or distracting oneself from the situation) separately to the research on other forms of emotion-focussed coping noting that while the evidence is mixed with regard to avoidance-focussed coping emotion-focussed coping in general is associated with poor outcome. They reach a similar conclusion to that of Steed and argue that the type of coping which will work best depends on the situation. In particular, problem-focussed coping, while generally adaptive, may be counter-productive if the stressful situation encountered is not amenable to change (Kohn & O'Brien, 1997; Lazarus & Folkman, 1984). While there is some evidence that problem-focussed coping is most effective in situations that are amenable to change (Steed, 1995), studies have failed to demonstrate it is counter-productive in situations not amenable to change (Conway & Terry, 1992; Steed, 1995).

While emotion-focussed coping seems to be of limited effectiveness, it has been argued that some forms of emotion-focussed coping (eg, cognitive reappraisal, accepting unalterable circumstances, seeking social support) are more adaptive than others (eg, self-blaming, ventilation, escapism) (Fondacaro & Moos, 1987; Kohn & O'Brien, 1997; Lazarus & Folkman, 1984; Schaefer & Moos, 1992). Similarly, it has been argued that problem-focussed coping is more multidimensional than it is often portrayed (Billings & Moos, 1981; McCrae, 1984). Billings and Moos (1981) divided active (problem-focussed) coping into cognitive and behavioural methods. They defined active-cognitive coping as "attempts to manage one's appraisal of the stressfulness of the event, such as 'tried to see the positive side of the situation'" (p. 141) Active-behavioural coping was defined as "overt behavioural attempts to deal directly with the problem and its effects" (p. 141). Greater use of either active coping strategy was associated with less stress.

If one were to reformulate Liebling's (1992) assertion that self-harmers are poor copers in terms of the research findings just outlined, one would predict that self-harmers would be less likely than other prisoners to engage in problem-focussed coping, active-cognitive coping (positive reinterpretation and acceptance) and seeking social support and are more likely to engage in other forms of emotion-focussed coping. In addition, one would predict that self-harmers would rate the effectiveness of their coping efforts less highly than non-self-harmers.

The objective of this study was to examine the coping strategies employed by prisoners who have self-harmed, and to determine whether, and in what way, their coping strategies differed from the coping strategies employed by prisoners who have not self-harmed.

2. METHODS

2.1. Design

This study employed a simple quasi-experimental design. The types of coping strategy employed by a group of prisoners who self-harmed in the Western Australian prison system were compared to those used by a matched comparison group comprising prisoners who denied ever having self-harmed in prison and for whom there was no record of ever having self-harmed in prison.

2.2. Identification of Self-Harm Incidents

Self-harm incidents were identified from the Situation Reports which are submitted by all prisons in Western Australia on a daily basis to a central data management unit. Among other information on critical incidents and prison security, these reports cite any incident of prisoner self-harm that has occurred over the preceding 24 hours. The research team was notified each day of all self-harm incidents reported. The prisoner who had self-harmed was interviewed within three days of the incident. For the purposes of this study a self-harm incident was defined as any occasion in which a prisoner intentionally engaged in behaviour which either resulted in injuries, or was likely to have resulted in, self-inflicted injury. This definition enabled the inclusion of those prisoners who attempted suicide without resultant injuries (eg, asphyxiation, hanging).

2.3. Participants

Ninety one prisoners were reported to have self-harmed over the nine month period in which data were collected. Eighty two of these were interviewed, one was released from prison within 24 hours of the incident, two were considered by medical staff to be unfit for interview due to their disturbed mental state, and six declined to participate. For each prisoner who self harmed a comparison prisoner was drawn from the same area of the prison (mainstream, protection, medical facility, separate confinement). These comparison prisoners were matched for race, custodial status (remanded or sentenced) and age (within two years of date of birth) and there was no indication that they had ever self-harmed in prison (from prison file, medical file or self-report). Where there were more than one prisoner who matched on these criterion variables, the one who was closest on date of birth was selected. Of the 82 prisoners who were interviewed regarding their first self harm incident during the period of data collection, a matched comparison prisoner was available for 71. The mean age was 24.7 for the self-harm group (SD = 5.49, ranging from 19 to 41) and 24.9 for the comparison group (SD = 5.59, ranging from 19 to 42). Other demographic details are outlined in Table 1.

2.4. Procedure

Prisoners were either sent or escorted to the interview room by Unit staff. The interviewer introduced himself, briefly explained the purpose of the study, and answered any

Table 1. Demographic details

Variable	Self-Harm		Comparison	
	n	%	*n*	%
Gender				
Male	64	90.1	64	90.1
Female	7	9.9	7	9.9
Incarceration status				
Remand	30	42.3	30	42.3
Sentenced	41	57.7	41	57.7
Race				
Caucasian	44	62.0	44	62.0
Aboriginal	24	33.8	24	33.8
Asian	3	4.2	3	4.2

questions raised by the prisoner concerning the interview or the study in general. Prisoners who consented to being interviewed were then asked to sign a written consent form.

2.5. Measures

A mix of qualitative and quantitative self-report data was collected within four areas: descriptive data regarding the most significant recent stressor, the level of distress experienced in response to this stressor, the coping strategies employed to deal with this stressor, and the effectiveness of these strategies in reducing distress.

2.5.1. The Most Significant Recent Stressor. Participants were asked to list the stressors experienced by them over the past week and then to identify which of these stressors had been the most stressful. A period of one week allowed a reasonable time for the occurrence of a meaningful stressor for the comparison group, without being too long an interval to allow an adequate recollection of events. For the self-harm group it was also important to sample from a time period which covered the days prior to the self-harm incident. Having identified their most significant recent stressor, participants then indicated how much control they felt they had over this situation (no control at all, a little control, quite a bit of control), whether it was an expected event (totally unexpected, half expected, totally expected), whether the stressor was a single event or an ongoing situation, and whether they had experienced this stressor, or something very similar, in the past.

2.5.2. Level of Distress. A 7-point scale (ranging from not at all distressing to extremely distressing) was used to measure the degree of distress participants reported having experienced in response to their main stressor.

2.5.3. Coping Strategies. The specific coping strategies employed in response to this stressor were then identified using a modified version of Stone and Neale's (1984) measure of daily coping. This measure employs a partly qualitative and partly quantitative approach to gathering data on coping behaviour. Stone and Neale identified eight broad coping strategies, each defined not by the specific behaviour involved but by the intended function of that behaviour (p. 897):

1. Distraction—diverted attention away from the problem by thinking about other things or engaging in some activity.
2. Situation redefinition—tried to see the problem in a different light that made it seem more bearable.
3. Direct action—thought about solutions to the problem, gathered information about it, or actually did something to try and solve it.
4. Catharsis—expressed emotions in response to the problem to reduce tension, anxiety, or frustration.
5. Acceptance—accepted that the problem had occurred, but that nothing could be done about it.
6. Seeking social support—sought or found emotional support from loved ones, friends, or professionals.
7. Relaxation—did something with the implicit intention of relaxing.
8. Religion—sought or found spiritual comfort and support.

Participants indicate whether or not they have used each type of strategy with reference to a specified stressor. If they have, they are then required to describe the particular action or thought enacted. Stone and Neale's subjects completed this measure on a daily basis providing data on their "most bothersome event or issue of the day" (p. 897).

Three main modifications to Stone and Neale's (1984) measure were made. First, information was sought pertaining to the past week rather than the past day. Secondly, Stone and Neale's eighth type of strategy, religion, was not included as this was thought to overlap too much with the other categories. For example one could pray not only to find spiritual comfort but also to ventilate emotions, as an acceptance strategy, or as part of the problem-solving process. Finally, given the low literacy levels displayed by many prisoners, the measure was administered orally rather than as a pencil and paper questionnaire, with the interviewer reading the definition to the prisoner and then writing his or her response. Similarly, the wording for some of the definitions was simplified somewhat. The definitions used in this study are outlined in Appendix A.

After collecting data on each of these seven types of strategies participants were asked if there was anything else they had done to try and handle the identified stressor. Responses given to this last question were then checked against each of the seven types of strategy, asking the participant if the objective of the strategy fitted any of these functions (i.e., was it aimed at distraction, was it an attempt to gain social support, etc.).

2.5.4. Coping Effectiveness. Finally participants were asked to rate on a 7-point scale (from not at all to totally) the extent to which their overall coping response had reduced their level of distress.

3. RESULTS

The results are presented for each of the four data areas: the most significant stressor experienced in the past week, the level of distress experienced in response to it, the coping strategies employed to deal with it, and the effectiveness of these strategies. A number of additional analyses are then conducted controlling for differences between the self-harmers and the comparison group which may have influenced coping behaviour and resulted in spurious differences emerging between the two groups.

3.1. The Most Significant Recent Stressor

3.1.1. Type of Stressor. The stressors identified by participants were examined for recurring themes and a coding system was devised based on these themes. As can be seen in Table 2, there were several differences between the two groups in terms of the type of stressor they cited. Most notably, no comparison prisoner cited bullying or psychological symptoms whereas these categories accounted for one in five of the self-harm group. For the self-harm group, the most common type of stressor was being isolated from family or other supports (which was three times as common for this group than for the comparison group). The most common type of stressor cited by the comparison group was some routine aspect of general prison life (which was three times as common for this group as for the self-harmers). Definitions for each of the categories of stressor are outlined in Appendix B.

3.1.2. Other Data Pertaining to the Main Stressor. The groups differed with regard to the perceived controllability of their stressor, with 84% of the self-harm group and 66% of the comparison group indicating they had no control ($\chi^2 = 7.81$, df = 2, p < .05), and

Table 2. Type of stressor experienced

Type of stressor	Self-harm		Comparison	
	n	%	*n*	%
Court/legal	9	12.7	12	16.9
Actual bullying or standover	5	7.0	0	—
Personal safety concern	0	—	3	4.2
Minor conflict with other prisoners	1	1.4	8	11.3
Specific regime restriction	5	7.0	5	7.0
Progression concern	3	4.2	5	7.0
General prison issue	5	7.0	15	21.1
Relationship problems	8	11.3	3	4.2
Isolated from family/supports	14	19.7	5	7.0
Worrying how family are coping	8	11.3	10	14.1
Psychological/psychiatric symptom	8	11.3	0	—
Other	5	7.0	5	7.0

Note n = 71 for each group.

with regard to whether the stressor had been anticipated or not, with 49% of the self-harm group and 30% of the comparison group indicating it was completely unexpected (χ^2 = 6.50, df = 2, p < .05). The groups did not differ with regard to previous experience of this or a similar stressor (51% of self-harmers and 48% of comparisons), or whether the stressor was an ongoing situation rather than a single event (93% of self-harmers and 89% of comparisons indicated it was ongoing).

3.2. Level of Distress

One-way ANOVA showed that the self-harm group gave a higher rating of their distress levels than did the comparison group (F = 67.8, df = 1,140, p < .001). The mean rating for the self-harm group was 6.55 (SD = 0.89), while the mean for the comparison group was 4.39 (SD = 2.02).

3.3. Coping Strategies

Chi-squared tests were used to determine whether the two groups differed in their use of each of the eight coping strategies measured. Table 3 sets out the proportion of each group who employed each type of coping strategy and the results of these Chi-squared tests. A lower proportion of the self-harm group employed situation redefinition, acceptance and direct action. While there was a tendency for a greater proportion of comparison prisoners employing each coping strategy, the other five strategies did show significant effects.

3.4. Coping Effectiveness

One-way ANOVA showed that the self-harm group rated the effectiveness of their coping response lower than the comparison group (F = 69.9, df = 1,140, p < .001). The mean rating for the self-harm group was 2.86 (SD = 1.73), while the mean for the comparison group was 5.27 (SD = 1.71).

Table 3. Number of self-harmers and comparisons who used
each type of coping strategy

Type of coping	Self-Harm		Comparison		χ^2
	n[a]	%	n[a]	%	
Distraction	58	81.7	64	90.1	2.01
Positive reinterpretation	29	40.8	54	76.1	18.12***
Direct action	40	56.3	55	77.5	7.16**
Catharsis	48	67.6	55	77.5	1.73
Acceptance strategies	27	38.0	56	78.9	24.39***
Seeking social support	52	73.2	57	80.3	0.99
Relaxation strategies	37	52.1	40	56.3	0.26
Other	12	16.9	11	15.9	0.05

Note: df = 1 for all chi-squared tests. A one-tailed Fisher's Exact Test was used as it was hypothesised that each type of strategy would be used by a smaller proportion of the self-harm group than the comparison group.
[a]n indicates observed frequency, that is how many of the 71 participants in each group who indicated that they had used that type of coping strategy.
** p < .01, *** p < .001

3.5. Re-Analyses Controlling for Level of Distress and Situation Factors

Further analyses were performed comparing the coping strategies used by each group while controlling for each of the following variables: type of stressor experienced, perceived control over the stressor, the extent to which the stressor was expected and the degree of distress reported. Table 4 outlines the results from these analyses. Consistent with the results obtained using all participants, in each re-analyses of the data a lower proportion of self-harmers used situation redefinition and acceptance strategies. Self-harmers used direct action less often than did the comparison group, and with proportions similar to that obtained using all participants: about three quarters of the comparison group and about half of the self-harm group. With the reduced sample sizes in these analyses, and the resultant loss of statistical power, some of the Chi-squared tests just failed to reach significance.

The only new finding to emerge from these analyses was that more of the comparison group (30 of the 32, 94%) than the self-harm group (17 of the 25, 68%) used distraction strategies when only those participants facing common stressors were used (χ^2 = 6.43, p < .05). Given that this was the only analysis which produced a significant effect for any of the five coping strategies which were not significant on the original analyses, and the large number of exploratory Chi-squared tests which were conducted, this finding is best regarded as spurious.

4. DISCUSSION

Prisoners who had self-harmed in the past three days differed from prisoners who had not self-harmed in prison in the type of situation identified as the most stressful event in the preceding week and the types of coping strategies employed in response to that stressor. Specifically, fewer of the self-harm group reported using situation redefinition, acceptance and direct action. These differences were still found when level of distress,

Table 4. Differences between self-harmers and comparisons in coping strategies used when controlling for other variables which differed between the two groups

Controlling for	Type of coping	Self-harm		Comparison		χ^2
		n^a	%	n^a	%	
Level of distress[b]	Positive reinterpretation	23	39.0	17	73.9	8.08**
	Direct action	32	54.2	17	73.9	2.67[‡]
	Acceptance strategies	24	40.7	15	65.2	4.00*
Common stressor[c]	Positive reinterpretation	8	32.0	27	84.4	16.3***
	Direct action	13	52.0	24	75.0	3.26[‡‡]
	Acceptance strategies	10	40.0	25	78.1	8.61**
Controllability[d]	Positive reinterpretation	23	39.0	34	73.9	12.7***
	Direct action	31	52.5	34	73.9	5.01*
	Acceptance strategies	19	32.2	39	84.8	28.9***
Stressor expected[e]	Positive reinterpretation	15	44.1	36	76.6	8.92**
	Direct action	21	61.8	38	80.9	3.63[‡‡‡]
	Acceptance strategies	14	41.2	37	78.7	11.9***

Note: df = 1 for all chi-squared tests. A one-tailed Fisher's Exact Test was used as it was hypothesised that each type of strategy would be used by a smaller proportion of the self-harm group than the comparison group.
[a]n indicates observed frequency, that is the number of participants in each group who indicated that they had used that type of coping strategy.
[b]Includes only those participants who rated their level of distress as 6 or higher (n = 59 for self-harm group and n = 23 for comparison group).
[c]Includes only those participants who were facing stressors which were common to both groups, ie, court/legal, specific regime restriction, progression concerns, and worry about family (n = 25 for self-harm group and n = 32 for comparison group).
[d]Includes only those participants who indicated they had no control over their stressor (n = 59 for self-harm group and n = 46 for comparison group).
[e]Includes only those participants who indicated that their stressor was at least somewhat expected (n = 34 for self-harm group and n = 47 for comparison group).
* p < .05, ** p < .01, *** p < .001, [‡] p = .08, [‡‡] p = .06, [‡‡‡] p = .05

type of stressor, controllability of the stressor and whether the stressor was expected or not were held constant. Furthermore, the self-harm group rated their overall coping response as less effective than did the comparison group. These findings are consistent with the predictions outlined in the introduction to this paper, with one exception: the prediction that self-harmers would be less likely to seek social support was not supported by the data. The three types of coping strategy that were used less often by the self-harm group have all been shown to be more effective more often than other types of coping strategy and are generally regarded as adaptive (Billings & Moos, 1981; Kohn & O'Brien, 1997; Schaefer & Moos, 1992; Steed, 1995).

One limitation of the data, however, is that we have a description of what they did (within each of a number of coping categories), but nothing to indicate how well the strategies were executed, and no index of the quality of the overall coping response. Participant X could have used some direct action strategies, some distraction strategies, and some cathartic strategies, and participant Y the same, yet these two prisoners may have differed markedly in how well they implemented these strategies, or in how appropriate their specific strategies were for their particular stressor. To illustrate this point consider the prisoner who described how he "paid out" on the officers in his unit so as to "ruin their day and make them feel as bad as I do. He surmised that staff would thus gain an appreciation of how bad he felt and would then become more sympathetic toward him and assist him to change his circumstances. This prisoner was coded as having employed a direct action strategy, but it is unlikely that his chosen strategy would have worked.

At least three main interpretations can be placed on the results of this study: (1) there is something different about the individuals in the self-harm group; (2) there is something different about the situations faced by the self-harm group which was not detected in this study; and (3) a failure to use what Billings and Moos (1981) termed active coping (either cognitive or behavioural) increases the likelihood of self-harming behaviour. Each of these will be discussed in turn.

We have termed the first explanation the vulnerable person model: that there is something different about prisoners who self-harm which leads them to become more distressed by their circumstances, limits their ability or inclination to use certain types of coping strategies (direct action, situation redefinition and acceptance) with a resultant poor outcome in terms of stress reduction, and also causes them to self-harm. There are a number of possibilities as to the nature of this vulnerability: personality disorder, mental illness, low self-esteem, impulsivity, learned helplessness, and so on. Further research being undertaken with this same sample of prisoners may shed some light on this issue. Previous research has found some evidence of vulnerability among prisoners who have self-harmed (Bonner, 1992) but it is not clear whether the key factor is a state of vulnerability or a more permanent trait-like vulnerability. In either event, the implication of this explanation is that one should identify vulnerable individuals and implement management strategies which compensate for their vulnerability and psychological interventions to reduce their vulnerability.

The second explanation is that there are differences in the stressful situations faced by prisoners who self-harm compared to other prisoners which were not discernible by the crude typology of stressors employed in this study. For example, one prisoner facing a court/legal stressor may be remanded for sentencing and worrying whether he will get a six month prison term or some form of community based sentence while another prisoner is remanded for trial on two counts of wilful murder which he claims to be innocent of but is terrified that he may be found guilty (and is likely to be in custody for well over 12 months before the trial begins). There may be other differences in the general circumstances surrounding those prisoners who self-harm compared to other prisoners which the data presented here were unable to control for and unable to detect. The implication from this explanation is that one should identify the situations, or situational characteristics, that increase the likelihood of self-harm, and then prevent such situations from arising.

The third explanation is that a failure to employ situation redefinition, acceptance and direct action in one's overall coping response which is less effective in reducing distress (hence the lower coping effectiveness and the higher distress levels seen in the self-harm group) which increases the likelihood that a prisoner will self-harm. This explanation is consistent with Liebling's (1993) suggestion that "coping skills courses" (p. 405) be conducted for prisoners as one component of a comprehensive suicide prevention programme. Our data, however, comprised self-reports of coping behaviour for one point in time and current coping strategies do not necessarily indicate usual strategies (coping style). A failure to employ what are seen to be the more productive types of coping strategy on this occasion does not necessarily mean that these individuals are deficient in their coping skills. It is possible that the self-harmers usually cope better (more in line with their non-self-harming peers) but for whatever reasons they coped poorly on this particular occasion. Nonetheless, the data are still consistent with there being a link between poor coping and self-harming behaviour. The nature of this link is, however, difficult to determine as the area does not lend itself well to experimental investigation. One cannot subject a sample of prisoners to an extreme chronic stressor, instructing one half to use certain coping strategies and the other half not to, while holding all other variables constant, and see which group provides the largest number of self-harm incidents. The best that can be done is to gather correlational data from a variety of perspectives looking for consistency across studies to provide some indication of the link between coping behaviour and self-harm. It is vital that future research includes longitudinal studies if any conclusions regarding the direction of causality are to be reached.

It may be that two, or even all three, of these explanations are valid. Perhaps the prisoners who are most likely to self-harm are vulnerable individuals who find themselves in particular types of stressful circumstances and who fail to employ productive coping strategies. With the present limited empirical knowledge base it is best for prison administrators, and others charged with the responsibility for preventing suicide and self-harm in prison, to act as if each of these explanations has some merit. This would lead to a three pronged approach to suicide prevention in prisons: the development of methods for identifying and managing vulnerable prisoners; minimising the occurrence of those situations which have been found to precipitate suicide attempts; and to assist prisoners to handle situations which cannot be prevented by training them in the use of the more effective coping strategies (direct action, situation redefinition, and acceptance).

The only firm conclusion that can be drawn from this study is that prisoners who have recently self-harmed are less likely to have been using active cognitive coping strategies (situation redefinition and acceptance) and problem-solving strategies (direct action) than are prisoners with no history of self-harm in prison. While this provides the first direct evidence of a link between coping behaviour and self-harm in prison, further research is required before the nature of this link can be understood and specific recommendations for preventing self-harm in prison can be made.

REFERENCES

Aldwin, C. M., & Revenson, T. A. (1987). Does coping help? A reexamination of the relation between coping and mental health. *Journal of Personality and Social Psychology, 53*, 337–348.

Billings, A. G., & Moos, R. H. (1981). The role of coping responses and social resources in attenuating the stress of life events. *Journal of Behavioral Medicine, 4*, 139–157.

Bonner, R. L. (1992). Isolation, seclusion, and psychosocial vulnerability as risk factors for suicide behind bars. In R. W. Maris, A. L. Berman, J. T. Maltsberger & R.I. Yufit (Eds.), *Assessment and prediction of suicide* (pp. 398–419). New York: Guilford Press.

Bonner, R. L., & Rich, A. R. (1990). Psychosocial vulnerability, life stress, and suicidal ideation in a jail population: A cross-validation study. *Suicide and Life Threatening Behavior, 20*, 213–224.

Conway, V. J., & Terry, D. J. (1992). Appraised controllability as a moderator of the effectiveness of different coping strategies: A test of the goodness of fit hypothesis. *Australian Journal of Psychology, 44*, 1–8.

Fondacaro, M. R., & Moos, R. H. (1987). Social support and coping: A longitudinal analysis. *American Journal of Community Psychology, 15*, 653–673.

Kohn, P. M., & O'Brien, C. (1997). The situational response inventory: A measure of adaptive coping. *Personality and Individual Differences, 22*, 85–92.

Lazarus, R. S., & Folkman, S. (1984). *Stress, appraisal and coping*. New York: Springer.

Liebling, A. (1992). *Suicides in prison*. London: Routledge.

Liebling, A. (1993). Suicides in young prisoners: A summary. *Death Studies, 17*, 381–409.

Liebling, A., & Krarup, H. (1993). *Suicide attempts and self-injury in male prisons*. Cambridge: Institute of Criminology, Cambridge University.

McCrae, R. R. (1984). Situational determinants of coping responses: Loss, threat, and challenge. *Journal of Personality and Social Psychology, 46*, 919–928.

Schaefer, J. A., & Moos, R. H. (1992). Life crises and personal growth. In B. N. Carpenter (Ed.), *Personal coping: Theory, research, and application* (pp. 149–170). Westport, CT: Praeger.

Steed, L. G. (1995). *The relationship between personality, coping flexibility, and psychological outcomes of stressful episodes*. (Doctoral dissertation, Curtin University of Technology, Western Australia).

Stone, A. A., & Neale, J. M. (1984). New measure of daily coping: Development and preliminary results. *Journal of Personality and Social Psychology, 46*, 982–906.

APPENDIX A. DEFINITIONS OF THE COPING STRATEGY TYPES USED IN THIS STUDY

1. Distraction—distracting yourself from the problem by thinking about other things or doing something to take your mind off it.
2. Situation redefinition—tried to see the situation in a different light that made it seems more bearable (thought about it in a way that made it not so bad).
3. Direct action—thought about solutions to the problem, or did something to try and solve it.
4. Catharsis—expressed how you were feeling and let your feelings out so that you would feel less tense or frustrated (anxious, depressed, angry, or whatever).
5. Acceptance—accepted that the situation had happened but that nothing could be done about it.
6. Seeking social support—sought or found emotional support from loved ones, friends (either mates in prison or friends on the outside), or professionals.
7. Relaxation—did something to make yourself feel relaxed.

APPENDIX B. DEFINITIONS OF TYPES OF STRESSOR

1. Court/legal—any aspect of court or legal proceedings
2. Actual bullying or standover—being subjected to malicious teasing, physical assaults (no matter how minor), or threats of assault.
3. Personal safety concern—worry about one's personal safety, perceiving other prisoners as intimidating or threatening, but without any experience of actual bullying.
4. Minor conflict with other prisoner/s—arguments with other prisoners without actual or threatened violence, dislike of other prisoners with whom one has to mix.
5. Specific regime restriction—loss of some privilege/s (eg, contact visits, access to recreation facilities) as a result of being subjected to some form of disciplinary regime (includes being placed in separate confinement), unwanted transfer to another prison or failure to obtain a transfer that one had applied for.
6. Progression concerns—setbacks in regard to, or worry about prospects of, obtaining next step in one's sentence plan (eg, reduction in security rating, commencement of rehabilitation programme, work release, parole).
7. General prison issue—any routine aspect of daily prison life not covered by any of the preceeding categories (eg, being locked up at night, particular rules or procedures, bored with the routine, missing things on the outside, lack of privacy).
8. Relationship problems—problems in one's relationship with one's spouse or partner, including actual ending of the relationship or worrying that this may occur.
9. Isolated from family/supports—not getting visits or personal contact from some (or even all) of their family or other social supports.
10. Worrying about how family are coping—worrying about how one's imprisonment is impacting on the rest of the family. This category does not include relationship problems (as defined above) or "missing" one's family.
11. Psychological/psychiatric symptoms—specific experiences which may be symptomatic of some psychological or psychiatric disorder (eg, hearing voices, flashbacks or nightmares of past traumatic events, dissociative experiences). Anxious or depressed feelings were not included here. Rather the prisoner was questioned as to what he/she was feeling anxious or depressed about and their response identified the stressor (which was coded into another category). A stressor was only coded into this category if it was the specific event which gave rise to their distress and was not a response to some other stressful event which had occured in the past week.
12. Other—any stressor which was not codable into any of the above categories. There was no discernable theme connecting these stressors and as such a meaningful category could not be established.

26

ATTEMPTED SUICIDES IN ANKARA IN 1995[*]

I. Sayil, O. E. Berksun, R. Palabirikoglu, A. Oral, S. Haran,
S. Guney, S. Binici, S. Gecim, T. Yucat, A. Beder, H. Ozayar,
D. Buyukcelik, and H. D. Ozguven

Halit Ziya Sokak
28/5, Cankaya
Ankara, Turkey

1. INTRODUCTION

Since 1962, statistics of successful suicides have been available in Turkey[1].These statistics are collected sysematically by the State Institute of Statistics. However, suicide attempts have never been systematically registered. Our information about suicide attempts was from findings of some limited researches and from hospital records[2–9]. The only comprehensive research about epidemiology of suicide attempts was carried out by Ankara University Crisis Intervention Centre in Ankara in 1990[10].

The aim of this study was to replicate the research which was conducted in 1990, to find out the incidence of attempted suicide in Ankara in 1995, and to compare the results of 1990 and 1995.

2. METHOD

From 1 January 1995 to 31 December 1995, the records of the emergency rooms of 9 large hospitals which provide medical care to most of the population living in Ankara, were reviewed by our team. In this review, age, sex, marital status, education, method of suicide attempts, date and time of suicide were noted. The results were compared with the findings of the research which was conducted by us in 1990. The evaluation of the data was made through distribution of frequencies of all the data collected.

[*] This paper was originally published in Turkish language, as "Ankara Intihar Girisimleri Ostune Karsilastirmali Bir Calisma" in Kriz Dergisi, 5:1–5,1997.We are very grateful to the publisher for their kind permission to publish it again in English lanuguage.

Table 1. Suicide attempts by sex in 1990 and 1995 (n=2532)

Sex	1990 (%)	1995 (%)
Male	34.20	33.4
Female	65.80	66.6

3. RESULTS

In 1995, 2532 persons were recorded as attempted suicide cases between the ages of 12–90 years in the emergency records of Ankara Hospitals (median=22years). The attempted suicide rate was calculated to be 113 persons per 100,000 in Ankara population. The rate in 1990 was 107 persons per 100,000[10].

3.1. Distribution of Sex

Out of the 2532 cases, 1652 were female (66.6%) and 829 were male (33.4%) (Table 1). The male/female ratio of 1:2 implied that the sex difference was still important as in 1990[10].

3.2. Distribution by Age

Table 2 shows that the majority (56.8% and 65.7%) of suicide attempts occured in the 15–24 year old age group.

3.3. Suicide Attempts According to the Months of the Year and the Hours of the Day

In the distribution of the suicide attempts according to the months there was no significant difference. But, the suicide cases massed between the hours of 18.30 and 21.30 (21%) as found in 1990[10].

3.4. Methods of Suicide Attempts

The most common method of suicide attempt was self-poisoning or overdose in women and men. This method takes the first rank with 2144 subjects (88.3%) and self-cutting takes the second rank with 141 subjects (5.8%). The ratio of jumping, shooting and gas inhalation have increased in 1995 with respect to 1990[10] (Table 3).

Table 2. Suicide attempts by age group in 1990 and 1995 (n=2532)

Age	1990 (%)	1995 (%)
<14	4.10	3.5
15–24	56.76	65.7
25–34	25.35	20.2
35–44	9.21	6.2
45–54	2.21	2.5
55–65	1.11	0.9
>65	0.26	1.0

Table 3. Suicide attempts by method used
in 1990 and 1995

Methods	1990 (%)	1995 (%)
Drug overdose	88.22	88.3
Cutting	8.32	5.8
Hanging	0.37	0.8
Jumping	0.47	1.0
Shooting	0.05	0.9
Burning	0.05	0.1
Gas inhalation	0.68	1.4
Other methods	1.84	1.84

4. DISCUSSION

The registrations of suicide attempts in hospitals were found to be inadequate. This affects the reliability of the results obtained.

The attempted suicide rate was 107 persons per 100,000 in Ankara in 1990[10]. In this research, this rate has been found as 113/100,000. The results are similar in 1990 and 1995. However, in the last 5 years, 6 large private hospitals have been opened in Ankara. It is supposed that some of the suicide attempts were admitted to these hospitals. If these are added to the others, the suicide attempt rate, increases to 145/100,000. In this situation, from 1990 to 1995, attempted suicides in Ankara have been increased significantly.

The general findings show that suicide attempts are especially characteristic of the younger age groups (15–24 ages). If the results of the 1990 and 1995 researches are compared, it can be seen that suicide attempts in the 15–24 age group have increased from 57.8% to 65.7% of the total between 1990 and 1995..

In light of these results, it can be claimed that 15–25 age group is a continuously growing risk group. The most interesting change in the methods of suicide attempt is the increase of the suicide attempt with shooting. This can be explained by derestricting the sale of guns in recent years.

5. CONCLUSION

In the emergency rooms of the hospitals, a better registration system for attempted suicide is needed. Education of the emergency staff and a preventive programme for the risk groups are suggested.

REFERENCES

1. Intihar Istatistikleri, T C Basbankalik Devlet Istatistik Enstitusu (DIE) 1974–1995, DIE Matbaasi, Ankara
2. Kucur R, Aktan K (1987) Konya Merkez Ilcesi'nde 196 yilind suicide insidansi. XXIII. Ulusal Psikiyatri ve Norolojik Bilimler Kongresi Bilimsel Calismalari Kitabi sayfa 299–305, Onur Ofset, Istanbul
3. Gurgen F (1989) Diyarbakir kent merkezinde hava sicaklii ile homicide, suicide, yaralanma ve trafik kazasi olgularinin iliskisi: 1983–1987. Dicle Universitesi Tip Fakultesi Dergisi, 16(1): 12–17
4. Sonuvar B, Oktem F (1986) Cocuk ve genclerde intihar girismim. Toplum ve Hekim, Mart: 16–22
5. Aydin H ve ark (1988) Intihar davranisinin sosyodemografik ozellikleri XXIV. Ulusal Psikiyatri ve Norolojik Bilimler Kongresi Bilimsel Calismalari Kitabi sayfa 238–247, I Saypa, Ankara

6. Sayil I ve ark (1988) Psikotik hastalarla grup tedavisi uygulamalarinda intihar olgusunun izlenisi. XXIV. Ulusal Psikiyatri ve Norolojik Bilimler Kongresi Bilimsel Calismalari Kitabi sayfa 553–558, I Saypa, Ankara
7. Kucur R (1988) Konya'da intihar insidansi ve onleyici tedbirler. XXIV. Ulusal Psikiyatri ve Norolojik Bilimler Kongresi Bilimsel Calismalari Kitabi sayfa 249–256, II VDK, Ankara
8. Ozsahin (1988) Intihar girismim sonucu acil servise basvuranlar ustune bir calisma. XXIV. Ulusal Psikiyatri ve Norolojik Bilimler Kongresi Bilimsel Calismalari Kitabi sayfa 208–214, I Saypa Ankara
9. Palabiyikoglu R, Azizoglu S, Ozayar H, Ercan A (1993) Intihar girisiminde bulunanlarin aile islevlerinin degerlendirilmesi. Kriz Dergisi Cilt 1, Sayi 2 (69–75)
10. Sayil I, Oral A, Guney S, Ayhan N, Ayhan O, Devrimci H (1993) Ankara'da Intihar Girisimleri Uzerine Bir Calisma. Kriz Dergisi Cilt1 Sayi 2 (56–61)

27

SUICIDAL TENDENCY AMONG HEROIN DEPENDENT PATIENTS IN MALAYSIA

Habil Hussain

Department of Psychological Medicine
University of Malaya Medical Centre
Kuala Lumpur, Malaysia

1. INTRODUCTION

Evidence gathered from other studies noted that suicidal behaviour is commonly seen among heroin dependence patients (1,2). In fact, suicide has been recognised as a major cause of death among addicts (3). Unfortunately, suicidal behaviour among addicts are usually difficult to elicit and quite hidden from our daily clinical practices in Malaysia. Very often it is only recognised when patients had already died and are brought to hospitals for postmortem. In situations where a heroin addict might commit suicide, there are usually considerable problems in identifying the cause of death. This could be the reason why many of these cases are classified as accidental death rather than suicide (5).

With regard to the situation in Malaysia we still do not know exactly what is the pattern for suicidal behaviour among heroin addicts. There is no single study yet which could specifically look into this matter. Nevertheless, there is some evidence from media reports which show that suicides often occur among heroin addicts. In fact, information obtained from patients who come for treatment, also suggests that suicide is not uncommonly seen among heroin addicts.

There is some difficulty in understanding suicidal behaviour among this group of patients in Malaysia and this could be due to the way addicts are being dealt with. Government policy places heavy emphasis on addiction as an internal security problem and thus the development of medical and more open treatment centres for addicts has been restricted. Therefore, addicts who need treatment can only get it through a residential form of rehabilitation which emphasises a military approach and deemphasises psycho-medical principles. Lack of this psycho-medical approach in treatment programs is currently a barrier for us to identify and treat addicts who may suffer from psychological problems, including suicide tendency. Furthermore, drug rehabilitation centres are never without a stigma. For example, many addicts find it hard to be accepted back to their jobs and are most likely to face rejection from societies once it is known that they have received treat-

Suicide Prevention, edited by Kosky *et al.*
Plenum Press, New York, 1998

ment from a rehabilitation centre. Therefore, some addicts fear treatment from these centres. The fear to be admitted to rehabilitation centres has further compounded our difficulties to reach depressed addicts who may have a suicide tendency.

To make matters worse, Malaysian cultural views on both suicide and drug addiction are very negative. Many people still do not consider these conditions as health problems, but see them as due to moral decadence. Many still believe that the cause of these two conditions has to do with loss of faith and, therefore, they are considered as bad behaviour rather than as illnesses. They somehow get marginalised from help agencies and continue their agony alone by themselves.

2. RECENT STUDY

The study was done in an outpatient clinic in University Hospital Kuala Lumpur. This clinic is a general psychiatry clinic which also caters for heroin addicts who seek treatment. In treating heroin addicts this clinic has three treatment objectives; a) Stop if you can b) Be safe if you can't c) But finally stop from your heroin and other forms of addictions as well. There are two clinic sessions every week and an average of 10 heroin dependent patients are seen per clinic session.

The study to identify suicide behaviour among those heroin addicts was undertaken from January to 31 December 1996. The main aim of this study was to examine the extent and characteristics of suicidal behaviour among heroin addicts. The objective of the study was to plan treatment and preventive strategies in order to reduce the occurrence of suicide among this group of patients.

Table 1. Sociodemographic data of the suicidal heroin addicts

	N	%
Age group		
<19	1	2
20-29	14	28
30-39	15	30
40 and over	20	40
Marital status		
Single	28	56
Married	20	40
Separated/divorced	2	4
Race		
Malay	22	44
Chinese	18	36
Indian	9	18
Other	1	2
Educational level		
Primary	6	12
Secondary	42	84
Tertiary	2	4
Employment status		
Unemployed	20	40
Unskilled job	11	22
Skilled worker	12	24
Business	6	12
Administrator	1	2

The study was carried out using a clinical interview technique. Variables collected included demographic, duration of heroin use, the use of other drugs and whether there was suicidal tendency. Those patients who were suicidal were asked the following questions:

- a. suicidal ideation, reasons and duration
- b. suicidal attempt, reasons and duration
- c. method used to attempt suicide
- d. help seeking behaviour

3. RESULTS

A total of 133 cases were interviewed for the above study. Out of these 50 (37.6%) expressed some form of suicidal tendencies. Forty seven (94%) were males with mean age of 35 years. Details of their sociodemographic data can be found in Table 1.

4. NATURE OF ADDICTION

The majority had a past history of using other drugs, most were still using more than one drug besides heroin. Cannabis and aramine (ephedrine) were noted to be very commonly used. Only one person used benzodiazepine. (Refer Table 2.)

5. NATURE OF ATTEMPT

Out of the 50 patients who reported tendencies to commit suicide, 20 (40%) of them had a past history of attempted suicide. Two popular methods used in their attempts were overdose and poisoning, either with benzodiazepine or with heroin. Eight of them also tried physical methods like hanging and cutting wrists. The most common reason why they wished to end life was due to difficulties they encountered related to drug use. These included poor relationships with family members or with others and the withdrawal symptoms they experienced when they abstained from heroin. Only 3 (6%) claim that they were depressed. These patients claimed that their suicidal tendency was present even prior to the use of heroin. Another three patients in this study wanted to die after learning that they were HIV positive.

In terms of getting help to overcome their suicidal intention, only 4 (8%) sought help immediately after their attempted suicide. Out of these four patients who went to seek

Table 2. Nature of addiction

Variables	N	%
Duration of heroin use		
< 5 years	11	22
6–10 years	14	28
11 and over	25	50
Use of other drugs		
Cannabis	16	32
Polydrugs	12	24
Ephedrine	4	8
Benzodiazepines	1	2

such help, three of them were admitted to hospital, while one was getting treatment in a general practice clinic. None of them told about their suicidal tendencies to the doctors who had treated them. Common reasons given why they do not tell others about their suicidal intention included not knowing that others could help them to deal with their problems and also fearing that their problems with heroin may be reported to authorities. Another peculiarity in this study was that none got any form of professional help which targeted their suicidal intention. Even those three patients whose attempts were serious enough to warrant emergency treatment were apparently denied professional help in dealing with their suicidal tendencies after treatment.

6. DISCUSSION

As can be seen from Table 3, Malaysian heroin addicts are at risk for suicidal behaviour, but their suicidality is hidden. therefore, the first issue in helping these suicidal addicts is how to identify them. In a Malaysian context there are several reasons why suicidal addicts remain hidden to treatment agencies. First and foremost this is due to national policy which is still not in favour of treating heroin dependent patients in an open community health service. This policy has lead to under-development of community and hospital counselling services which have a less stigmatised approach to treating addiction problems. It has also lead to lack of interest among health workers to either learn more about the subject or to have special interest in treating these kinds of patients. This lack of interest has been the main reason why many health workers, including many doctors in Malaysia, are still very negative towards addicts. In fact, many doctors try not to have any contacts with heroin addicts, because they either feel fearful of becoming involved or they feel helpless to treat patients who suffer from it.

The lack of health centres with conducive treatment programs for Malaysian addicts has resulted in rejecting health workers even when they contact them. It is more difficult for Malaysian doctors to elicit history of heroin use and suicidal tendencies from these patients even when we have high index of suspicion to such possibilities. The main reason

Table 3. Nature of suicidal intent among 50 heroin addicts seen in University Hospital, Kuala Lumpur

Variables	N	%
Suicidal ideas	30	60
Previous attempts	20	40
Methods used		
Overdose/poisoning	7	14
Hanging/cutting	8	16
Multiple methods	5	10
Reason to die		
Heroin related problems	44	88
Depression	3	6
HIV positive	3	6
Help agencies contacted		
Hospitals	3	6
Clinics	1	2
Family history of suicide		
Present	4	8
Absent	46	92

for this is because patients fear that doctors might get angry if they are to reveal their involvement with drugs.

Lack of health workers and chronic financial problems to develop more health services are other barriers which obviously need to be addressed. As far as Malaysia is concerned, issues like addiction and suicide are still relatively new public health problems. Being a developing country we still have not overcome our 'old diseases', like vector born diseases such as Dengue Fever. Hence, the recent introduction of these to new 'diseases' is another burden for our health system. Therefore, it may take some time before we can finally cope with them.

It is common to see a doctor in a government clinic treating at least 60 patients a day. So, one can imagine what type of help they can provide, even if they know their patients are suffering from heroin addiction and worse still, suicide tendencies. Another unfortunate reality is that many who suffer from these conditions come from a low social economic background, whereby the possibility of getting early help from health professionals might not be easy, due to financial constraints, cultural barriers and the lack of health services near their home.

Community services like Befrienders and drop in centres have been known to play some part in managing these patients, but again, this form of service is not well developed yet. Another problem for the existing health centres is a lack of coordination between them and hospitals.

REFERENCES

Haastrup S, Jepsen PW. Seven years follow-up of 300 young drug abusers. Acta Psychiatr. Scand. 70:503–509:1984

Facy F, Rosch D, Angel P, Touzeau D, Cordonnier P, Petit F. Drug addicts attending specialised institutions: Toward a drug addiction data bank? Drug and Alcohol Dependence. 27:43–50:1991

Puschel K. Drug related death: an update. Forensic Science International. 62:121–128:1993

Cheng T. Medical hazard of drug abuse. Singapore Medical Journal 2 June. 341–346:1979

28

THE PSYCHOPHYSIOLOGY OF SELF-MUTILATIVE BEHAVIOUR

A Comparison of Current and Recovered Self-Mutilators

Kerryn L. Brain, Janet Haines, and Christopher L. Williams

Psychology Department
University of Tasmania
GPO Box 252-30, Hobart, Tasmania, 7001, Australia

1. TENSION REDUCTION

The tension reduction model of self-mutilation has proposed that behaviours such as self-cutting and burning are effectively tension reducing (Favazza, 1989; Simpson, 1975). This model has indicated that it is these tension reducing qualities of self-mutilation that serve to reinforce the act and establish it as an habitual behaviour. Using a guided imagery methodology, the specific reinforcement processes of self-mutilation have been delineated and the tension reduction pattern that has been reported in the clinical literature, has been empirically verified (Haines, Williams, Brain & Wilson, 1995).

In one study, self-mutilating prisoners were interviewed regarding the details of a previous self-mutilative episode. This information was used for the construction of personalised guided imagery scripts. Script information was presented in stages to allow accurate identification of the specific reinforcement processes that the act provides. In the first stage, the environment in which the behaviour occurred and the circumstances, thoughts and feelings prior to self-mutilation were imaged. In the second stage, the approach to the behaviour was described. This included a detailed description of the events, thoughts and feelings leading up to the point of self-mutilation. The incident stage described the actual act of self-injury and the thoughts and feelings that accompanied that behaviour. The final stage of the imagery script detailed the events immediately following self-injury, and the thoughts and feelings experienced at that time. At the incident stage, when the actual act of self-injury was imaged, an immediate and significant reduction in arousal was evident. This was compared with a significant increase in psychophysiological arousal when accidental injury was imaged. Results of this study indicated that the self-mutilative behaviour is reinforced by this reduction in psychophysiological arousal

Suicide Prevention, edited by Kosky *et al.*
Plenum Press, New York, 1998

(Haines et al., 1995) and that this tension reduction pattern is unique to injury that is self-inflicted. Results demonstrated no significant differences between the self-mutilation group and a control group with no history of self-mutilation in terms of psychophysiological and psychological responses to control imagery scripts depicting accidental injury, anger and neutral events. This has indicated that individuals who self-mutilate respond appropriately to events that are experienced by most people.

Using this guided imagery methodology, it was also possible to identify the psychological states during the act of self-mutilation. Individuals were asked to rate how they were feeling during each stage of self-mutilation imagery on a number of different dimensions related to the phenomenology of self-mutilation. Results indicated a tension reduction pattern for psychological response to self-mutilation. That is, self-mutilating prisoners reported that the act of self-mutilation made them feel better. However, this reported reduction in negative feeling did not occur significantly until the consequence stage of imagery, after the act of cutting was complete. This result represented a lag between the reduction of physiological arousal and reported negative feeling (Haines et al., 1995). Individuals who self-mutilate often are unable to provide an explanation for their own self-mutilative behaviour (Favazza & Conterio, 1989; Simpson, 1976; Walsh & Rosen, 1988). Results of this study indicated that it is the alteration of psychophysiological arousal that operates to reinforce the behaviour, rather than the emotional response (Haines et al., 1995).

The aim of the current investigation was to determine whether the tension reduction pattern to self-mutilation depicted in the incarcerated sample is generalisable to a broader population of individuals who self-mutilate. It was hypothesised that the lag between the reduction in psychophysiological and psychological arousal would be replicated in a community sample of self-mutilation participants.

In clinical research it is not always practical to have access to participants who are currently engaging in problem behaviours. Clinicians may be reluctant to encourage their clients to participate in research that is not directly involved with a current treatment programme. Some people may simply not be well enough to participate in intensive research.

From a methodological point of view, it was of interest to determine the efficiency of a guided imagery methodology in the retrospective investigation of clinical behaviour. No significant difference in the strength of the psychophysiological or psychological arousal response pattern to self-mutilation imagery between individuals who were currently engaging in the behaviour and a recovered sample of self-mutilation participants was expected.

1.1. Method

1.1.1. Participants. Thirty-five individuals with a history of self-mutilation participated in this investigation. The self-mutilation group was categorised according to whether participants were currently self-mutilating (n=15) or had not self-mutilated for more than 6 months (n=20).

1.1.2. Materials. Visual Analogue Scales (VASs) (McCormack, Horne & Sheather, 1988) were used to determine participants' subjective response to imagery. VAS scores (from 0 to 100) represented this response on seven bipolar dimensions that related to the phenomenology of self-mutilation. These were, relaxed/tense, relaxed/anxious, calm/angry, unafraid/afraid, happy/sad, normal/unreal, and relieved/uptight (Haines et al., 1995). A higher score on these dimensions represented a more negative experience.

Measurement of psychophysiological responses was facilitated using Chart 3.4 on a Macintosh Quadra 840AV computer linked to a MacLab/8 Data Acquisition System. Recordings were made at 1mm/s-1, with a sampling frequency of 200 sample/s-1. Measurements were taken for finger pulse amplitude (FPA), electrocardiograph (ECG) integrated via cardiotachometer to obtain a mean heart rate (HR), respiration (RESP) and skin conductance level (SCL). These measures were selected to incorporate a range of psychophysiological responses to account for the idiosyncratic nature of participants' responses to imagery (Fleming & Baum, 1987).

1.1.3. Procedure. Participants were interviewed regarding an incident of self-mutilation they could clearly recall. Using this personalised information, imagery scripts were constructed comprising of four distinct stages: 1) setting the scene (a description of the environment in which the incident occurred and the context of the situation); 2) approach to the behaviour (description of events immediately preceding the incident); 3) the incident (details of the actual event as it occurred); and 4) the consequence (description of the events immediately following the incident and the resolution phase). (Guidelines for the construction of imagery scripts are available by request from Christopher L. Williams.)

Participants attended a recording session where the imagery script was presented while psychophysiological responses to imagery were measured. Participants were asked to close their eyes while a one minute pre-imagery baseline recording was taken prior to the presentation of the four stage imagery script. Participants were asked to keep their eyes closed while the imagery script was presented. Each stage was of approximately 60 seconds in duration and there was a 10 second pause between stages during which participants were permitted to open their eyes. Following script presentation, participants completed VASs rating their subjective responses to each stage of that script. To facilitate this process, participants were reminded of key elements of each stage prior to rating that stage.

1.1.4. Transformation and Scoring of Psychophysiological Data. Scores were extracted for a 30 second pre-imagery baseline recording and for a 30 second period of each stage of the imagery script. This scoring period was generally taken 15–20 seconds into each stage and was based on script content. This scoring method has been used successfully in previous research (Brain, Haines, & Williams, 1997; Brain, Haines, Williams, Stops & Driscoll, 1996; Brain, Williams & Haines, 1996; Driscoll, Brain, Williams, & Haines, 1997; Driscoll, Williams & Haines, 1996; Haines, Brain & Williams, 1997; Haines et al., 1995; McLaren, Haines & Williams, 1996; Williams, Haines & Brain, 1995).

Mean psychophysiological responses were calculated for HR and SCL. Mean number of breaths per minute were used for RESP. Change scores were calculated for FPA by subtracting the scores obtained during each stage from baseline and dividing by the baseline measure. Results were analysed using analyses of variance (ANOVAs) with a Huynh-Feldt correction. Tables detailing means and standard deviations are available from the authors on request.

1.2. Results

1.2.1. Total Sample Psychophysiological Response to Self-Mutilation Imagery. For the total sample, significant between stage differences for the self-mutilation script were demonstrated for all of the psychophysiological measures, FPA, $F(3,99) = 9.57$, $p < .001$; HR, $F(3,102) = 12.35$, $p < .001$; RESP, $F(3,96) = 4.76$, $p < .01$; SCL, $F(3,51) = 2.91$, $p < .05$. A

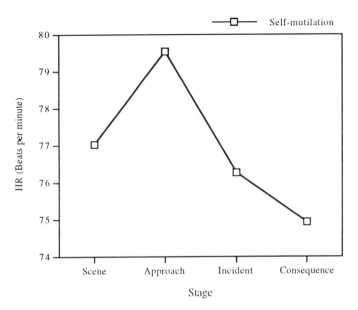

Figure 1. Pattern of arousal depicted across the four stages of the self-mutilation script for the total sample for heart rate.

significant increase in psychophysiological arousal from stage 1 to stage 2 was demonstrated for HR, $F(1,3) = 10.29, p < .01$; and RESP, $F(1,3) = 4.82, p < .05$. Arousal decreased significantly at stage 3 when actual self-injury was imaged for all measures, FPA, $F(1,3) = 12.10, p < .01$, HR, $F(1,3) = 17.62, p < .001$; RESP, $F(1,3) = 7.47, p < .01$; SCL, $F(1,3) = 7.98, p < .01$. This reduction in psychophysiological arousal was maintained at stage 4 when the immediate consequences of the act of self-mutilation were imaged. This arousal reduction pattern to self-mutilation imagery is illustrated in Figure 1.

1.2.2. Total Sample Subjective Response to Self-Mutilation Imagery. Significant between stage differences were demonstrated for 6 of the VAS measures were demonstrated, relaxed/tense, $F(3,102) = 11.93, p < .001$; relaxed/anxious, $F(3,102) = 9.76, p < .001$; calm/angry, $F(3,102) = 9.70, p < .001$; happy/sad, $F(3,102) = 2.92, p < .05$; normal/unreal, $F(3,102) = 7.76, p < .001$; relieved/uptight, $F(3,102) = 11.26, p < .001$. The VAS measure unafraid/afraid was the exception.

Reported negative feeling increased significantly from stage 1 to stage 2 for relaxed tense, $F(1,3) = 10.69, p < .01$; relaxed/anxious, $F(1,3) = 10.48, p < .01$; calm/angry, $F(1,3) = 6.80, p < .05$; unafraid/afraid, $F(1,3) = 4.75, p < .05$; happy/sad, $F(1,3) = 4.44, p < .05$; normal/unreal, $F(1,3) = 7.82, p < .01$. Reported negative feeling decreased significantly during stage 3 for relieved/uptight only, $F(1,3) = 4.04, p < .05$. During stage 4, reported negative feeling decreased significantly for, relaxed/tense, $F(1,3) = 20.02, p < .001$; relaxed/anxious, $F(1,3) = 15.55, p < .001$; calm/angry, $F(1,3) = 12.84, p < .001$; happy/sad, $F(1,3) = 4.19, p < .05$; normal/unreal, $F(1,3) = 7.41, p < .01$; relieved/uptight, $F(1,3) = 12.04, p < .001$.

As for the psychophysiological dependent variables, a pattern of tension reduction during self-mutilation was evident for subjective measures. However, a significant reduction in subjective response generally did not occur until stage 4, after cutting had been

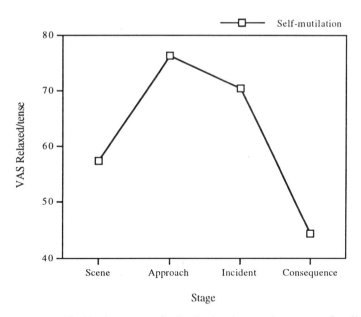

Figure 2. Pattern of subjective response for the visual analogue scale measure: relaxed/sense.

completed. This response pattern is illustrated in Figure 2. This lag between psychophysiological and subjective reduction in arousal to self-mutilation imagery has been demonstrated previously (Haines et al., 1995)

1.2.3. Comparison between Current and Recovered Groups' Response to Self-Mutilation Imagery. Group (current, recovered) × Stage (scene setting, approach, incident, consequence) ANOVAs were conducted to determine any difference in the strength of the arousal pattern associated with self-mutilation imagery between the current and recovered groups.

No significant differences between the current and recovered groups' psychophysiological responses to self-mutilation imagery were demonstrated.

Significant Group × Stage interactions were evident for 6 of the VAS measures, relaxed/tense, $F(3,99) = 6.20$, $p < .001$; relaxed/anxious, $F(3,99) = 5.34$, $p < .01$; calm/angry, $F(3,99) = 10.15$, $p < .001$; and unafraid/afraid, $F(3,99) = 5.43$, $p < .01$; happy/sad, $F(3,99) = 3.07$, $p < .05$; uptight/relieved, $F(3,99) = 4.45$, $p < .01$. Normal/unreal was the exception. *Post hoc* analyses indicated that current self-mutilation participants reported significantly more negative feelings than the recovered participants at stage 1 of the self-mutilation script for calm/angry, $F(1,33) = 7.17$, $p < .01$; and happy/sad, $F(1,33) = 8.36$, $p < .01$. Current self-mutilation participants also reported significantly higher levels of negative feeling that the recovered group at stage 2 for happy/sad, $F(1,33) = 5.50$, $p < .05$. Of particular note is the result that current self-mutilation participants reported significantly lower levels of negative feeling at stage 3 of the self-mutilation script than the recovered participants for relaxed/tense, $F(1,33) = 8.83$, $p<.01$; relaxed/anxious, $F(1,33) = 12.65$, $p < .001$; calm/angry, $F(1,33) = 5.05$, $p < .01$; and relieved/uptight, $F(1,33) = 5.91$, $p < .05$.

Figure 3 depicts the different subjective response patterns of the current and recovered groups to self-mutilation imagery for the VAS measure relaxed/tense.

It was of particular interest that for the recovered group, reported negative feelings did not decrease significantly until stage 4, when the consequences of self-injury were

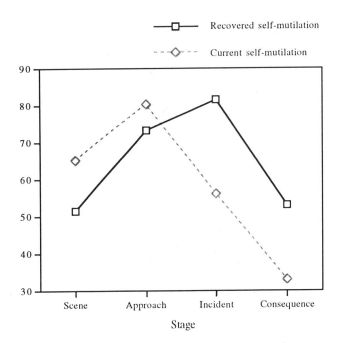

Figure 3. Comparison between current recovered groups to self mutilation images on VAS measure: relaxed/sense.

imaged, relaxed/tense, $F(1,3) = 18.83$; $p < .001$; relaxed/anxious, $F(1,3) = 22.37, p < .001$; calm/angry, $F(1,3) = 17.00, p < .001$; and uptight/relieved, $F(1,3) = 13.38, p < .001$. However, for current self-mutilation participants, reported negative feelings decreased significantly during stage 3 for relaxed/tense, $F(1,3) = 6.94$, $p < .01$; relaxed/anxious, $F(1,3) = 5.98, p < .01$; calm/angry, $F(1,3) = 15.07, p < .001$; unafraid/afraid, $F(1,3) = 5.64, p < .05$; and relieved/uptight, $F(1,3) = 12.76$, $p < .001$. These feelings continued to decrease at stage 4. This continued decrease was significant for relaxed/tense, $F(1,3) = 6.23, p < .05$.

1.3. Discussion

Results of this study have indicated that the tension reduction pattern to self-mutilation imagery that has been previously identified in an incarcerated sample of self-mutilators is generalisable to a broader population of individuals who self-mutilate. Initial analyses replicated the lag between the reduction of psychophysiological arousal and psychological distress that has been demonstrated previously (Haines et al., 1995). These results suggested that it is the reduction in psychophysiological arousal that serves to reinforce the behaviour rather than the emotional response to the act.

Comparisons between the responses of self-mutilation participants who were currently self-mutilating and a recovered self-mutilation group were conducted initially to determine the efficacy of a guided imagery methodology in charting the processes of a behaviour in which a person is no longer engaging. These results have clarified the reinforcement qualities of self-mutilation.

For those participants who had not engaged in the behaviour for more than six months, the previously described lag between the reduction of psychophysiological arousal and psychological tension was demonstrated. That is, the recovered group did not report a reduction in negative feeling until the consequence stage of imagery, after cutting was imaged. However, for those who were currently engaging in the behaviour, the act of self-mutilation was immediately psychophysiologically and psychologically reinforcing.

The results of this study have clarified the reinforcement qualities of the self-mutilative act. For those who are currently engaging in the behaviour, an appropriate cognitive interpretation of the psychophysiological state that self-injury provides is evident. However, results have indicated that the feelings associated with the act of self-injury are cognitively reinterpreted when self-mutilation is no longer part of an individuals' behavioural repertoire. But the psychophysiological reinforcement properties of the self-mutilative act remain the same.

Because the reinforcement qualities of self-mutilation are so strong, it is unlikely that individuals stop self-mutilating because the behaviour no longer works to reduce tension. It is more likely that an alteration in symptomatology leads to a reduced need to engage in the behaviour. Working on this premise, an examination of the symptomatology currently reported by the current and recovered self-mutilation groups was completed.

2. SYMPTOMS REDUCTION

The phenomenology of self-mutilation has been well documented (e.g., Haines et al., 1995; Simpson, 1975). Reports have indicated that the feelings that precede self-mutilation typically include depression, anger and increasing intolerable tension or anxiety (Simpson, 1975). As this distress continues to escalate, transition into a state of depersonalisation may occur (Feldman, 1988; Simpson, 1975; Winchel & Stanley, 1991). It has been suggested that in this depersonalised state individuals experience a marked decrease in impulse control and are unable to resist the urge to self-mutilate (Pattison & Kahan, 1983; Waltzer, 1968). It has also been suggested that it is this depersonalised state that allows painless self-injury (Simpson, 1976). With the sight of blood, repersonalisation occurs and tension is reduced (Haines et al., 1995; Simpson, 1976).

Research has indicated that the quality of mood that precedes self-mutilative behaviour is not qualitatively different from the individuals' long standing affective traits (Simeon, Stanley, Frances, Mann, Winchel & Stanley, 1992). The aim of the current study was to clarify the association of the phenomenology of the self-mutilative act with the long standing affective traits associated with the behaviour.

Most of the research concerned with the symptomatology associated with self-mutilation has been conducted with psychiatric inpatient populations using psychiatric control groups as a comparison. Researchers have interpreted self-mutilation as a marker of severity of particular disorders (Simeon, Stanley et al., 1992). It follows from this view that self-mutilative behaviour would cease if the symptoms associated with the disorder were effectively treated.

This investigation systematically compared the symptoms currently experienced by individuals who were presently self-mutilating with those who were no longer engaging in the behaviour. It was expected that recovered self-mutilation participants would report lower levels of symptomatology than those who were currently self-mutilating.

2.1. Method

2.1.1. Participants. Twenty one individuals who were currently self-mutilating and 25 individuals who had not self-mutilated for more than 6 months participated in this investigation. Participants were recruited from community clinics, private psychological practice and the University of Tasmania undergraduate population.

2.1.2. Materials. The following scales were selected to measure the symptomatology that has been reported to be associated with the phenomenology of self-mutilation: The Symptom Check List 90 Revised (SCL-90-R; Derogatis, 1983), the Beck Hopelessness Scale (BHS; Beck & Steer, 1988), the Beck Anxiety Inventory (BAI, Beck & Steer, 1990), the Beck Depression Inventory (BDI; Beck & Steer, 1987), the State Trait Anxiety Inventory (STAI, Form Y; Spielberger, 1983), the Dissociative Experiences Scale (DES, Bernstein & Putnam, 1986), the Hostility and Direction of Hostility Questionnaire (HDHQ; Caine, Foulds & Hope, 1967) and the Eysenck Impulsiveness Questionnaire (Eysenck &McGurk, 1980).

A self-mutilative behaviour checklist devised by the authors was used to determine history of self-mutilation as well as history of help-seeking behaviour and medication. The Schedule of Recent Experience (Holmes, 1988) was used to determine the degree of recent negative life events.

The Reasons for Living Inventory (RFL-48; Linehan, Goodstein, Nielsen & Chiles, 1983) and the Modified Scale for Suicidal Ideation (MSSI; Miller, Norman, Bishop & Dow, 1986) were included to measure suicidal thoughts and coping ideas related to suicide because, although self-mutilation is typically not a suicidal act, individuals who self-mutilate do attempt suicide and have reported feelings of suicidal ideation and hopelessness (Walsh & Rosen, 1988; Favazza & Conterio, 1989).

2.1.3. Procedure. The self-mutilative behaviours checklist was completed during an interview with participants. In addition, current and recovered self-mutilation participants were asked to complete other scales with regard to degree of symptomatology they were currently experiencing.

2.2. Results

2.2.1. Description of Sample. The total sample of participants had deliberately injured themselves a median of 32 times (range = 1–350) over a mean period of 60.4 months (SD = 75.73 months, range = 2 weeks to 30 years). Cutting was the most frequently reported method of self-mutilation (93.5%). Participants also had hit objects (60.9%), engaged in self-burning (39.1%), wound excoriation (26.1%), skin abrading (21.7%), self-hitting (21.7%), inserting objects under the skin (19.6%), self-biting (8.7%), and ingesting solid objects (2.2%). There were no significant differences between the current and recovered self-mutilation groups in the types of injuries inflicted, or the duration of self-mutilative behaviour.

One significant difference between current and recovered self-mutilation participants was noted for reported frequency of self-mutilative behaviour. Results depicted a significantly higher frequency of self-biting for the current group (t = 48.5, df = 2, p < .001). Current self-mutilation participants had bitten themselves a mean of 100 times (SD = 0) and the recovered self-mutilation group reported a mean of 3 incidents of self-biting (SD = 2.83). Inspection of the raw data indicated that this result was due to one currently self-mutilating participant who habitually bit his fingers and finger-nails until they bled.

The majority of self-mutilation participants had never sought help for coping with or modifying their self-mutilative behaviour (71.7%). Those that did seek help (28.3%) did not do so until a mean of 31.6 months after the initial episode of self-mutilation (SD = 65.11, range = 0, i.e., within hours of the initial self-mutilation episode, to 19 years). There was no significant difference in help seeking behaviour between the current and recovered self-mutilation groups.

Of the total number of participants, 34.8% reported currently taking medication, most commonly selective serotonin reuptake inhibiting antidepressants (37.5%), mono-amine oxidase inhibitors (31.3%) and antianxiety agents (25.0%). No significant differences between current and recovered self-mutilation participants were evident with regard to current medication.

2.2.2. Symptomatology. Results indicated that the current and recovered self-mutilation groups barely differed with regards to the level of symptomatology they were currently experiencing. Mean and standard deviations for both groups for all scales are available on request. No significant differences between current and recovered self-mutilation participants were evident for the BHS, BAI, BDI or the STAI. Scores for both groups on these measures were within the mild to moderate ranges of symptom severity. No significant difference between current and recovered self-mutilation participants was evident for dissociative experiences as measured by the DES. Both groups indicated substantially higher levels of dissociative experiences that the median score for normal subjects in the original sample (Burnstein & Putnam, 1986). In addition, no significant difference between current and recovered groups was demonstrated for the Eysenck Impulsiveness Questionnaire. No difference between the groups in terms of negative life events as measured by the Schedule of Recent Experience was noted. Both groups reported a high number of recent life events. No between group differences for the MSSI were noted. In fact, extremely low scores for both groups were noted for this measure indicating suicidal ideation was minimal for both groups.

Figure 4 depicts current and recovered groups' responses for the sub scales and global scales for the SCL-90-R.

No significant differences between the groups were evident for any of the SCL-90-R subscales. Mean scores for the Obsessive–Compulsive, Interpersonal Sensitivity, Depres-

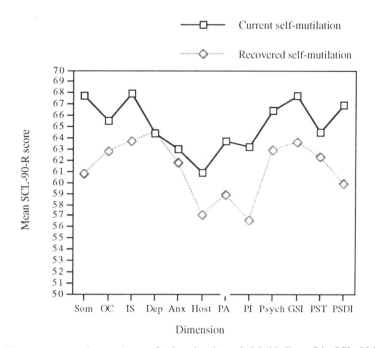

Figure 4. Current v recovered groups' scores for the subscales and global indices of the SCL-90-R subscales.

sion and Psychoticism subscales reached clinical significance as defined by Derogatis (1983) for both groups. Mean scores for Phobic Anxiety and Paranoid Ideation were above the cut off for caseness for the current self-mutilation group only but these scores did not differ significantly from the mean scores of the recovered group on these measures. No significant difference between groups was evident for the Global Severity Index (GSI) or the Positive Symptom Total (PST) for the SCL-90-R. The GSI for both the current and recovered groups was indicative of the presence of psychological maladjustment. However, current self-mutilation participants did report significantly higher levels of distress regarding the presence of these symptoms as measure by the Positive Symptom Distress Index (PSDI) (Fisher PLSD = 5.92, $p < .05$) than the recovered group. In addition, mean PSDI reached a level indicating clinical significance for the current self-mutilation group only.

There were a few other factors that distinguished the current and recovered self-mutilation groups. For the HDHQ, current self-mutilation participants reported significantly higher scores for a measure of total hostility (Fisher PLSD = 4.29, $p < .05$) and for the urge to act out hostility subscale (Fisher PLSD = 1.28, $p < .05$). In addition, the current group scored significantly lower than the recovered group for the Survival and Coping Beliefs subscale of the RFL-48 (Fisher PLSD = 0.55, $p < .05$) and the fear of suicide subscale (Fisher PLSD = 0.56, $p < .05$). Lower scores on these subscales are indicative of an inability to generate coping ideas related to suicide and a low fear of suicidal acts.

2.3. Discussion

It was hypothesised that current self-mutilation participants would report significantly higher levels of symptomatology than the recovered group. Results did not support this hypothesis. No significant differences between current and recovered self-mutilation groups were demonstrated for most symptomatology measures. In addition, the level of symptomatology that participants reported was generally of clinical significance. These results have indicated that the recovered self-mutilation group had not necessarily recovered from the symptoms that have been associated with self-mutilative behaviour. It follows that it is possible to effectively treat the symptom of self-mutilation without significantly altering the level of symptomatology a person is experiencing.

Both self-mutilation groups demonstrated elevated scores on the empathy subscale of the Eysenck Impulsiveness Questionnaire. This has indicated that individuals with a history of self-mutilative behaviour may be particularly sensitive in terms of sharing the perceived emotional experiences of others. In fact, self-mutilating individuals have been described as emotionally labile and as having a tendency to overreact to negative experiences (Simpson, 1976; Zweig, Paris & Guzder, 1994).

There were a few factors that distinguished the groups. On the HDHQ, the current group scored significantly higher on the measure of total hostility, in particular the urge to act out hostile feelings. In addition, the current self-mutilation group were significantly less able to generate coping ideas related to suicide and reported feeling significantly less fearful of the suicidal act. Mean scores on these measures have indicated that current self-mutilation participants' attitude to suicide could best be described as ambivalent.

It was of particular interest that although the current and recovered groups did not differ significantly in number of current symptoms or the degree of symptomatology they were presently experiencing, the current group were significantly more distressed regarding the presence of these symptoms. These differences between the groups could not be accounted for by differences in level or type of current medication, help seeking behaviour or number of recent negative life events. In fact, both groups reported recently experiencing a high number of recent negative life events. The factors that alter the level of distress reported by self-mutilating individuals remains unclear.

3. CONCLUSIONS

It is clear from the results of this investigation that people cut themselves because of the reinforcing nature of the reduction in psychophysiological arousal and psychological tension that the act provides. Results also have indicated that the psychophysiological reinforcement that the act provides is maintained even when the individual is no longer engaging in the behaviour. Therefore, it is unlikely that people stop cutting themselves because the behaviour no longer provides the desired relief from tension.

The result of these studies have demonstrated that individuals who have recovered from self-mutilative behaviour may not necessarily have resolved the symptoms associated with self-mutilation. However, they may be significantly less distressed regarding the presence of these symptoms than individuals who are currently self-mutilating. The factors that alter this level of distress remain unclear. It seems that self-mutilative behaviour can be effectively controlled without significantly changing the level of symptomatology a person is experiencing. Therefore, the question is not why do individuals cut themselves, but why do they stop.

REFERENCES

Beck, A.T., & Steer, R.A. (1987). Manual for the revised Beck Depression Inventory. San Antonio, TX: The Psychological Corporation.
Beck, A.T., & Steer, R.A. (1988). Manual for the Beck Hopelessness Scale. San Antonio, TX: The Psychological Corporation.
Beck, A.T., & Steer, R.A. (1990). Manual for the Beck Anxiety Inventory. San Antonio, TX: The Psychological Corporation.
Bernstein, E.M., & Putnam, F.W. (1986). Development, reliability, and validity of a dissociation scale. Journal of Nervous and Mental Disease, 174, 727–735.
Brain, K.L., Haines, J., & Williams, C.L. The psychophysiology of self-mutilation: A comparison of current and recovered self-mutilators. Paper presented at The XIX Congress of the International Association for Suicide Prevention, Adelaide, March, 1997.
Brain, K.L., Williams, C.L., & Haines, J. The psychophysiology of self-mutilation: Evidence of tension reduction. Paper presented at The 23rd Annual Experimental Psychology Conference, Perth, April, 1996.
Brain, K.L., Williams, C.L., Haines, J., Stops, D., & Driscoll, C. The influence of imagery ability on the response to personalised guided imagery. Paper presented at The 6th Australian Psychophysiology Conference, Hobart, December, 1996.
Caine, T.M., Foulds, G.A., & Hope, K. (1967). Manual of the Hostility and Direction of Hostility Questionnaire (HDHQ). London: University of London Press.
Derogatis, L.R. (1983). SCL-90-R. Administration, scoring and procedures manual-II. Towson, MD: Clinical Psychometric Research.
Driscoll, C., Brain, K.L., Williams, C.L., & Haines, J. A comparison of the tension reduction of self-poisoning and self-mutilation. Paper presented at The XIX Congress of the International Association for Suicide Prevention, Adelaide, March, 1997.
Driscoll, C., Williams, C.L., & Haines, J. The psychophysiology of self-poisoning. Paper presented at The International Congress on Stress and Health, Sydney, October, 1996.
Eysenck, S.B.G., & McGurk, B.J. (1980). Impulsiveness and venturesomeness in a detention center population. Psychological Reports, 47, 1299–1306.
Favazza, A.R. (1989). Why patients mutilate themselves. Hospital and Community Psychiatry, 40, 137–145.
Favazza, A.R., & Conterio, K. (1989). Female habitual self-mutilators. Acta Psychiatrica Scandinavica, 79, 283–289.

Feldman, M.D. (1988). The challenge of self-mutilation: A review. Comprehensive Psychiatry, 29, 252–269.

Fleming, I., & Baum, A. (1987). Stress: Psychobiological assessment. In J.M. Ivancevich & D.C. Ganster (Eds.), Job stress: From theory to suggestion (pp117–140). New York: Hawthorn Press.

Haines, J., Brain, K.L., & Williams, C.L. Self-cutting: Factors associated with tension reduction. Paper presented at The XIX Congress of the International Association for Suicide Prevention, Adelaide, March, 1997.

Haines, J., Williams, C.L., Brain, K.L., & Wilson, G.V. (1995). The psychophysiology of self-mutilation. Journal of Abnormal Psychology, 104, 471–489.

Holmes, T.H. (1988). Schedule of recent experience. In M.D. Davis, E. Robbins Eshelman, & M. McKay (Eds.), The Relaxation and Stress Reduction Workbook (pp. 4–8). New Harbinger Publications, Inc. Oakland, CA.

Linehan, M.M., Goodstein, J.L., Nielsen, S.L., & Chiles, J.A. (1983). Reasons for staying alive when you are thinking of killing yourself: The reasons for living inventory. Journal of Consulting and Clinical Psychology, 51, 276–286.

McCormack, H.M., Horne, D.J., & Sheather, S. (1988). Clinical applications of visual analogue scales: A critical review. Psychological Medicine, 18, 1007–1019.

McLaren, S.J., Haines, J., & Williams, C.L. The psychophysiological and psychological responses of police officers to work situations. Paper presented at The International Congress on Stress and Health, Sydney, October, 1996.

Miller, I.W., Norman, W.H., Bishop, S.B., & Dow, M.G. (1986). The modified scale for suicidal ideation: Reliability and validity. Journal of Consulting and Clinical Psychology, 54, 724–725.

Pattison, E.M., & Kahan, J. (1983). The deliberate self-harm syndrome. American Journal of Psychiatry, 140, 867–872.

Simeon, D., Stanley, B., Frances, A., Mann, J.J., Winchel, R., & Stanley, M. (1992). Self-mutilation in personality disorders: Psychological and biological correlates. American Journal of Psychiatry, 149, 221–226.

Simpson, M.A. (1975). The phenomenology of self-mutilation in a general hospital setting. Canadian Psychiatric Association Journal, 20, 429–434.

Simpson, M.A. (1976). Self-mutilation. British Journal of Hospital Medicine, 16, 430–438.

Spielberger, C.D. (1983). Manual for the State-Trait Anxiety Inventory (STAI-Form Y). Palo Alto, CA: Consulting Psychologists Press.

Walsh, B.W., & Rosen, P.M. (1988). Self-mutilation. Theory, research and treatment. New York: Guilford Press.

Waltzer, H. (1968). Depersonalization and self-destruction. American Journal of Psychiatry, 125, 399–401.

Williams, C.L., Haines, J., & Brain, K.L. The psychophysiology of the binge-purge cycle. Paper presented at the Second International Conference on Eating Disorders, London, April, 1995.

Winchel, R.M., & Stanley, M. (1991). Self-injurious behaviour: A review of the behaviour and biology of self-mutilation. American Journal of Psychiatry, 148, 306–317.

Zweig, F.H., Paris, J., & Gudzer, J. (1994). Psychological risk factors for dissociations and self-mutilation in female patients with borderline personality disorder. Canadian Journal of Psychiatry, 39, 259–264.

29

HAVE BIOLOGICAL STUDIES OF SURVIVORS OF SUICIDE ATTEMPTS INFLUENCED OUR MANAGEMENT?

Lil Träskman-Bendz, Margot Alsén, Gunnar Engström, Åsa Westrin, and Mats Lindström

The Lund Suicide Research Center
Department of Clinical Neuroscienc
Lund University, Lund, Sweden

INTRODUCTION

Patients with mood disorders have long been known to have monoaminergic dysregulation (Schildkraut, 1965; Lapin & Oxenkrug, 1969; Siever & Davis 1985; Harro & Oreland 1996; Van Praag, 1996). The heterogeneity of depressive disorders has recently been discussed by Halbreich and Lumley (1993). It is essential to note that a large part of people have depressed mood associated with social dysfunction and suicidality without fulfilling criteria of mood disorders according to conventional systems of classification.

The current neurochemical theories of biological correlates of suicidal behaviour principally involve the serotonergic system. The finding of an association between serotonin disturbance and suicidality is very robust and has opened up the possibility for a search for other biological variables that may also be related to suicidal behaviour as such (rather than to any particular psychiatric diagnostic category). Among such variables may be mentioned catecholamines, cortisol and some other hormones, as well as several neuropeptides. Few data are avialable about the role of catecholamines. Monoamines have neuromodulating effects on the endocrine axes, such as the hypothalamus-pituitary-adrenal (HPA) axis, and a dysfunction may be reflected through abnormal secretion of steroids as an effect of stressors (Dinan, 1996).

1. SEROTONIN

1.1. The Association between CSF 5-HIAA and Suicidality

Serotonin has a role in complex adaptive behaviour such as social behaviour and impulsivity. When measured in the cerebrospinal fluid (CSF), the serotonin metabolite

Suicide Prevention, edited by Kosky *et al.*
Plenum Press, New York, 1998

5-hydroxyindoleacetic acid (5-HIAA) is an indirect measure of serotonergic transmission in the brain. There is no detailed understanding of the stipulated deviance of serotonin in suicidal, impulsive, and/or aggressive individuals.

However, there is evidence that CSF 5-HIAA reflects frontal lobe serotonin (Stanley, Träskman-Bendz, & Dorovini-Zis, 1985). The frontal lobes are used for planning of future activities. A deviant coupling between the frontal lobes and amygdala seems to play an essential role for divergent socialisation (Bechara, Tranel, Camasio, & Damasio, 1996).

Studies of 5-HIAA in lumbar cerebrospinal fluid drawn from psychiatric patients, have shown that those patients who made a suicide attempt or who later committed suicide, had lower concentrations of the metabolite than the remainder. This association has been reproduced in well over 20 studies, including a meta-analysis (Lester, 1994), and it appears to cut across conventional diagnostic boundaries. Determination of CSF 5-HIAA may have a place in the clinical assessment of suicide risk, as increased mortality occurs within the first year after the index suicide attempt (Nordström, Samuelsson, Åsberg, Träskman-Bendz, Åberg-Wistedt, Nordin, & Bertilsson, 1994). Lower levels may predict lesser suicide.

Studies of behaviour and biological variables in free running monkeys offer possibilities for comparisons with humans. Pharmacological manipulations of serotonergic transmission affect aggressiveness and social function in monkeys, and in humans, suicidality and aggression covary with measures of serotonergic function.

The influence of hereditary and environmental factors could be measured from adoption studies of rhesus-monkeys. Soon after birth, about 90% of the variance of CSF 5-HIAA in monkeys can be explained by heredity. This percentage decreases with increasing age. (Higley, Thompson, Champoux, Goldman, Hasert, Kraemer, Scanlan, Suomi, & Linnoila, 1993).

1.2. Other Markers of Serotonergic Activity

Since lumbar puncture is a cumbersome procedure in routine clinical practice, other markers of serotonin function, which are more accessible markers are needed. Among factors associated with serotonergic function, several have shown associations with suicidal behaviour. These include platelet markers such as monoamine oxidase (MAO) activity or ligand-binding to some serotonin (5-HT) receptors. The serotonin system displays an astonishing heterogeneity with regard to different receptors. To date 15 serotonergic receptors have been described. These receptors are critically involved in the mediation of behavioural stress-response, and are presumably dependent on the serotonergic tone. 5-HT2 receptors are located postsynaptically, and when activated they induce phosphoinositide hydrolysis.

Challenge tests may provide a functional assessment of serotonin neurons. Such tests involve administration of a drug such as a releaser of fenfluramine, the 5-HT1A agonist flesinoxan, or a precursor like 5-hydroxytryptophan (5-HTP). In these tests, changes of endogenous substances (such as prolactin or cortisol) which are controlled by serotonergic neurons are induced.

Apart from the well established fenfluramine-prolactin studies described by Coccaro, Siever, Klar, Maurer, Cochrane, Cooper, Mohs, and Davis (1989), Mann, McBride, Malone, DeMeo and Keilp (1995) recently found blunted responses in young suicide attempters who were hopeless, had high suicidal intent and borderline personality disorder.

D,l-fenfluramine has a mixed action on serotonin and catecholamines, while d-fenfluramine has no catecholaminergic effects. D-fenfluramine challenge caused attenuated cortisol-responses in patients with major depression, and this response was especially marked in suicidal patients (Cleare, Murray, & O'Keane, 1996). Enhanced cortisol-responses in suicidal depressives were previously found after challenge with the precursor 5-HTP (Meltzer, Perline, Tricou, Lowy, & Robertson, 1984). Similarly cortisol-responses after paroxetine to healthy individuals were associated with impulsivity as well as 5-HT2A mediated calcium-responses in platelets after 5-HT (Reist, Helmeste, Albers, Chhay, & Tang, 1996).

Pitchot, Ansseau, Gonzalez-Moreno, Lembreghts, Hansenne, Wauthy, Reel, Jammaer, Rapart, and Sulon (1995) tried the 5-HT1A agonist flesinoxan in major depressed patients. The mean delta cortisol responses were significantly lower in those with a history of suicide attempt, who also had lower temperature responses.

The time-perspective of serotonin and suicidality was elucidated in a study, in which patients were rated as *acute* suicidal and compared with those with *anamnestic* (previous) suicidality. Those with acute suicidality had the lowest levels of 5-HT in spinal fluid (Becker, Laakman, Baghai, Kuhn, Pfeifer, & Kauert, 1996). In contrast to discussions in other articles on 5-HT as trait-dependent, 5-HT was in this case regarded as a state marker. State and trait were discussed recently in a study by Verkes, Fekkes, Hengeveld, Vand der Mast, Tuyl, and Van Kempen (1996). Platelet 5-HT and 3H-paroxetine binding was studied repeatedly the year after an index suicide attempt. High 5-HT then represented trait for suicidality, while a high affinity constant for 3H-paroxetine changed after the suicide attempt like a state marker.

2. CATECHOLAMINES

Pathologic aggressiveness and suicidality have been correlated positively with high CSF levels of 3-methoxy-4-hydroxyphenylglycol (MHPG), the main noradrenaline (NA) metabolite. When measured in urine, the ratio between NA and adrenaline (A) was high in aggressive individuals, while in suicidal patients this ratio was low according to a couple of studies (for a review, see Gerra, Zaimovic, Avanzini, Chittolini, Giucastro, Caccavari, Palladino, Maestri, Monica, Delsignore, & Brambilla, 1997)

Challenge studies include growth hormone (GH) responses to clonidine (an alfa-2 agonist) or apomorphine (a dopamine-agonist). In suicidal men with major depressive disorder, there were increased GH responses to apomorphine, but not to clonidine according to a recent study (Pitchot, Hansenne, Gonzalez-Moreno, Wauthy, & Ansseau, 1995).

3. MONOAMINES AND STRESS

Suicidal individuals often have difficulties in coping with stress. One possible correlate with this psychological failure could be the fact that longterm stress induces a profound decrease of dopamine (DA) in the nucleus accumbens. Acute exposure to stress produces time-dependent biphasic alteration in DA release in the mesolimbic system, and the initial increase of DA is probably related to arousal. Since the ascending NA-ergic pathways have been implicated in brain mechanisms underlying attention and arousal, it is not surprising that they are involved in the stress response. Acute stressful situations increase the metabolism of NA in the cerebral cortex. (for a review, see Harro & Oreland, 1996).

Anxiety, anger and arousal are key phenomena related to stress, and in many cases leading to depressed mood. According to Van Praag (1996), there is a subgroup of depressives, who are sensitive to stress. Like in depressed suicide attempters, these patients have low concentrations of CSF 5-HIAA.

4. GLUCOCORTICOIDS

The involvement of the Hypothalamic-Pituitary-Adrenal-axis in the control of suicidal behaviour/aggression and impulsivity has been investigated, but the results are inconclusive. However, a consistent association between completed suicide and nonsuppression of cortisol after dexamethasone has been shown in a meta-analysis by Lester (1992).

There are indications that dexamethasone has serotonergic effects, for example, enhanced prolactin responses after tryptophan-administration have been reported in individuals whom in addition were given dexamethasone (Träskman-Bendz, Haskett, & Zis, 1986). Thakore and Dinan (1995) reported normalised prolactin-responses to fenfluramine after successful antiglucocorticoid treatment with ketoconazole of depressed patients. They suggested an association between hypercortisolemia and serotonergic subsensitivity.

Aggressiveness in subjects with psychiatric disturbances, mainly personality disorders, is negatively correlated with plasma cortisol and beta-endorphin levels as well as urinary free cortisol (for a review, se Gerra *et al*, 1997). Low cortisol plasma levels have been found in abusive and suicidal alcoholics (Bergman & Brismar, 1994), and similarly low urinary cortisol was reported in impulsive suicide attempters with alcoholism (Engström, Alling, Oreland, & Träskman-Bendz, 1996).

5. IMMUNE STUDIES

Altered immunological function represents a significant observation made previously in the study of possible etiologic and pathophysiological factors for psychiatric disorders. For example, increased immunoglobulin G with affinity for DA (DA-IgG) has been reported in CSF from psychotic patients (Bergquist, Bergquist, Axelsson, & Ekman, 1993). Similarly, a study of suicide attempters shows high levels of DA-IgG, indicating that autoimmune mechanisms involving the dopaminergic neurotransmitter system could be of pathophysiological importance in psychiatric disorders connected to an attempt of suicide (Bergquist, Träskman-Bendz, Lindström, & Ekman, submitted for publication).

Another example of activation of the immune system in psychiatric disorders was reported by Nässberger and Träskman-Bendz (1993), who found high plasma levels of the soluble interleukin-2 receptor (S-IL-2-R) in suicide attempters compared to controls without psychiatric disease. These levels were not changed when patients were treated with an antidepressive or other drugs, or when the acute phase was compared with clinical remission. Thus, elevated S-IL-2-R may be a trait marker of suicidality, or of phenomena related to suicidality.

The interleukins act as signal substances in the communication between cells of the immune system. In another study from Ireland (Keeley, 1996), preliminary findings show that not all suicide attempters have pathological S-IL-2-R values, but a subgroup of repeat attempters have significantly increased levels.

6. LIPIDS

Epidemiological data have highlightened the possible associations between low cholesterol and suicidal behavior. In a sample of totally 52000 men and women, Lindberg,

Råstam, Gullberg, and Eklund (1992), reported more violent deaths in male subjects with low cholesterol levels, and Muldoon, Manuck, and Matthews (1990) reported more violent deaths in males with low cholesterol levels when performing a meta-analysis of six cholesterol lowering primary prevention trials. However, there are also a number of epidemiological studies which could not find any links between low cholesterol levels and violent or suicidal behaviour (Smith, Shipley, Marmot, & Patel, 1990; Irribarren, Reed, Wergowske, Burchfiel, & Dwyer, 1995). Furthermore, the association between low cholesterol and low serotonergic activity in humans have so far not been proved, and Engström, Alsén, Regnéll and Träskman-Bendz (1995), could not find any convincing associations between total serum cholesterol and CSF 5-HIAA in a sample of suicide attempters. In some recently performed placebo controlled trials of cholesterol lowering agents, no increase in accidents or suicide were found (see Law, 1996). However, in trials of cholesterol lowering drugs, patients with a history of psychiatric illnesses are most often excluded, and it is still possible that vulnerable individuals, e.g. with a dysfunctional central serotonergic system, could have an increased risk for suicide after lowering the cholesterol levels.

7. CONCLUDING REMARKS

An understanding of the relationship between the psychobiology of suicidal behaviour, stress and mood is an important scientific and public health issue. The introduction of preventive programmes should therefore include a careful evaluation of the expected psychological as well as the physical effects.

From *monoamine studies* we have learnt that all three monoamines are more or less involved in suicidal behaviour. There are survival analytic studies indicating that a low CSF-5-HIAA could predict further suicidal behaviour rather soon after the sampling procedure. As serotonergic measures so far have shown associations with certain temperament and personality traits, they have been regarded as biochemical trait markers. However, recent studies from Germany and Holland have called this issue in question, as CSF serotonin-concentrations and findings from platelet paroxetine-binding differed between those with actual (ongoing) suicidality as compared to those with anamnestic suicidality. Findings of a dysfunctional serotonergic system in subgroups of suicidal individuals must mean that these patients need a special attention and probably for a longer period of time, maybe at least three years according to our own follow-up investigations (Johnsson Fridell, Öjehagen & Träskman-Bendz, 1996).

One problem when considering prescription of antidepressants, is that most of them induce a decrease of both CSF 5-HIAA and MHPG (Potter, Scheinin, Golden, Rudorfer, Cowdry, Calil, Ross, & Linnoila, 1985). Why then, do not (all) patients become suicidal during treatment? Our hypothesis is that seriously suicidal individuals have a monoaminergic imbalance (Träskman-Bendz, Alling, Oreland, Regnéll, Vinge, & Öhman, 1992). One important action of antidepressants is probably then to restore the interaction activity of monoamines to normal.

Still, some early studies show that some low CSF 5-HIAA patients seem to be resistant to treatment with conventional antidepressants (Träskman, Åsberg, Bertilsson, Cronholm, Mellström, Neckers, Sjöqvist, Thorén, & Tybring, 1979).

We have learnt from studies of the 5-HT1A and 5-HT2 receptors that these could be essential not only for depression but also for suicidal individuals. Therefore it would be of interest to study the "antisuicidal" effects of drugs specifically acting on these receptors.

Furthermore, as events of the 5-HT2 receptors involve phosphatidylinositol-metabolism, maybe inositol -treatment in combination, or alone, could be of interest. The 5-HT2 receptor is also interesting when discussing biological effects of lithium, which at least in epidemiological studies could be regarded as preventing suicide (Ahrens, Mueller-Oerlinghausen, Schou, Wolf, Alda, Grof, Grof, Lenz, Simhandl, Thau, Vestergaard, Wolf, & Möller 1995). Lithium causes increases of CSF 5-HIAA (Regnéll *et al,* unpublished).

Another agent causing increases in CSF 5-HIAA is the serotonin precursor 5-HTP (Van Praag, 1981), which has not yet been tried specifically as an anti-suicidal agent. The serotonin-releaser, fenfluramine was however tried in a small study of seriously suicidal and self-destructive individuals in Michigan, and ratings of suicidal ideation showed decreases in several of the patients (Meyendorff, Jain, Träskman-Bendz, Stanely, & Stanley, 1986).

Chronic administration of antidepressants result in desensitisation of the 5-HT1A autoreceptor resulting in increased 5-HT neurotransmission responsible for the clinical response. Antagonism of 5-HT1A combined with serotonergic acting antidepressants leads to immediate and sustained increases of extracellular 5-HT in cortex or hippocampus. The above mentioned findings from the flesinoxan-challenge test and from stress research make it tempting to try this 5-HT1A paradigm not only in treatment-resistant depressed patients, but also in suicidal ones.

As suicidal individuals use dysfunctional coping strategies in stressful situations or when socialising, individual and familial psychological interventions seem to be extremely important. In a biological sense, antagonists of *cortisol* production or cortisol release could theoretically be of interest when treating these patients (Arana, Santos, Laraia, McLeod-Bryant, Beale, Rames, Roberts, Dias, & Molloy, 1995; Thakore & Dinan, 1995).

The possible causality between *cholesterol* and violent death has not yet been proven. More interest in vulnerable persons' eventual reactions to cholesterol-lowering drugs and dietary matters is warranted.

Recent advances in brain imaging in human subjects should bring us a new era with more possibilities to understand biological research, which in turn will offer us a still better understanding of biological events in suicidal people and thus help us develop alternative preventive strategies (Ågren, Reibring, Hartvig, Tedroff, Lundqvist, Bjurling, & Långström, 1993; Mann *et al.*, 1996).

ACKNOWLEDGMENTS

Our studies are supported by the Swedish Medical Research Council 8319-10A, the Söderström König Foundation, the Kock Foundation and the Sjöbring Foundation.

REFERENCES

Ågren, H., Reibring, L., Hartvig, P., Tedroff, L., Lundqvist, H., Bjurling, P., Långström, B. (1993). Monoamine metabolism in human prefrontal cortex and basal ganglia. PET studies using [beta-11C]L-5-hydroxytryptophan and [beta-11C]L-DOPA in healthy volunteers and patients with unipolar major depression. *Depression 1,* 71–81.

Ahrens, B., Mueller-Oerlinghausen, B., Schou, M., Wolf, T., Alda, M., Grof, E., Grof, P., Lenz, G., Simhandl, C., Thau, K., Vestergaard, P., Wolf, R., Möller, H.J. (1995). Excess caridovascular and suicide mortality of affective diosorders may be reduced by lithium prophylaxis. *J. Affective Disorders, 33,* 67–75.

Arana, G.W., Santos, A.B., Laraia, M.T., McLeod-Bryant, S., Beale, M.D., Rames, L.J., Roberts, J.M., Dias, J.K., Molloy, M. (1995). Dexamethasone for the treatment of depression: a randomized, placebo-controlled, double-blind trial. *Am. J. Psychiatry, 152(2),* 265–267.

Bechara, A., Tranel, D., Camasio, H., Damasio, A.R. (1996). Failure to respond autonomically to anticipated future outcomes following damage to prefrontal cortex. *Cereb Cortex, 6(2)*, 215–25.

Becker, U., Laakman, G., Baghai, T., Kuhn, K., Pfeifer. B., Kauert, G. (1996). Reduced CSF 5-HT; a state marker for acute suicidality. Abstract, Sixth European Symposium on Suicide and Suicidal Behaviour.

Bergman, B., Brismar, B. (1994). Hormone levels and personality traits in abusive and suicidal male alcoholics. *Alcohol. Clin. Exp. Res., 18*, 311–316.

Bergquist, J., Bergquist, S., Axelsson, R., Ekman, R. (1993). Demonstration of immunoglobulin G with affinity for dopamine in cerebrospinal fluid from psychotic patients. *Clin. Chim. Acta., 217*, 129–142.

Bergquist, J., Träskman-Bendz, L., Lindström, M., Ekman, R. Suicide-attempters having immunoglobulin G with affinity for dopamine in cerebrospinal fluid. *Manuscript submitted.*

Cleare, A.J., Murray, R.M., O'Keane, V. (1996). Reduced prolactin and cortisol responses to d-fenfluramine in depressed compared to healthy matched control subjects. *Neuropsychopharmacology, 14(5)*, 349–354.

Coccaro, E.F., Siever, L.J., Klar, H.M., Maurer, G., Cochrane, K., Cooper, T.B., Mohs, R.C., Davis, K.L. (1989). Serotonergic studies in patients with affective and personality disorders. *Arch. Gen. Psychiatry, 46*, 587–599.

Dinan, T.G. (1996). Noradrenergic and serotonergic abnormalities in depression: stress induced dysfunction? *J. Clin Psychiatry, 57, Suppl 4*, 14–18.

Engström, G., Alsén, M., Regnéll, G., Träskman-Bendz, L. (1995) Serum lipids in suicide attempters. *Suicide and Life-Threatening Behavior, 25*, 393–400.

Engström,G., Alling, C., Oreland, L., Träskman-Bendz, L.(1996). The Marke-Nyman Temperament (MNT) scale in relationship with monoamine metabolism and corticosteroid measures in suicide attempters. *Archives of Suicide Research, 2*, 145–159.

Gerra, G., Zaimovic, A., Avanzini, P., Chittolini, B., Giucastro, G., Caccavari, R., Palladino, M., Maestri, D., Monica, C., Delsignore, R., Brambilla, F. (1997). Neurotransmitter-neuroendocrine responses to experimentally induced aggression in humans: influence of personality variable. *Psychiatry Research, 66*, 33–43

Halbreich, U., Lumley, L.A. (1993). The multiple interactional biological processes that might lead to depression and gender differences in its appearance. *J Affect. Disord., 29*, 159–173.

Harro, J., Oreland, L. (1996). Depression as a spreading neuronal adjustment disorders. *Eur. Neuropsychopharmacol., 6*, 207–223.

Higley, J.D., Thompson, W.W., Champoux, M., Goldman, D., Hasert, M.F., Kraemer, G.W., Scanlan, J.M., Suomi, S.J., Linnoila, M. (1993). Paternal and maternal genetic and enviornmental contributions to cerebrospinal fluid monoamine metabolites inrhesus monkeys (Macaca mulatta). *Arch. Gen. Psychiatry, 50(8)*, 615–623.

Iribarren, C., Reed, D.M., Wergowske, G., Burchfiel, C.M., Dwyer, J.H. (1995). Serum cholesterol level and mortality due to suicide and trauma in the Honolulu heart program. *Archives of Internal Medicine, 155 (7)*, 695–700.

Johnsson Fridell, E., Öjehagen, A., Träskman-Bendz, L. (1996). A 5-year follow-up study of suicide attempts. *Acta Psychiatr Scand, 93*, 151–157.

Keeley, H. The mark of a suicide.(1996). Abstract, Sixth European Symposium on Suicide and Suicidal Behaviour.

Lapin, I.P., Oxenkrug, G.F. (1969). Intensification of the central serotonergic processes as a possible determinant of the thymoleptic effect. *Lancet, 1*, 132–136.

Law,M. (1996). Commentary: Having too much evidence (depression, suicide, and low serum cholesterol). *B Ml J, 313*, 580–581.

Lester, D. (1992). The dexamethasone suppression test as an indicator of suicide: a meta-analysis. *Pharmacopsychiat.,25*, 265–270.

Lester, D. (1995). The concentration of neurotransmitter metabolites in the cerebrospinal fluid of suicidal individuals: a meta-analysis. *Pharmacopsychiat., 28*, 45–50.

Lindberg, G., Råstam, L., Gullberg, B., Eklund, G.A. (1992). Low serum cholesterol concentration and short term mortality from injuries in men and women. *B.M.J.,305*, 277–279.

Mann, J.J., McBride, P.A., Malone, K.M., DeMeo, M., Keilp, J. (1995). Blunted serotonergic responsivity in depressed inpatients. *Neuropsychopharmacology, 13(1)*, 53–64.

Mann, J.J., Malone, K.M., Diehl, D.J., Perel, J., Nichols, T.E., Mintun, M.A. (1996). Positron emission tomographic imaging of serotonin activation effects on prefronal cortex in healhty volunteers. *J. Cerebral Blood Flow and Metabolism, 16*, 418–426.

Meltzer, H.Y., Perline, R., Tricou, B.J., Lowy, M., Robertson, A. (1984). Effect of 5-hydroxytryptophan on serum cortisol levels in major affective disorders II. Relation to suicide, psychosis and depressive symptoms. *Arch. Gen. Psychiatry, 41*, 379–387.

Meyendorff, E., Jain, A., Träskman-Bendz, L., Stanley, B., Stanley, M. (1986). The effects of fenfluramine on suicidal behavior. *Psychopharmacol. Bull., 22(1)*, 155–159.

Muldoon, M.F., Manuck, S.B., Matthews, K.A. (1990). Lowering cholesterol concentrations and mortality: a quantitative review of primary prevention trials. *B.M.J., 301*, 309–314.

Nässberger, L., Träskman-Bendz, L. (1993). Increased soluble interleukin-2 receptor concentrations in suicide attempters. *Acta Psychiatr. Scand., 88*, 48–52.

Nordström, P., Samuelsson, M., Åsberg, M., Träskman-Bendz, L. Åberg-Wistedt, A., Nordin, C., Bertilsson, L. (1994). CSF 5-HIAA predicts suicide risk after attempted suicide. *Suicide and Life-Threatening Behavior,* 24(1), 1–9.

Pitchot, W., Ansseau, M., Gonzalez-Moreno, A., Lembreghts, M., Hansenne, M., Wauthy, J., Reel,C., Jammaer, R., Rapart, P., Sulon, J (1995), The flesinoxan 5-HT1A receptor challenge in major depression and suicidal behavior. *Pharmacopsychiatry, suppl. 2,* 91–102.

Pitchot, W, Hansenne, M., Gonzalez-Moreno, A., Wauthy, J., Ansseau, M. (1995). Bases biologiques du comportement suicidaire: approche neuroendocrinienne et psychophysiologique du role des catecholamines. *Acta Psychiatr. Belg. 95(4–5),* 210–233.

Potter, W.Z., Scheinin, M., Golden, R.N., Rudorfer, M.V., Cowdry, R.W., Calil, H.M., Ross, R.J., Linnoila, M. (1985). Selective antidepressants and cerebrospinal fluid. Lack of specificity on norepinephrine and serotonin metabolites. *Arch. Gen. Psychiatry, 42,* 1171–1177.

Reist, C., Helmeste,C., Albers, L. Chhay, H., Tang, S.W. (1996). Serotonin indices and impulsivity in normal volunteers. *Psychiatry Res. 60(2–3),* 177–184.

Schildkraut, J.J. (1965). The catecholamine hypothesis of affective diosrder: a review of supporting evidence. *Am. J. Psychiatry, 122,* 509–522.

Siever, L.J., Davis, K.L. (1985). Overview: toward a dysregulation hypothesis of depression. *Am. J. Psychiatry 142,* 1017–1031.

Smith, G.D., Shipley, M.J., Marmot, M.G., Patel, C. (1990). Lowering cholesterol concentrations and mortality. *B.M.J., 301,* 552

Stanley, M., Träskman-Bendz, L., Dorovini-Zis, K. (1985). Correlations between aminergic metabolites simultaneously obtained from human CSF and brain. *Life Sci., 37,* 1279–1286.

Thakore, J.H., Dinan, T.G. (1995). Cortisol synthesis inhibition: a new strategy for the clinical and endocrine manifestations of depression. *Biol. Psychiatry, 37(6),* 364–368.

Träskman-Bendz, L., Haskett, R., Zis, A.P. (1986). Neuroendocrine effects of L-tryptophan and dexamethasone. *Psychopharmacology, 89,* 85–88.

Träskman-Bendz, L., Alling, C., Oreland, L., Regnéll, G., Vinge, E., Öhman, R. (1992). Prediction of suicidal behavior from biologic tests. *J. Clin. Psychopharmacol., 12(2), Suppl.,* 21–26.

Träskman, L., Åsberg, M., Bertilsson, L., Cronholm, B., Mellström, B., Neckers, L., Sjöqvist, F., Thorén, P., Tybring, G. (1979). Plasma levels of chlorimipramine and its demethyl metabolite during treatment of depression. *Clin. Pharmacol. Ther., 26,* 600–610.

Van Praag, H.M. (1981) Management of depression with serotonin precursors. *Biol. Psychiatry, 16(3),* 291–310.

Van Praag, H.M. (1996). Serotonin-related, anxiety/aggression-driven, stressor-precipitated depression. A psychobiological hypothesis. *Eur. Psychiatry, 11,* 57–67

Verkes, R.J., Fekkes, D., Hengeveld, M.W., Van der Mast, R.C. Tuyl, J.P., Van Kempen, G.M.J. (1996) Platelet serotonin, 3H-paroxetine binding and recurrent suicide attempts: A one-year follow up study. *Eur.Neuropsychopharmacol. 6, Suppl.4*

30

SUICIDE INTERVENTION IN RURAL WESTERN AUSTRALIA

A Preliminary Report

Samar Aoun[1] and Tricia Lavan[2]

[1]WA Centre for Rural Health and Community Development
Edith Cowan University
[2]South West Regional Mental Health Team
Bunbury, Western Australia

INTRODUCTION

The effectiveness of suicide intervention programs in reducing the rates of suicide or attempted suicide, has been difficult to ascertain (Commonwealth Department of Human Services 1995, Canadian Task Force 1990, Shaffer et al 1988, Barraclough et al 1977 and Deykin et al 1986). Such evaluative studies were methodologically inadequate or they have used non-comparable outcome measures. or were difficult to interpret conclusively.

In Australia, recent efforts in suicide prevention have been focusing on suicide attempts. They constitute one of the largest and most readily identifiable risk factors for completed suicide (Silburn et al 1991) and are an important opportunity for suicide prevention which is immediately available to clinical services (Clinical Health Goals & Targets 1994).

Hamilton et al (1994) at the WA Research Institute for Child Health undertook to evaluate the intervention strategies set up in one Perth hospital for a group of patients attending emergency departments following attempted suicide. The efficacy of the intervention was assessed by comparing this group to a control group in another hospital where such intervention strategies were not set up. While preliminary outcomes from the initial six months follow-up are encouraging, the evaluation will have to span over a few years to be conclusive.

Australian data for attempted suicides are limited and relate mostly to hospitalisation following attempted suicide. The difficulty experienced in Australia in producing reliable measures of attempted suicide is common to other countries. The issue is multi-faceted, and involves complexities in definition, reporting and social factors. Davis and Kosky (1991) reported that official rates for attempted suicide underestimate the extent of the problem in the community by 67 per cent, as not all cases require a hospital admission. It has been estimated that for every completed suicide, there are between 30 and 40 suicide attempts (Davis and Schrueder 1990). The latest official figures in W.A. (Health Dept of WA 1994) suggest a ratio of 1:10 of deaths from completed suicides to hospitalisations for attempted suicide. Silburn et al (1991) reported a ratio of completed to attempted suicide of 1 to 21 for youth under the age of 25, and a risk for a repeated attempt among this group as high as 33 per cent.

The broad aim of this study was to assess the efficacy of an intervention program designed to reduce hospital admissions for repeated suicidal attempts in a rural community in the south west of Western Australia. We considered that individuals who are at-risk of deliberately harming themselves are an important group to include in the intervention program. Also individuals who attempt suicide but who are not hospitalised need to be included in the intervention program.

METHODOLOGY

Setting

The study was conducted in the Bunbury Health Service (South West Region of Western Australia) which services a population of 40,000 in the primary catchment area and its regional hospital and regional mental health team are also servicing a secondary catchment area in the south west of a population of 67,600. The total geographical spread amounts to 23,682 sq.kms.

All people who presented with a suicidal attempt, or were identified to be at risk of harming themselves, were offered the special intervention. However at the hospital level, complete data is only available on patients admitted to the Bunbury Regional Hospital, the main hospital in the district.

Intervention Program

The intervention program consisted of employing a suicide intervention counsellor, setting up a hospital protocol of best practice, professional and community education.

The Suicide Intervention Counsellor. The position of the suicide intervention counsellor (SIC) was created in November 1996, and incorporated into the existing South West Regional Mental Health Team. The role of the SIC was to provide an outreach approach to individuals identified of being at-risk of or having attempted suicide, for both hospitalised and non-hospitalised cases in the south west health district. Referrals are made by accident and emergency department staff, ward staff, the attending doctor or. community organisations.

The main tasks of SIC is risk estimation, crisis management recommendations, establishment of a therapeutic alliance with the person, coordinating adequate follow-up and appropriate longer term treatment and improving liaison between community-based organisations and treatment agencies.

Patients are seen by SIC within 48 hours of admission and are followed up intensively for an initial period of six weeks after discharge from hospital, or community referral. Family and friends are involved with the patient's consent and are offered support and education. The management of the patients is planned with other health professionals and support agencies. Close contact and feedback are maintained with the referring agent.

The Hospital Protocol of Best Practice. A standardised hospital approach to dealing with cases of deliberate self-harm was developed, in order to implement referrals to the suicide intervention counsellor and to systematically record the information needed to measure outcomes.

The Bunbury Regional Hospital protocol states that the care of individuals, who attempt deliberately to harm themselves or attempt to take their own lives will be enhanced through improved:

- case identification and systematic recording of data
- psycho-social assessment and treatment within 48 hours of admission
- follow-up after discharge
- staff development and training.

Professional and Community Education. Another aspect of the role of the SIC is to provide the community with information on how to access the service, information about intervention strategies and to promote awareness of indicators and risk assessment. Several presentations have targeted the general practitioners, the nursing and accident and emergency staff at the hospital, community health nurses, school teachers and psychologists, youth agencies, social security staff, family and children services.

Subjects

To date, a total of 122 patients were followed up by the suicide intervention counsellor for a period of one year, from November 1995 to October 1996. Thirty six out of these 122 patients were referred from the Bunbury Regional Hospital ward. The rest were from community referral sources.

RESULTS

Characteristics of Subjects

Sixty three percent of patients were females. Males predominate below 24 years of age. Females predominate in the middle age groups. The age of the patients ranged from 12 to 55 years, with a mean of 30 years (SD=11.9)

For those over 15 years of age, there is an over-representation in the defacto, separated and divorced groups compared to the general population (six-fold in the separated and two-fold in divorced and defacto). The proportion unemployed in the sample (31.3%) is three-fold greater than the proportion in the general population, and 24.1% of women had home duties. Australian-born patients were over represented compared to the overseas-born Australians.

Forty percent of patients in the sample attempted suicide, while 60% were considered at risk of deliberately harming themselves. Gender differences were not significant between the two groups.

For those who harmed themselves, the most common method was an overdose (73.2%) followed by cutting (14.6%). Overdose is the chosen method for the majority of females, while more men have used cutting. Drugs or alcohol were involved in 34.5% of the cases who are at risk and 59.5% of those who have attempted.

Precipitating stresses related to relationship problems with partner/divorce/separation were (46.3%), relationship problems with parent or other family member were

(16.8%) and problems resulting from sexual abuse were (11.6%). Half of the patients seen by the counsellor had a current diagnosis of depression, and a third suffered from other mental disorders.

Referral and Follow-Up

One half of patients referred to SIC were from hospitals in the district. A third of all patients were referred by hospital staff and another third by community organisations. Doctors referred 20% of the patients and psychiatrists 8%. Most of those who attempted were referred from the hospital, and the majority of those at risk (71%) were referred from the community. However, 35% of patients who attempted suicide were not hospitalised.

Follow-up arrangements were undertaken by the counsellor alone in 22% of cases, in conjunction with a GP in 28% and in conjunction with a psychiatrist in 23% of cases.

Occurrence of Deliberate Self-Harm

Thirty seven percent of patients had previous attempts. For those who attempted deliberate self-harm, nearly one quarter had one previous attempt and another quarter had at least 2 previous attempts (ranging up to 14 previous attempts). For non attempters who were at risk, just over one quarter had at least 1 previous attempt.

For those with previous attempts and a current attempt, 42% had attempted in the previous year, and a further 17% in the previous two years. Nearly one third of those at-risk had made an attempt within the previous year.

For the 62 patients who were admitted to a hospital in the south west, the length of stay at the hospital varied between 1 and 38 days, with a mean length of stay of 6 days. The total cost for hospital stay for all patients was about $223,200.

Comparison between Those Who Were Referred to SIC and Those Who Were Not

Forty nine patients were admitted to the ward of the Bunbury Regional Hospital for suicidal behaviour and not referred to SIC. They were referred to, as follows: psychiatrist (24.5%), a member of the mental health team (22.4%), a mental hospital (20.4%), a psychiatrist in conjunction with the mental health team (14.3%), General Medical Practitioners (4.1%), without a follow-up plan (10.2%) and other (4.0%).

This group differed from those referred to SIC in terms of having higher proportions of males, aboriginals and overseas-born, and a slightly shorter length of stay at the hospital. This latter may be attributed to the significant proportion transferred to a metropolitan mental hospital after a one-day stay at the regional hospital.

DISCUSSION

The preponderance of females who were referred to SIC is in line with health department data (Serafino et al 1996) and other local studies (Silburn & Zubrick 1991, Williams et al 1996). As women tend to use less violent methods than men, their chances of surviving serious suicide attempts are greater than men, particularly because of advances in intensive-care medical technology (Hassan 1995). Evaluation studies from the USA indicate that it is young women who benefit mainly from intervention programs, as it is evident from the significant decrease in their suicide rates, in communities who established centres for crisis and suicide intervention (Miller et al 1984, cited in Neimeyer and Pfeiffer 1994). Young white females were the most frequent callers to these centres. In this study, more women are followed-up through the high intervention approach, which might have a beneficial impact on this subgroup of the local population.

The age distribution of self-harm patients also follow reported patterns in that the young age group 15–24 had the highest proportions of those who attempted or were considered at risk, followed by the age group 25–34. After the age of 34, the proportions with attempts decline, while more persons at risk come to the attention, possibly because the older age groups, predominantly women, seek help in good time, or because of their previous records which alert the referring agencies.

The referral patterns to the suicide intervention counsellor reflect the good liaison between the treatment/follow-up service and the referring sources such as the hospital staff, the community, the GPs and the psychiatrist. In turn the counsellor has collaborated with these referral sources for the treatment of those patients. The most frequent collaborating arrangements were with a general medical practitioner, a psychiatrist or a community organisation. It is important to highlight the significant proportions at risk (71% of those at-risk) who are detected by these referral sources. Likewise, 35% of those who attempted have not been hospitalised.

The proportion of patients who received care according to the protocol of best practice amounted to 42% of a total of 85 hospitalised patients. Those patients who were not referred to SIC were either transferred to a metropolitan mental hospital (20%), or were old clients of the mental health team, and therefore continue to be followed-up by the same members of the mental health team or the treating psychiatrist.

CONCLUSION

Suicide is a final outcome of diverse disorders, risk exposures and secular influences, both social and economical. Given that these influences have their origin outside the health system, hospital services can only partially contribute to the reduction of the overall suicide rates. The Suicide Intervention Counsellor is one means of facilitating closer bonds between hospitals, clinical services, the community and patients.

ACKNOWLEDGMENTS

This study has been funded by the Southern Health Authority. The authors would like to thank staff involved in this project in the Bunbury Regional Hospital.

REFERENCES

Barraclough, B.M., Jennings, C. & Moss, J.R. (1977). Suicide prevention by the Samaritans. *Lancet* 24, 868–870.
Canadian Task Force on the Periodic Health Examination (1990). *Canadian Medical Association Journal*, 142 (11), 1233–1238.
Commonwealth Dept of Human Services and Health. (1995). *Youth suicide in Australia: A background monograph*. Australian Government Publishing Service.
Commonwealth Dept of Human Services and Health. (1995). *Here for life: A national plan for youth in distress*. Australian Government Publishing Service.

Davis, A.T. & Kosky, R.J. (1991). Attempted suicide in Adelaide and Perth: Changing rates for males and females, 1971–1987. *Medical Journal of Australia*, Vol. 154, 666–85.

Davis, A.T. & Schrueder, C. (1990). The prediction of suicide. *Medical Journal of Australia*, Vol. 53, 552–4.

Deykin, E.,Hsieh, C., Joshi, N.& Mcnamarra, J. (1986). Adolescent suicidal and self-destructive behavior: Results of an intervention study. *Journal of Adolescent Health Care*, 7,88–95.

Dobson, S., Penman, A. & Eighty-two others. (July 1994*). Clinical Health Goals and Targets for Western Australia, Vol. 1.* First report of the Western Australian task force on state health goals and targets. Perth: Health Dept of Western Australia.

Hamilton, T., Silburn, S., Zubrick, S., Cook, H. & Acres, J. (1994*). Facilitating management of suicidal patients between hospitals and the community: A perspective from the emergency department.* Paper presented at the National Conference on the Public Health significance of suicide prevention strategies. Canberra: Public Health Association.

Hassan, R. (1995). *Suicide explained: The Australian experience.* Melbourne: Melbourne University Press.

Hawton, K. & Fagg, J. (1988). Suicide, and other causes of death, following attempted suicide. *British Journal of Psychiatry*, 152, 359–366.

Hawton, K., O'Grady, J., Osborne, M. et al (1982). Adolescents who take overdoses: Their characteristics, problems and contacts with helping agencies. *British Journal of Psychiatry,* 140, 118–123.

Neimeyer, R., & Pfeiffer, A. (1994). Evaluation of suicide intervention effectiveness. *Death Studies*, 18:131–166.

Serafino, S., Swensen, G. & Thomson, N. (June 1996*). Attempted suicide in Western Australia (1981–1993).* Occasional paper / 79. Perth: Health Information Centre, Health Dept of WA.

Shaffer, D., Garland, A., Gould, M., Fisher, P. & Trautman, P. (1988). Preventing teenage suicide: A critical review. *Journal of American Academy Child and Adolescent Psychiatry*, Vol. 27, No. 6, 675–87.

Silburn, S., Zubrick, S., Hayward, L. & Reidpath, D. (1991*). Attempted suicide among Perth youth.* Youth suicide steering committee. Perth: Health Dept of WA.

Swensen, G., Serafino, S. & Thomson, N. (January 1995*). Suicide in Western Australia (1983–1992).* Occasional paper / 65. Perth: State Health Purchasing Authority, Health Dept of WA.

Williams, B., Penhale, L. & Kelly, H. (1996*). Great Southern Suicide Prevention Project: Report on the first phase of data collection in regional and district hospitals and nursing posts.* Produced by the Southern Public Health Unit and the Great Southern Community Mental Health Services, Albany.

31

SUICIDE PREVENTION ON THE INTERNET

Graham Stoney[*]

E-mail: greyham@research.canon.com.au

1. INTRODUCTION

Computer networking and suicide prevention may seem poles apart, but the explosive growth of the Internet raises a number of interesting possibilities. This paper gives a brief introduction to some of the most popular services available on the Internet, and describes some of the growing array of suicide prevention and other crisis related resources available.

2. THE INTERNET

The Internet can be roughly described as a global, loosely organized series of inter-connected networks linking several million computers which are actively used by an estimated 50 million people worldwide. It provides services such as the World Wide Web, Electronic Mail, Usenet News and a vast array of information databases. The network originated in 1969 to connect computers at a number of universities and computer research establishments, and most of the users have traditionally been computer scientists, engineers or university students. Since its inception the network has doubled in size roughly every 9 months, and now has much broader appeal as the network has become available to more and more people from non-technical backgrounds who find its services useful.

With all that networking technology, it can be easy to forget that beneath it all, it is really a group of people communicating; not just computers -- so it is not surprising that the usual array of human problems arise, although the circumstances are somewhat unconventional. Computers can be extremely impersonal, but networked communication introduces a new set of social dynamics.

One of the key points to keep in mind is that the Internet's design is inherently decentralized: nobody owns it, runs it or controls it, and anyone who has a connection can

---

[*] Graham Stoney is a volunteer Youthline counsellor with Lifeline Western Sydney, part of a national crisis telephone counselling service in Australia. He works as a Computer Hardware/Software Engineer at Canon Information Systems Research Australia, and can be reached by electronic mail at greyham@research.canon.com.au.

generally provide or access whatever information and/or services they desire. Having said that, many of the "virtual communities" that exist on the Internet have a strong sense of how you're expected to act in their backyard and for the most part, the Internet functions as a co-operative venture.

My own involvement in suicide prevention on the Internet began after writing and publishing a number of articles via the Internet about suicide, based on my training and experience as a volunteer Youthline telephone counsellor with Lifeline Western Sydney (Arthur, 1995).

3. WORLD WIDE WEB

The first introduction to the Internet for many people is via the World Wide Web, yet it is only one of the many services available via the Internet, and is in fact a relatively recent innovation in the network's history. A good analogy to describe "The Web" is that of a global, distributed encyclopedia of information pages linked together via electronic cross-references. It is primarily an information retrieval service, where the user starts at a particular page of information and moves to other related pages by following the cross-references that they find interesting. The service is interactive in the sense that the user chooses which information they wish to browse next, but unlike other services such as Usenet News, the information flow is largely one-way and the reader is a relatively passive recipient of whatever content the author of the pages chooses to provide.

Anyone with access to a web server can provide information which most other Internet users can access via their Web browser, such as Netscape Navigator or Microsoft Internet Explorer. Each page typically provides information on a particular topic, along with links to other relevant pages which may be located anywhere on the globe. Like most information on the Internet, there is no central control over the information which is available, and The Web has no official table of contents or index. The vast quantity of information available can make finding relevant information difficult, so a number of sites provide "search engines" which allow users to search The Web for particular topic keywords. Two popular search engines are (Altavista) and (Yahoo).

Much of the information available is provided by users simply because they found the topic in question interesting or useful, and wanted to share the information with others. Other information is provided by organisations or corporations according to their own objectives, or as a public service provided in return for "free advertising" viewed by users who choose to visit their page on the Net. As a result, the information available covers the full spectrum of usefulness, quality and accuracy, and it is generally up to the user to discern which information they find helpful. For example, a search on the word "suicide" will yield information both on suicide prevention, and on various ways to take your own life. There is already a large and growing number of pages related to the topic of suicide prevention: at the time of writing, a simple search via (Altavista) revealed about 3000 pages containing references to "suicide prevention." A number of organizations and individuals active in the field of suicide prevention are already providing quality information on suicide prevention via The Web.

4. ELECTRONIC MAIL

Electronic mail is the computer equivalent of the post office, but dispensing with the paper and pens. Correspondence is private and typically between two individuals. In general any user connected to the Internet can send mail to any other user, provided the sender knows the recipient's E-mail address. Ironically, the impersonal nature of computers acts as a positive here: sending or receiving E-mail is much less threatening than talking to someone in person or even on the phone. The lack of physical presence of the other person can make an E-mail "conversation" less threatening, and each person may take as long as they wish to formulate a thoughtful reply, unlike in a telephone conversation. For these reasons, people often find that they are much more easily able to express themselves in an E-mail message, although it does also carry the same limitations as any written communication.

5. MAILING LISTS

Mailing lists are a variation on E-mail, which provide a forum where a group of people with a common interest can hold informal discussions. Messages are addressed to the mailing list, rather than to an individual, and are broadcast to every member of the group. There is still a degree of privacy in the sense that only members of the list can read the messages, although the recipient is a group rather than an individual. Some mailing lists have restricted membership and the owner of a mailing list is free to enforce whatever policy decisions they like.

There literally thousands of public mailing lists available from computers all over the Internet, covering all sorts of topics from rock bands to religion (Da Silva, 1996). Anyone with a computer running the appropriate software can set up and run a mailing list, which other people around the globe may join if they are sufficiently interested. Over the last few years, I've started three lists relevant to suicide prevention, which are hosted by one of the machines where I work.

5.1. The Suicide-Prevention Mailing List[†]

After being contacted via E-mail by a number of other people interested or involved in suicide prevention, I started the suicide-prevention mailing list in November, 1994. It provides an informal forum for discussions related to suicide prevention in general, and particularly about the use of the Internet in suicide prevention work.

It currently has around 100 members from a wide variety of backgrounds, and includes quite a number of volunteer workers and staff from different crisis hotlines around the globe.

5.2. The Suicide-Support Mailing List Feedback

From members of the suicide-prevention mailing list suggested that there was a need for a group dedicated to supporting suicidal people, and to provide an emotionally supportive environment where people could share their story, no matter how desperate it may be. This led me to start the suicide-support mailing list in February 1995, which has slowly grown to over 80 members, and has a regular stream of messages from people sharing their experiences.

[†] To join the suicide-prevention mailing list, send E-mail to majordomo@research.canon.com.au containing "subscribe suicide-prevention" in the message body.

Messages on this mailing list are sometimes quite depressing, as members share their stories and often talk about how much they would like to escape their situation via suicide. However, most messages to the group are supportive of other members, and the group essentially runs itself most of the time. Occasionally, the topic of discussion needs to be gently steered away from ways-to-kill-yourself back to reasons-not-to.

5.3. The Suicide-Survivors Mailing List

The friends and family members of people who have died by suicide (termed "survivors") often carry terrible grief, which is complicated by the circumstances surrounding their loved one's death. Survivors can find support groups where they can relate to other people in similar circumstances extremely beneficial, so in June 1995, I set up the suicide-survivors mailing list to provide such an environment on the Internet.

Although the background of the various group members is quite diverse, the suicide-survivors group is extremely supportive as many members can relate deeply to the pain experienced by the others and so the group has a surprisingly positive tone, even though the personal stories are heartbreaking. At times the grief expressed in the stories of some group members can be quite overwhelming, so some members have found it necessary to take time out and leave the group at times when the burden of other people's pain starts making it more difficult to cope with their own.

Shortly after setting it up I ran an informal recovery program in the group addressing a particular theme every couple of weeks, but for the most part mailing lists have no formal program and members join and leave as they see fit, and there are currently around 90 members.

5.4. Real People, Real Lives

Now the idea of seeking emotional support from a computer network may seem rather odd, but keep in mind that behind all the screens and keyboards are real people, with real lives. Some people may be in desperate situations where they feel unable to discuss their feelings face to face with those around them, and find posting a message on a mailing list much less threatening.

6. USENET NEWS GROUPS

News groups provide a truly public discussion forum where any message posted is broadcast to make it accessible from virtually every other machine connected to the Internet (Moraes, 1995). There are well over ten thousand public groups distributed worldwide, each addressing a particular topic. To make the system manageable, the groups are organized into a hierarchy, and in most groups anyone may post a message or contribute to the discussion. A number of self-help groups exist which provide a public electronic support community where people are often remarkably open about discussing personal problems which other readers can relate to.

"soc.support.depression" is a hierarchy of groups where sufferers of depression often talk openly about their feelings, what's happening in their lives, the side effects of anti-depressant drugs they may be using, and thoughts of depression and/or suicide. Each group tends to develop its own prevailing culture and many of the "soc.support" and "alt.support" groups can create a very strong sense of community where regular readers and contributors often feel both a part of, and supported by, the group. Contributors often go into surprising detail about their problems considering that they are broadcast publicly to millions of machines across the world, but once again its electronic nature can make this less threatening than in a face to face or support group context.

"soc.support.depression.crisis" is a news group with a similar charter to the suicide-support mailing list, so there is some degree of overlap, although the messages on the mailing list are significantly more private since it is distributed much less widely.

"alt.suicide.holiday" is a more controversial group where regulars openly discuss various suicide methods and previous suicide attempts in what sometimes appears as a search for the perfect, painless suicide method like a quest for the holy grail. It can sometimes be rather hostile, but once again, the group has a very strong and unique culture where regulars have a strong sense of community borne out of identifying with other people who feel that their life is so painful and worthless that they openly talk about wanting to kill themselves in a public forum. In an ironic twist, finding that other people feel the same way sometimes gives people hope to keep living, despite the outward preoccupation with suicide.

Because of their wide distribution and open nature, news groups are sometimes more hostile than mailing lists and not all responses are helpful or even well-intentioned. Unlike a mailing list, nobody owns or runs a news group, aside from some special groups which are moderated to keep discussions on-topic.

7. FREQUENTLY ASKED QUESTIONS — FAQS

One of the popular traditional information resources available on the Internet are "Frequently Asked Questions" postings (FAQs), distributed via the Usenet News service. Many news groups have one or more FAQs, which are posted regularly to the group and typically address questions which are raised frequently, and for which there is a well agreed upon answer. Contributions are often made by experts, professionals or interested lay people in the relevant field who regularly contribute to the group in question.

After posting a number of separate articles in a number of news discussions about suicide, I put together an unofficial Frequently Asked Questions posting on suicide (Stoney, 1994–1997a) based primarily on my training and experience at Lifeline. It addresses questions such as "Why do people attempt suicide?," "Are all suicidal people crazy?" and "Doesn't talking about suicide encourage it?," as well as listing risk factors and warning signs to help identify people who may be in crisis. Originally targeted at Australian University students, many of whom have Internet access through their University computer systems, the "Suicide FAQ" is now broader in scope, and has attracted responses from a variety of interested people around the world including suicide survivors and mental health professionals. It is posted regularly each month in groups such as "soc.support.depression.crisis" and "alt.suicide.holiday," and is accompanied by a list of other Internet crisis and emotional support resources, plus a number of national resources like Lifeline from various countries (Stoney, 1994–1997b).

8. CRISIS COUNSELLING VIA E-MAIL

After seeing the depth of hopelessness present in many of the postings on groups like "alt.suicide.holiday," the Samaritans of Cheltenham, UK set up a pilot E-mail based crisis service in July 1994 (Samaritans). After the success of a trial period, they have continued providing the service which is accessible worldwide for people who are depressed or suicidal by E-mailing to "jo@samaritans.org." The service is effectively the Internet equivalent of their telephone counselling service, from which it is staffed by volunteer counsellors with additional training. The Samaritans service is particularly interesting, as it could be an indication of the future for other suicide prevention and crisis telephone counselling services.

One point to note is that the Internet's decentralized, international nature makes it somewhat difficult or undesirable to offer a service which is limited to a specific geographical area. Most Internet users are located in the United States, so most of the users of the services described here are from outside Australia. For instance, the Samaritans E-mail service is accessible internationally and many users may be unaware that their correspondent is in another country.

9. WHAT ABOUT THE DRAWBACKS?

It's not all good news, of course, and I have some reservations about support groups such as the suicide-support mailing list. In any support group, there needs to be a balance between the emotional support gained from the group, and the progress that the individual makes towards resolving his or her problems outside the group. It's important to acknowledge that the sense of community fostered by a support group may actually hinder the resolution of the underlying problems, causing its members to remain stuck where they are, rather than encouraging them to move forward. This is particularly difficult to monitor on the Internet, where group members are free to come and go between various groups as they please, and may become overly invested in one or more support groups, to the detriment of their outside life. Regular contributors may get a strong secondary gain from telling their story in a context where many other readers can relate, and this sense of inclusiveness may be lost if they were to leave the group having truly recovered from or overcome their problems.

Usenet support groups such as "soc.support.depression.crisis" have no leader as such, and no mechanism for dealing with contributors which are hostile or disruptive. Even in an E-mail support group, the "owner" has very little information by which to assess people who request to join the group. There is also no way to monitor or control the private E-mail interactions between group members, and when a dispute arises it can become extremely difficult to arbitrate between members who may not be willing to co-operate. Some group members have experienced a life history of what they perceive as unfair treatment, and arbitrating between hostile group members who are unwilling or unable to resolve their differences without excluding one or both from the support group can be extremely difficult.

A strong precedent exists in the real world for support groups for suicide survivors, but not for groups containing people who are actively suicidal interacting with each other. Whether the members of an electronic support group will make progress without some formal structure remains to be seen, although a general theme in many of the postings is that hearing similar stories to their own has made them feel less isolated, and isolation is a key risk factor in suicide attempts. However, loneliness is also a recurring theme in many of the stories in the various online support groups, and the ability to make and maintain close personal relationships is very much a "people skill" which interaction with computers isn't likely to help develop.

There are also ethical questions concerning counselling via E-mail, although the parallel with telephone crisis services is close enough that the same principles regarding privacy, anonymity and confidentiality in telephone work could be applied without a great deal of change. The issue of hoax messages is a much more severe on a news group or mailing list though, since there are not even verbal cues to help identify whether the message is factual or not, and not all users take the topic seriously. This makes it almost impossible to accurately assess the suicidality of a contributor based on any single message. There is also the issue of privacy and responsibility: many genuinely suicidal contributors to the suicide-support mailing list or alt.suicide.holiday news group would be extremely angry if another group member took any action (such as to call the emergency services, for example) in response to a message saying that they were thinking of, or planning to attempt suicide.

Measuring the true effectiveness of online support groups in helping people live more effectively is difficult since there is little direct evidence of their true experiences in "real life" beyond the stories they choose to tell the group. People come and go for a variety of reasons and are often never heard of again, so there is very little feedback in terms of how the group has impacted their life. Whether a group member lived happily ever after or perhaps completed suicide, it is unlikely that the news would propagate back to the group in any event. However, people join online support groups through their own volition, and many members are thankful for the opportunity to participate. If we believe that people should be empowered to choose the means of support that best suits them, and have the resources to make decisions which are in their own best interests, then the majority of feedback from online support group members suggests that such groups are beneficial. Certainly not everyone who joins such a group will benefit, and we need to be realistic enough to admit that some may be harmed by the experience; but the feedback suggests that most members consider the groups to be beneficial and this is why they remain in them.

10. THE FUTURE

The Internet continues to grow as electronic communication costs continue to fall and more and more people have mainstream access to the network. In many ways, there are a mixture of different cultures present on the Internet, and certainly a wide diversity of backgrounds and points of view. This raises both new challenges and new opportunities for suicide prevention organisations regarding their involvement. The question of how heavily organizations should be involved, and what path would be most appropriate is uncertain. Networks such as the Internet could potentially have a greater impact on our lives than the telephone or television, but whether it is an appropriate vehicle for often-scarce resources or the most effective way to proceed still remains to be seen. Some individuals and organizations have taken the first steps, and indeed this paper has only scratched the surface of what is already available, let alone what could happen in the future.

REFERENCES

Altavista. Altavista Internet Search Engine. http://altavista.digital.com/
Arthur, J. (1995). Lifeline Australia Internet home page. http://www.chem.usyd.edu.au/~arthur_j/lifeline/lifeline.html
Da Silva, S. (1996). Publicly Accessible Mailing Lists. http://www.neosoft.com/internet/paml
Moraes, M. (1995). Welcome to Usenet!. ftp://rtfm.mit.edu/pub/usenet/news.answers/usenet/welcome/part1

Samaritans. The Samaritans Internet home page. http://www.compulink.co.uk/~careware/samaritans/

Stoney, G. (1994–1997a). Suicide — Frequently Asked Questions. ftp://rtfm.mit.edu/pub/usenet/news.answers/suicide/info

Stoney, G. (1994–1997b). Suicide — Internet & International Crisis Resources and Information. ftp://rtfm.mit.edu/pub/usenet/news.answers/suicide/resources

Yahoo. Yahoo Internet Search Engine http://yahoo.com/

32

SKILLING KEY WORKERS

The Implementation of a Youth Suicide Prevention Project in Belgium

K. Andriessen,[*] P. Cosyns, G. Verthriest, and T. Veys

Centrum ter Preventie van Zelfmoord
Kasteleinsplein 46, 1050 Brussel, Belgium

The objective of the project is to prevent suicidal behaviour of young people through the setting up of a local network and the specific training of selected key persons in and around the school. Target key persons are teachers, pupil counsellors, welfare and health workers and educators in institutions for young people. The project started at the end of 1991 and was implemented within 3 years in the region of Turnhout (380,000 inhabitants). Since the end of 1994, the project runs without state funding. Development included sensitization of the youth key persons, screening of schools (N=63. Pupils ages 12 to 18, N=20,000), health and welfare services (N=37), and the presentation of a consensual document on suicide as it is specific for the area. Important findings were: that every school can be confronted with suicidal behaviour, but only a few schools include this in their health policy; that schools are in a position to detect and/or to refer suicidal youth, but this does not seem to be a common practice.

The step by step implementation of the local structure is based on maximising informal and formal relations and professional backgrounds of key persons. Evaluation by all participants focused on influences of the project on: the key persons themselves detecting and counselling suicidal youth, the organisations involved, and networking in the area.

1. INTRODUCTION

In December 1991 the Suicide Prevention Centre (Centrum ter Preventie van Zelfmoord) started with the development of a youth suicide prevention project, at the request of the Department of Special Juvenile Support of the Ministry of the Flemish Community

---

[*] Correspondence to: Mr Karl Andriessen, Centrum ter Preventie van Zelfmoord, Kasteleinsplein 46, 1050 Brussel, Belgium.

Suicide Prevention, edited by Kosky *et al.*
Plenum Press, New York, 1998

(Bestuur Bijzondere Jeugdbijstand van het Ministerie van de Vlaamse Gemeenschap). Two important tendencies had generated the need for such a project: At the end of the eighties the official Belgian death statistics confirmed the dramatic increase, especially in the young, of suicide as cause of death.. Public attention was aroused and authors in the field of suicidology stressed the need for prevention initiatives[1].

At the same time, the tasks of the local Services for Special Juvenile Support (SJS, Comite voor Bijzondere Jeugdzorg, N=20) were rearranged. The Department aimed at introducing preventive work in their local SJS Services. Suicide prevention was one of the subjects chosen by these services. For the first time in the Flemish region it was possible to develop and to implement a local suicide prevention project. Funding was granted by the Ministry for 3 years.

2. METHODS

Analysis of the SJS Services showed their initial need for:

- detailed data on suicide and overall mortality in their community;
- basic information on suicide and its prevention;
- inviting the SJS Services to a symposium;
- contacts with professionals in the field of suicide prevention;
- workshops and training for the counsellors and their colleagues from other services;
- a preventive project applicable in their community.

Basic principles concerning suicide, a concept of prevention[2], objectives of the project, and a strategy for implementation with 3 years were outlined. A board of representatives of the Services watched over the development.

2.1. Objective

To prevent suicidal behaviour of young people by setting up of a local network of selected key persons. Target key persons were teachers, pupil counsellors, welfare and health workers and educators in institutions for young people.

The choice to focus the project on the school community was based on our experiences in working with schools and on the evidence in the literature[3-10]. Schools consider themselves able to detect suicidal ideation or behaviour, but they experience a lack of knowledge and skills to lend first aid to the suicidal students. This can be countered by specific training. But, on the other hand, suicide prevention is absolutely not a task solely for schools. A network sustains prevention initiatives within the community.

2.2. Phases of Implementation

- Training of youth key persons.
- Screening of schools, health and welfare services
- Actual implementation of the local project.
- Evaluation by the participants.

2.3. Training of Key Persons

Basic information included statistical data on suicide (Table 1–2), road accidents and overall mortality per local region. Discussion of these data also dealt with the spectrum of non-lethal suicidal behaviour. Data were updated each year.

Table 1. Suicide mortality in Belgium and in the Flemish region — all ages

All ages	per 100,000 Inhabitants		% of all deaths	
	Belgium	Flemish region	Belgium	Flemish region
1989	19.34	16.85	1.79	1.70
1990	19.05	16.42	1.82	1.68
1991	18.07	15.50	1.73	1.60
1992	18.74	15.75	1.80	1.62
1993		17.63		1.80
1994		18.88		1.99
1995		18.58		1.95

Source: NIS ('89-'92) + cel Gezondheidsindicatoren, Vlaamse Gemeenschap ('93–'94).

Suicide, quantitatively, does not seem to be a major youth problem. However, suicide is the second cause of death after road accidents for the 10–24 age group. In 1994, for the age group of 10–19 year olds, in the Flemish region, there was an average of one suicide a week, an incidence of 1 suicide to 7 deaths by other causes. Only 5 years ago this ratio was 1 to 10.

When broadening our perspective of the continuum of suicidal behaviour, it is important to state that many youngsters have suicidal thoughts, wishes and plans. These covert ideas are usually unknown to key persons.

Research on self-reported suicidal behaviour in adolescents allows us to make a rough estimation of its frequencies . Data from Netherlands' surveys in the nineties showed that between 2.2 and 5.7% of pupils between ages 12–18 reported at least one suicide attempt. Suicidal thought during the past 12 months were reported by 11.3 to 20.1% of the pupils[11], and contemplating suicide was reported by 22.9%. Some surveys in Canada and the United States estimate the prevalence of suicide attempts between 2.2 and 20% and suicidal ideation between 15 to 53%[12]. The authors suggest that the variation in results are due to age and sex variation in the research groups, and different interpretations of words as 'ending your life,' 'suicide attempt.' Only recently similar research was conducted in Belgium[13]. Of the 2,209 pupils in the survey, who attend secondary schools in Brussels, 34% reported ever having had suicidal ideation at some time in their life, of these 9% more than once. Six percent reported one suicide attempt and another 2% more than one.

Table 2. Suicide mortality in Belgium and in the Flemish region — 10–19 year age group

	Ages 10–19 years					
	per 100,000 Inhabitants				% of all deaths	
	Belgium		Flemish region			
	Male	Female	Male	Female	Belgium	Flemish region
1989	6.50	1.26	5.52	1.65	8.96	8.26
1990	5.21	1.44	4.26	1.67	8.26	7.14
1991	3.56	0.65	2.96	0.56	5.23	4.41
1992	5.64	1.97	4.62	0.85	10.02	8.23
1993			6.58	2.59		12.45
1994			9.08	0.29		13.64
1995			6.61	2.60		14.80

Source: NIS ('89-'92) + cel Gezondheidsindicatoren, Vlaamse Gemeenschap ('93–'94).

If we extrapolate these self-reported data for the Flemish region, we estimate that of the 550,000 youngsters between ages 12–18 years, 33,000 attempted suicide and another 11,000 more than once.

More detailed analysis of (unpublished) data in this research shows a significant correlation between pupils who attempted suicide and illegal absence from school. These findings are in accordance with other authors[14,15] saying that the most vulnerable pupils are probably not reached by school-based preventive activities.

Thinking about life and death is considered as a necessary part of the psychological development. But when this occurs too often or is intensified by stressors and decreased problem-solving abilities, the risk of suicidal behaviour increases. The local SJS Services mostly deal with vulnerable and multi-problem youngsters and their families, and with suicidal clients[16].

2.4. Symposium

Through the distribution of statistical data, awareness of the importance of the suicide problem was increased. However, epidemiological data do not mention the possible motivations for suicidal behaviour, nor do they explain the occurrence or guide you in dealing with it. A symposium: 'See you tomorrow...maybe" discussed these approaches by exploring experiences from the counsellor's point of view, as well as that of the suicidal person. The counsellors of the SJS Services, and their colleagues from other services, attended the symposium.

2.5. Initial Training of Counsellors

Following the symposium we started a training programme for the counsellors of the SJS Services. Our preparation was based on information from other training programmes and manuals[17–23]. The programme was conducted by the team from the Suicide Prevention Center during 3 separate days with a follow-up after six months. One hundred and forty key workers participated in 15 groups. The program focused on experiences and attitudes of the participants. Initially this was met with some resistance. Afterwards it was found necessary. The aim was to increase expertise through gaining knowledge about suicide prevention and crisis intervention, recognising signs, acquiring counselling skills, active intervention and referral possibilities. Discussions were often focused on the worker's own attitude towards dead and suicide. When evaluating this program, awareness by the worker of their own attitude, was found to be a basic element in helping.

2.6. Screening of Schools, Health, and Welfare Services

The screening was the first step in preparing the implementation in the local area. The objective was to reach the key persons, to know their thoughts on, and experiences with suicide, their preventive initiatives, to introduce the project and to arouse their interest in it.

A written questionnaire was sent to all 63 schools (20,000 pupils aged 12–18) concerning the past 5 years activity. Seventy percent responded. All 37 health and welfare services were telephoned for a structured interview.

Important findings were that:

- every school can be confronted with suicidal behaviour, but not all schools include this in their health policy as a specific target;

- suicidal behaviour occurs in schools with a health policy, as well as in schools without one;
- schools are in the position to detect suicidal youths, but they report less suicide attempts than are expected from statistical data;
- schools have contacts to whom they can refer suicidal youths, but they tend to keep cases to themselves: they refer suicidal youths less than they do other troubled pupils.
- services see more suicidal youngsters than schools do. Only a few of these youngsters were referred by a school;
- suicidal ideation or attempts are not systematically registered;
- none of the services have specialised team members for suicide prevention;
- help for suicidal persons depends on the setting and the professional background of the staff;
- a lot of the services have a waiting list for counselling, but most state that they give priority to crises;
- crisis intervention is mainly oriented to medical settings.

An important issue that came up was in the relationship between schools, health and welfare services. They are willing to cooperate with each other, but their respective views of each other, and how to help suicidal young people, do not always match. Getting acquainted with each other by focussing[24,25] on the mutual problem of youth suicide could be the key in installing a prevention network.

3. IMPLEMENTATION OF THE LOCAL PROJECT

The results of the screenings were incorporated in a consensual document[26] on suicide as it is specific for the area. The document was discussed at two meetings to which all contacted persons and the local press had been invited. Actual implementation of the step by step structure (Figure 1) was initiated during these meetings: the structure was proposed together with a call for participation.

The implementation of the programme was based on maximising existing structures, developing informal relationships and improving the professional expertise of key per-

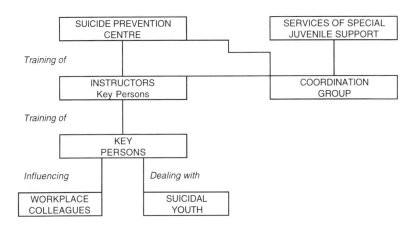

Figure 1. Local structure.

sons[27]. Two instructors trained groups of key persons during 3 days training with follow-ups after 6 months. Emphasis was put on knowledge about suicide, one's own attitude towards death and suicide and training of helping skills. The programme is based on evaluation of the initial training[28–30].

After the training, participants received a package containing 20 different thematic modules for talking with youngsters about suicide, their emotions, thoughts and attitudes concerning suicide. The material has an educational approach and is not suited for crisis interventions or therapeutical purposes[31].

The local coordination, the training facilities, follow-up and the organisation of a yearly congress (oriented on counselling or therapeutical issues) were arranged by the co-ordination group, which consisted of the instructors and a representative from the Suicide Prevention Center.

4. FOLLOW UP WITH THE PARTICIPANTS

4.1. Trainees

The trainees evaluate the program at the end of the third day and again after six months. All trainees felt better prepared to deal with suicidal youth. They were less afraid and were more confident in their abilities. They were more aware and attentive to troubled youth. Detection improved and at the same time they could put their qualities into perspective: there was no infallible help.

The flow of incoming information varied from one setting to another. The flow improved when more than one person of the same school or service attended the training: there was more feedback and reflection. The trainees were consulted by colleagues in schools for problematic situations. Some distributed copies of their manual. Trainees recommended their colleagues to attend the training, which some did. Trainees felt encouraged by their principals in their work.

Only a few of the trainees used the package of 20 modules to talk with youngsters. Reasons given for this were that the modules were not ready to use; the teacher had to work them out; they were also aware that you cannot walk into a classroom unprepared and talk about suicide.

After the training, no new suicide preventive initiatives or health policies were installed in schools or services. Trainees were satisfied with the attention that the programme drew to referring at risk students to health services. But, waiting lists in therapeutical settings were felt to be important obstructions for referral.

When discussing a specific youngster, the trainees turned first to a colleague who also attended the training, or to an instructor from the programme. Trainees and instructors were also consulted by key persons who had never attended the training.

Some trainees found it interesting to organize more than one follow up meeting. They would appreciate feedback in some kind of permanent training. Most trainees asked for more participants from hospitals and therapeutical settings.

4.2. Coordination Group

The instructors feel strengthened by their initial teaching. They relied on their comprehensive instructors' manual. At the same time they recognised a need for supervision by the Suicide Prevention Center. The instructors agreed with the trainees' suggestion to attract more medical and therapeutical settings to the network. At the same time, the group was aware of the importance of keeping in touch with school principals. The instructors were in touch with the target key persons. For the SJS Service, which is the pivot in the area, their project provided a means for constructive dialogues with the school communities. This was important with regard to the prevention assignment.

5. DISCUSSION

The preparatory phase was exhaustive and took two years. This enabled us to get acquainted with our local partners and facilitated the actual implementation, which was effected within one year. The Department of Special Juvenile Support considered then that their objective of developing a model prevention project had been completed.

The pivot service in the area is a vital link in the implementation process. The Service of Special Juvenile Support of Turnhout is well-known and respected for its services. This was very important for gaining the trust of schools with different religious or ethical affiliations. For the same reason it is beneficial that different key persons, who know the area well, coordinated the project.

Throughout western societies a wide variety of youth suicide preventive programmes have been developed. Most of these are curriculum-based school programmes that target all pupils with an education approach[32].

But only few programme evaluations[33,34] show significant gains in knowledge and in positive attitudes toward help seeking and intervening with troubled peers. Other consistent evaluations of these kinds of programmes[34,35] fail to find evidence or point out that in addition to positive effects[36,37], such as improved knowledge and abilities to cope, there is a solution.

The issue of suicide prevention can also be incorporated as a specific target within school health policies. In this way suicide can be related to a lot of causations and other 'deviant' behaviour[32,34,38] The project we developed is not curriculum-based. Emphasis was put on skilling[35,36] key persons and integrating them in a network of school and health and welfare services. The goal was to improve their awareness for early suicide detection, first aid counselling and referral. The only research we found on measuring the skills key persons[39] (general practitioners) within a network[40] showed a significant beneficial effect on the suicide rate. Repetition of the program seems a condition for long term effects to be maintained.

6. CONCLUSIONS

Different aspects of the development and implementation of a local youth suicide prevention project are given. Experiences and evaluations of other relevant projects are taken into account. Our approach to suicide and its prevention tries to meet actual expectations regarding suicide prevention in school communities.

Implementation of the programme took three years—the first two being preparation with the key workers and services. Participants felt enriched by the training programme and their contacts in the local network.

Upgrading referral possibilities, by including more therapeutical settings within the network, is needed. The integration of suicide as a specific target in school health policies remains an important issue for further development.

REFERENCES

1. Moens GFG, Aspects of the epidemiology and prevention of suicide. Leuven: University Press, 1990
2. Vandenabbeele N. Zelfmoordpreventie en initiatieven in Vlaanderen (Suicide prevention and initiatives in Flanders). Arch Public Health 1993; 51: 345–358
3. Kienhorst CMW, Broese van Groenou MI. Opvang van suicidale leerlingen. Over de mogelijkheden en onmogelijkheden. In: Wolters WHG, Diekstra RFW, Kienhorst CMW, editors. Suicidaal gedrag bij kineren en adolescenten, Baarn: Ambo, 1987: 107–114
4. De Heus P, Diekstra RFW, Van der Leeden BI. Suicidaal gedrag van leerlingen in het voortgezet onderwijs. 1 Hoe gaat de school om met suicidaal gedrag? 2 Wat voor taken heeft de school volgens leraren? In: Wolters WHG, Diekstra RFW, Kienhorst CMW editors. Suicidaal gedrag bij kinderen en adolescenten, Baarn: Ambo, 1987: 84–105
5. Van den Bout J, Kienhorst I. Omgaan met suicidale leerlingen. Tijdschrift voor Jeugdhulpverlening 1988; 16: 337–342
6. Mulder A, Methorst G, Diekstra R. Prevention of suicidal behaviour in adolescents. The role and training of teachers. Crisis 1989; 10(1): 36–51
7. Spano NA. To be or not be. Adolescent suicide: a statewide action plan. New York: State Senate, 1988
8. Ryerson DM. A proposal for the development of a high school based youth services program. South Bergen: Mental Health Center and Hackensack High School, 1987
9. Report of the National Conference on Youth Suicide. Community response to a national tragedy. Washington DC: Youth Suicide National Center, 1985
10. Poland S. Suicide intervention in the schools. New York: Guilford Press, 1989
11. Kienhorst I, De Wilde EJ. Suicide attempts in adolescence. 'Self report' and 'Other report.' Crisis 1995; 16(2); 59–62,65
12. Diekstra RFW, Kienhorst CMW, De Wilde EJ. Suicide and suicidal behaviour among adolescents. In: Rutter M, Smith DJ, editors: Psycosocial disorders in youg people. Chichester: John Wiley & Sons, 1995: 688–698
13. De Clercq M, Vranckx A, Navarro F, Piette D Onderzoek naar de geestelijke gezondheid van jongeren uit het secundair onderwijs in het Brussels Hoofdstedelijk Gewest. Brussel: Overlegplatform voor Geestelijke Gezondheid & ULB, 1996
14. Shaffer D, Garland A, Vieland V, Underwood M, Busner C. The impact of curriculum-based suicide prevention programs for teenagers. J Am Acad Child Adolesc Psychiatry 1991; 30: 588–596
15. Hawton K. Suicide and attempted suicide among children and adolescents. Beverly Hills: Sage, 1986: 69–87, 129–137
16. Tot morgen ... misschien. Verslag van een denkdag over jongeren en zelfdoding, 01.04.92. Brussel: Ce trum ter Preventie van Zelfmoord & Ministerie van de Vlaamse Gemeenschap, 1993
17. Methorst GJ, Kerkhof AJFM. Omgaan met depressief en suicidaal gedrag van jongeren, deel 1 en 2. Leiden: Rijksuniversiteit, 1991
18. Mulder AM, Methorst GJ, Diekstra RFW. Sh=uicide preventie in het voortgezet onderwijs. Bijscholingsprogramma voor leerkrachten. Handboeck voor prgramma-begeleiders. Leiden: Rijksuniversiteit, 1989
19. Suicide prevention and coping. A manual for teachers, counsellors and administrators. Calgary Alberta: Alberta Education, 1987
20. Suicide prevention program for California Public Schools. Cacramento: California State Department of Education, 1987
21. Lang WA, Ramsay RF, Tanney BL, Tierney RJ. California suicide intervention training workshop. Workshop organizer's guide. California: Department of Mental Health, 1987
22. Berkan WA. Suicide Prevention: a resource and planning guide. Madison, Wisconsin Department of Public Instruction, 1986
23. Raymond S. Suicide prevention program in school: a community based approach. Montreal: Suicide Action Montreal, 1985
24. Vettenburg N. Welzijnswerk en onderwijs. Mogelijkheden en moeilijkheden in de samenwerking. Deel 1. Leuven: Onderzoeksgroep Jeugdcriminologie & vzw Majong, 1991
25. Hillen M. Bereidheid tot samenwerking met de welzijnssector bij leerkrachten in het secundair onderwijs. Welwijs 1993; 4(3): 28–31
26. Regionale suicidaliteitsnota. Brussel: Comete voor Bijzondere Jeugdzorg Turnhout, Sint-Niklaas & Centrum ter Preventie van Zelfmoord, 1992
27. Andriessen K, Verthriest G, Veys T "...en wat met zelfmoord?" Schets van een project. Welwijs 1995; 6(3): 32–38

28. Crabtree G. A basic manual on intervention with persons at risk of self harm. Texas: Abilene MHMR Center, 1993

29. Rollez A. Ta vie j' m' en mele. Prevention du suicide a l'Universite de Montreal. Volume 2. Universite de Montreal: Table de Prevention du suicide, 1992.

30. Saul D. Let's Live! A school based suicide awareness and intervention program. Inservice guide ant teachers' resource manual. British Colobia: Council for the family, 1992

31. "20 manieren om zelfmoord te ... bespreken in klas of groep." Brussel: Centrum ter Preventie van Zelfmoord & Ministerie van de Vlaamse Gemeenschap, 1995

32. Garland A, Zigler E. Adolescent suicide prevention. Current research and policy implications. Am Psychologist 1993; 48(2): 169–182

33. Kalafat J, Elias M. An evaluation of a school based suicide awareness intervention. Suicide Life Threat Behav 1994; 24: 224–233

34. Ploeg J, Ciliska D, Dobbins M, Hayward S, Thomas H, Underwood J. A systematic overview of adolescent suicide prevention programs. Can J Public Health 1996; 87(5): 319–324

35. Vieland V, Whittle B, Garland A, Hicks R, Shaffer D. The impact of curriculum-based suicide prevention programs for teenagers: an 18 month follow-up. J Am Acad Child Adolsc Psychiatry 1991; 30: 811–815

36. Crabtree C, Baum D, Hennig C. Summary on research findings on adolescent suicide intervention. Paper on 'Mental health CPR for adolescents' 1993. Montreal: XVIIth IASP Congress, 1992

37. Orbach I, Bar-Joseph H. The impact of a suicide prevention program for adolescents on suicidal tendencies, hopelessness, ego identity and coping. Suicide Life Threat Behav 1993; 23: 120–129

38. Dryfoos JG. Adolescents at risk: a summation of work in the field, programs and policies. J Adolesc Health 1991; 12: 630–637

39. Rutz W, von Knorring L, Walinder J. Frequency of suicide on Gotland after systematic postgraduate education of general practitioners. Acta Psychiatr Scand 1989; 80: 151–154

40. McDaniel W, Rock M, Grigg J. Suicide prevention at a United States Navy Training Command. Military Medicine 1990; 155: 173–175

41. Rutz W, von Knorring L, Walinder J. Long-term effects of an educational program for general practitioners given by the Swedish Committee for the prevention and treatment of depression. Acta Psychiatr Scand 1992; 85: 83–88

33

PARASUICIDE AND SUICIDE PREVENTION PROGRAMME

An Experience in Kuala Lumpur

Habil Hussain

Department of Psychological Medicine
University of Malaya Medical Centre, Kuala Lumpur, Malaysia

1. INTRODUCTION

It has been noted that although the numbers of parasuicide and suicide cases has increased steadily in Malaysia, an awareness in prevention, especially at a national level, is still minimal. The topic on prevention, of suicide has, on many occasions, been confined to certain services where people have an interest in a related subject. Unfortunately, their numbers are still very small. Even if one took a look at health care settings throughout Malaysia, awareness pertaining to suicide and prevention was still not recognised at the same level as other public health problems.

Among the reasons why Malaysians still have strong denial of suicide could be their cultural orientation which strongly prohibits suicide. The cultural prohibition to suicide is further reinforced by official national attitudes which blame suicide as western disease. Ignorance about suicide is another reason for the development of these processes. The lack of understanding and ignorance about suicide among health workers has its own implications for preventive programmes on suicide in this country. For instance, community services which have a special interest in dealing with suicidal patients are almost negligible in numbers and the lack of such service has led to the excessive inflow of suicidal patients to health centres. Ignorance to the nature of suicide has often lead doctors and health workers to provide only medical and surgical treatments without any effort to help patients overcome their psychological distress. There have also been times when health workers have ridiculed patients who have come to get help from them after their attempted suicide.

In acknowledging the above problems, my department was prompted to draw up a programme whereby doctors and supporting staff could become more aware of suicidal people and the proper way of handling these patients. The main objective of this programme is to help reduce suicide cases in the hospital and also to prevent reattempting

Suicide Prevention, edited by Kosky *et al.*
Plenum Press, New York, 1998

suicide among parasuicide cases. It also hoped to build a network with relevant community services so as to prevent suicide which happens in the community.

2. DEFINING THE RISK GROUP

Initial steps taken were to review studies related to suicidal attempts in the Klang Valley, where the University hospital is situated. All previous available local studies were hospital based and not community based. In these studies it was noted that young females who came from low socio-economic background were groups noted to be at risk for parasuicide. In studies where comparison between the three races were involved, Indians seem to be over represented and Malays were consistently noted to have lower rates of parasuicide. Nevertheless, if one looked at a yearly pattern of parasuicide admission rate, it could be clearly seen that there had been a gradual increase of parasuicide among Malays. Hence, the present belief that the Malays are protected against parasuicide is probably no longer true.

3. CAUSES OF PARASUICIDE

The complexities in the social factors contributing to suicide which is found in other countries, are similarly shared in Malaysia. There is no single causal factor which, so far, can be identified as predominant. What can be concluded, is that the cause of suicidal behaviour is multifactorial. Many attempters were experiencing psychosocial stresses prior to their attempt. These included difficult ineterpersonal relationships, financial difficulties, chronic and severe pain and job losses. Only a small proportion had been actually diagnosed as having major psychiatric conditions.

In a study done to determine vulnerability, it was noted that a significant proportion of parasuicides had a past history of an unhappy childhood. Several factors which contributed included early parental loss, and a past history of battered child syndrome. It was also noted that family and marital discord due, either to divorce or addicted parents, were vulnerability factors, which predisposed to adult parasuicide.

4. THE RISK OF SUICIDE

In a one year follow up study, it was noted that there was a definite risk of suicide for parasuicide cases that were admitted to the University Hospital Kuala Lumpur. Risk factors noted to correlate with those who repeated and those who died included high intention for suicide, underlying major psychiatric conditions and old age.

In daily practice, suicide risk is indicated by older age, male gender, high lethality methods and a stressful situation. However, there are wide individual variations which can modify this general risk, which needs to be taken into account as well. Failure to indicate this variation can result in high risk patients receiving no treatment or premature discharge from the hospital. Hence, the general rule given to all doctors who see parasuicide patients, is to admit them for a minimum period of twenty four hours observation.

5. MANAGEMENT PROBLEMS

Most often a situation is encountered when the patient's motives for attempted suicide were not clear. The fear of hospital, loss of face and the shame of bringing embarrassment to their families, were some factors which could further complicate our understanding in individual cases. The doctor's attitude and his or her attitude to parasuicide patients could also have a major influence in understanding the patient's actual intention. For example, if one assumes that parasuicide is nothing more than seeking attention and a cry for help, then one can be judgmental or careless in one's assessment. These attitudes could also indicate one's denial for discovering the patient's motivation for the parasuicide.

In attempting to understand cases of suicide at the University Hospital the following contributing factors were noted:

1. Failure, especially by medical staff in a non-psychiatric setting, to recognise early signs and symptoms which indicate suicide. This happened when parasuicide patients were admitted to non-psychiatric wards and were treated medically.
2. Staff were unable to notice the urgency of the patients' suicidal gestures.
3. Staff tried to manage difficult suicidal patients on their own without psychiatric referral.

Those who were noted to be particularly in need of training were nurses and doctors from non-psychiatric wards, medical students and student nurses. Recently, training has also been extended to private practitioners and volunteer groups like Befrienders, who have shown interest in the management of suicidal patients.

6. TRAINING MODULES

Our training is provided in both lecture form and clinical presentations. Topics covered include:

I. basic knowledge on how to identify early signs and symptoms of suicide;
II. probable causes;
III. common problems encountered in parasuicide patients, which include the patients refusal for admission, risk of reattempting suicide either in the ward or after discharge and the impacts on their families;
IV. basic counselling for suicidal patients, supportive psychotherapy and crisis intervention.

REFERENCES

Hussain H.: Study on eight-years pattern of parasuicide admission to University Hospital Kuala Lumpur presented in 1st Malaysian colloquium on depression 1995.

Murugesan G, Yeoh H: Demographic and psychiatric aspect of attempted suicide. Medical Journal Malaysia 1978; 23:102–12

Hussain H, Ganesvara T, Agnes L: Attempted suicide in Kuala Lumpur. Asia Pacific Journal of Public Health 1992;6:5–6

Hussain H, Hmann N: Family psychopathology and childhood experience of parasuicide in University Hospital Kuala Lumpur. Asian Journal of Psychiatry 1993;2:10–16

Hussain H, Ganesvaran T, Anges L: Assessing suicidal risk in parasuicide admitted to University Hospital Kuala Lumpur. Family Physician 1992;4:22–24

Hussain H: Health seeking behaviour of depressed parasuicide patients in primary health care clinic. Asian Medical Journal 1995;38:1–5

34

FOCUS GROUPS WITH YOUTH TO ENHANCE KNOWLEDGE OF WAYS TO ADDRESS YOUTH SUICIDE

Carolyn Coggan and Pam Patterson

Injury Prevention Research Centre
Department of Community Health
University of Auckland
New Zealand

1. INTRODUCTION

This paper illustrates the use of focus groups to enhance knowledge of ways to address youth suicide. The impetus for this study, which was one aspect of a programme of research focusing on youth suicide, was the statistics which show that New Zealand has the highest rate of reported youth suicide among industrialized (OECD) countries (World Health Organisation, 1993). In 1993, the male youth suicide rate was 39.9 per 100,000 and the female rate was 6.9 per 100,000. The New Zealand male youth suicide rate is three times higher than the United Kingdom rate in 1993. Over the period 1974 to 1993, the male suicide rate among 15–24 year olds in New Zealand has quadrupled (Disley & Coggan, 1996). In addition, suicide attempts which do not result in death are a significant concern resulting in approximately 1000 hospital admissions among young people aged 15–24 years (Coggan, Fanslow, Norton, 1995). Within New Zealand there is a higher rate of attempted suicide among females than males, which is similar to international trends (Coggan et al, 1995; Diekstra & Gulbinat, 1993).

While there is an extensive body of literature in the area of youth suicide (for example, Kachur, Potter, Powell, et al, 1995), no qualitative studies were found which incorporate young people's views on ways to address the issue. The qualitative research technique of focus group discussion has been identified as relevant in the formative stages of programme design and development (Pope & Mays, 1995; Murphy, Cockburn & Murphy, 1992). This is because focus group discussions explore a predefined topic, yet are open and flexible. It has also been suggested that the stimulating nature of the focus group discussion has the potential to yield more and richer information than do individual interviews (Morgan, 1988). However, when discussing suicide with young people, there is the

Suicide Prevention, edited by Kosky *et al.*
Plenum Press, New York, 1998

potential to normalise this behaviour (Beautrais, 1994; Goldney, 1989), although the effect of this is still somewhat controversial (Davidson, Rosenberg, Mercy, et al, 1989). Nevertheless, a major ethical decision to be resolved prior to proceeding with this study was: is it appropriate to discuss suicide with young people in any forum? After extensive consultation it was decided to proceed, with the following proviso: i) that groups be randomly selected but that the recruitment of individuals be voluntary; ii) that all individuals be provided with a debriefing session, and iii) that each participant be offered the opportunity of follow-up counselling.

The aim of this study was to ensure that young people had a "voice" in the design of intervention strategies to address youth suicide in the Auckland region of New Zealand. The specific objectives of the study were to describe: i) the pressures young people face; ii) whether suicide is an issue for young people; iii) the barriers to utilising existing services/resources; and, iv) what strategies could be introduced that would be appropriate and accessible for young people.

2. METHODS

A list of all potential groups representing young people (WHO definition: 15–24 years) within the Auckland region was compiled and stratified by geographical area. This list included: secondary schools; technical institutes; universities; and youth groups. From this list eight schools, two tertiary educational institutions and two youth groups were randomly selected. Organisations identified were personally contacted and all agreed to participate in the focus group discussions. The recruitment of individuals was voluntary and it was left to the organisation to recruit individuals to participate in the group discussions. Although organisations were given the ideal criteria for recruitment of individuals (same gender, age group and ethnic groupings) (Morgan, 1993), in some cases this did not occur. Several methods for the recruitment of individuals were adopted. These included: tertiary institutions placing posters calling for volunteers; an oral presentation in some schools' assemblies; and a combination of both of these for the youth groups. Publicity concerning the recruitment of volunteers stressed that the topic to be discussed was youth suicide prevention. All volunteers were provided with an information sheet prior to their agreeing to participate in the focus group discussions. The information sheet gave details of the subject and the purpose of the discussion, explained how the focus groups would operate and stressed the voluntary nature of the group.

All focus groups were conducted by the same person, a young, experienced group facilitator, able to relate well with youth. Sessions were held at a time and place convenient to the individual participants and the host organisations. Each participant completed a consent form and demographic profile at the beginning of the group discussion. The same interview schedule was used for each focus group although this operated as a flexible guide rather than a structured protocol. This interview schedule began with a general discussion on pressures faced by youth and ways to address these. It then moved on to a scenario 'A close friend has told you that they are thinking seriously of ending their life' and probes were used to obtain information on ways to reduce youth suicide. Each group discussion lasted approximately one-and-a-half hours and with the permission of the participants, all discussions were recorded on an audiotape. At the conclusion, a debriefing session was held and participants were supplied with a list of counselling services.

Immediately after each group discussion, tapes were fully transcribed. Transcriptions were read several times to allow researchers to develop agreement and an understanding of the 'themes' of responses. Two researchers working independently developed and applied codes to the data. Small subsets of these analyses were compared on a regular basis as a reliability measure (approximately 75% of codes were subject to reliability checks). In the event of a discrepancy the two researchers worked together to negotiate a settlement relating to 'what do we think this means.' This type of inter-researcher agreement helped to ensure the validity of the coding scheme (Patton, 1986). Once coding had been completed and all discrepancies resolved, the data was reduced to one set. Subgroup analysis was not possible because the voluntary nature of the groups resulted in the composition of some groups being mixed in terms of gender and ethnicity.

A word processing package was used to 'cut and paste' the relevant themes within the category headings of the interview schedule: pressures faced by young people; whether suicide was an issue for young people; barriers to the use of services/resources; and potential strategies to prevent youth suicide. Within each category, themes, including contradictory points of views were identified. Findings, together with pertinent quotations, were then organised into a draft report which was distributed to the participants, via the host organisations. This ensured that the information, as reported, accurately reflected the messages that had been conveyed. Following minor alterations, a report was prepared and disseminated to participants.

Ethical approval for this study was obtained from the University of Auckland Human Subjects Ethics committee.

3. FINDINGS

3.1. Focus Group Participants

Twelve focus groups were conducted. Group size ranged from eight to 16, with an average of 12 participants. In all, 140 young people took part in the study, ranging in age from 16 to 24 years (mean age 18.7). Sixty-four percent of participants described their ethnicity as European/Pakeha, 24% as Maori and 12% as Pacific Islands. Just over half of the participants were male (52%), with slightly more participants still attending school (59%).

Debriefing sessions followed each focus group discussion. All the participants indicated that they had enjoyed the experience and stated that they welcomed the opportunity to discuss the complexity of the issues surrounding suicide in such a safe and supportive environment. The use of the scenario was seen by all the participants as an excellent way of introducing the topic. None of the participants sought counselling as a result of their participation in the focus group discussions. Follow-up enquiries with the host organisations indicated that none of the participants appeared to have experienced any adverse effects.

3.2. Pressures Faced by Young People

The first question asked of each focus group was, 'What are some of the pressures young people face which may be different to children or older people?' There were a number of pressures that young people identified as being significant, specifically: i) negative societal perceptions of young people; ii) unrealistic expectations to do well in exams; iii) to conform to a particular body image; iv) to be a macho male; v) peer pressure: to take drugs, drink alcohol; vi) violence: physical/sexual abuse; vii) conflict between needing to be independent and forced dependency due to lack of jobs, money and material possessions; viii) existing in two cultures; ix) relationship difficulties: family, peer group, friends, boy/girl friends; x) sexuality difficulties: involving both homosexuality and heterosexuality; xi) emotional pressures: to be an adult and child at the same time.

No one pressure stood out as being overly important. Rather, it was suggested that it is the build-up of a number of pressures that leave young people feeling stressed and unhappy. This pressure seems to come from all angles — family, friends and media.

> "lots of expectations from everybody ... you must be either Elle Macpherson or Jean-Claude Van Damme, you must have perfect skin, you must be at least 6 feet 7"

Pacific Islands youth talked about the pressures of belonging to two different cultures. They lived in a European world but were expected to conform to the cultural norms of their families.

> "the Island ways are different to European ways, but they want you to do it the same way they were brought up"

The groups found that overall emotional pressures arose from the interaction of the many situations faced by young people.

> "sometimes it's endless problems that are building on one another ... it might be one particular thing that sets it off but it's lots of things building up"

3.3. Suicide: Is It an Issue for Young People?

The majority of young people, who participated in the focus group discussions, indicated that suicide was something that, at this point in their lives, they came in contact with. Suicide was something they talked about with friends and thought of when things went wrong. However, whereas issues surrounding sex were discussed in many different forums today, they felt that the issue of suicide was a hidden one. They felt that there was a need for more open dialogue on suicide between the youth themselves and educators, caregivers, politicians and others who work in the area.

> "it has to be an open subject now, it can't be just hidden, needs to come out in the open, the attitude of society has to change. People should know more about it, and it's happening ... people need to feel okay about having problems, I mean really dealing with the gut issues of what's going on instead of hiding them and sweeping them under the carpet"

Using the scenario technique, young people were then asked to identify what they considered to be the warning signs of a suicidal friend. Three themes emerged --- risk-taking behaviours, unusual actions and personality changes. Young people identified peers as wanting to harm themselves when they took risks with their lives by: jumping out of moving cars; getting in cars with drunken drivers who were "wasted off their face"; and overly heavy use of alcohol and drugs. Examples of unusual actions included: giving away prized possessions; talking about finalising things; seeing someone they had not seen for a long time; and self-mutilation. Personality changes, which were identified as the most common warning signs of a suicidal friend, included: depression; shutting off; crying; constant mood swings; false fronts: rarely happy over anything; and being withdrawn and uninterested in everything. Although all groups could identify perceived warning signs of suicidal friends they also indicated that sometimes it was hard to tell and often it was only on reflection, after a friend had attempted suicide, that the signs became obvious.

"sometimes you can't tell; they hide it really well ...the signs aren't always obvious"

3.4. Barriers to Utilising Existing Services/Resources

A number of barriers were identified which restricted young people making use of the existing services/resources that are available. The major barrier was a complete lack of knowledge of where or whom they could turn to in a crisis. Many participants stated that if they were going to tell anyone they were feeling suicidal it would be their closest friend. However, some participants stated that many young people were forced to cope alone with a very difficult situation. As a consequence, one of the coping mechanisms for young people in times of crisis is to "toke up" which, to them, relates to taking drugs and drinking alcohol simultaneously.

"they either hide in a bottle or drugs, anything that sort of alienates them so they don't feel like they're in their own body, this way they don't have to deal with the crap that's going on"

Participants stated that adolescence and young adulthood, were more often than not, difficult times for family dynamics and this created a barrier to utilising the resources available within families. For example, participants stated that family members were over protective and often judgemental. It was also stated that parents tended to trivialise the concerns of young people and that this often results in young people not confiding in their families at a crucial time in their lives. One participants recalled a sentence left in a note by a close friend of his who had recently committed suicide

"when I was here, did you realise I was one of your kids and precious"

Most young people knew very little about the existing services for youth who were feeling down and/or contemplating suicide. They had heard of places such as Youthline or Lifeline but knew very little of what they had to offer or how they were run.

" me myself I don't know many services, and besides, like school counsellors, or like my friends, or just a pastor or a minister or something, or a relative but there's not many organisations that I know of"

Another reason for not using services/resources was their friends' experiences of them. Participants indicated that young people would not use services/resources if their friends reported negative experiences of those services/resources. A negative experience by a friend or a friend of a friend was a strong barrier for subsequent referral. These negative experiences either with a professional, friend, or whanau (extended family), left a feeling of isolation among at-risk young people. Group participants stated that young people placed tremendous importance on trust. They wanted to be able to trust counsellors, their parents and church leaders. Often this trust was broken and this led to them and their friends not using many agencies in the area of helping young people.

"sometimes you can't trust them with problems ... at my last school no-one would ever go and see the counsellors because they used to tell everyone"

Another barrier identified by participants was that, amongst young people, there was an overall feeling that health professionals, such as doctors, psychiatrists and psychologists, were too impersonal, cost too much, and that it took too long to get an appointment. The feeling of just being a statistic or another case came across very strongly. Participants indicated that because you were there on an appointment basis there was insufficient time, which was reflected in the way you were treated. The young people felt health professionals were into "diagnosis" and dealing with the immediate rather than the underlying problems.

> "maybe there's not enough people like psychologists and psychiatrists ... but then maybe that's a good thing as they can really screw you up"

The final barrier identified by participants related to access problems due to the cost involved and/or lack of transport. For many young people, access to services that might be beneficial to them in a crisis situation were not easily attainable. This was due to the actual cost of the services and/or the indirect costs such as transport to and from services. For example, many young people did not have access to either their own transport or that of family members (due to their desire for confidentiality). Therefore they were restricted to using the public transport system or having close access so they could walk. As a consequence, participants argued for services which are accessible by a good public transport service or, alternatively, are close to where young people often go.

> "while health workers are a minimal part of your life, you don't get sick that often and, when you do, you can't afford to go, or alternatively you can't afford to get there."

3.5. Potential Youth Suicide Prevention Strategies

Four strategies for reducing suicide and promoting health and wellbeing among young people were highlighted by the group discussions. These have been organised under the following themes: information initiatives; education sector initiatives; health sector initiatives; and legislation issues.

3.5.1. Information Initiatives. There were a variety of ways that young people saw for transmitting information to all sectors of the community to inform them of the issues regarding youth suicide. Participants strongly argued that more information-type resources needed to be made available for youth and those who worked with them. Such messages could be disseminated through schools, by posters strategically placed where young people "hang out" and through the media of television and radio. It was felt that the media in various forms could play a high-profile role in getting the message across about suicide prevention among young people by being the vehicles by which young people received information on what to do and where to go if they were in need of help.

> "the media are part of everyone's life. It's part of society and the media could have a major part in educating everyone, like it would be the most valuable asset."

It was emphasised that any resources developed would need to include information on the warning signs as well as contain information on where to go for help. Posters/pamphlets were seen as good ways of obtaining information without having to identify yourself. They said that such information, if it is to be of any use to young people, needed to be displayed in areas including bus shelters, fast food outlets, and public toilets as these were identified as places young people frequently visited. Participants also favoured the use of large billboards around town to let their peers know of services that are available to them. It was stressed that any messages developed would need to be relevant to young people living in the 1990s.

However, it was seen as important that the issue of suicide not be over-dramatised thus leading to glamorization and that any resource developed which deals with suicide not be taken lightly.

> "they've got to stop making it really glamorous...I just read an article... about Kurt Cobain, and it just made him and his situation which in any other social area he'd be really down and out and on the streets and really a really sad depressing person, they turned him into a megastar that shot himself and I mean he has a lot of influence over thousands of teenagers in this world and that's really scary"

3.5.2. Education Sector Initiatives. Participants stated that as educational institutions are the place where the majority of young people spend a large part of their lives, what they learn here was going to have far-reaching effects. They therefore considered that it was an important place for young people to get positive messages about themselves. Consequently, all participants argued that there was an urgent need for educational institutions to introduce curriculum-based programmes that deal with the issues surrounding conflict resolution, overcoming depression, dangers of excessive substance abuse, stress, being happy, and ways of handling the emotional trauma of relationship breakups and coping with sexual orientation. Most participants stated that having a broad focus would probably do more to help to reduce the number of young people contemplating self-harm than programmes which concentrated only on suicide.

> "You've got to address it maybe as coping with stress or drugs or having high self-esteem as opposed to suicide"

While the majority of participants agreed that school-based programmes were needed, a large proportion of the focus group participants indicated that a general education programme which focused on the wider community was also important. It was felt that everyone needed to be aware that suicide was a problem and, as a consequence, a community awareness campaign which highlighted the warning signs and where to turn to for help was considered worthy of further investigation.

> "it's the education of the community as a whole, not necessarily just in schools, that is important"

3.5.3. Health Sector Initiatives. The general feeling among the groups was that there needed to be more people out there who specialised in young people's health who had the resources to promote the health status of youth. Specifically, the participants favoured a "one stop" concept for youth health which was friendly and which also provided "social support" as well as "medical treatment."

> "I mean if you've got a friend who you think is suicidal, is there anywhere you can take him which will assess the seriousness of his threats. It's easy if they have made a physical attempt but verbal threats are the ones we really need help with"

Most participants also believed that there was a real need for emergency department staff to be better trained in dealing with young people in times of crisis. They felt that emergency departments in hospital clinics are too busy to be able to deal with anything other than the practicalities of "treating" the physical symptoms. In addition, participants wanted facilities for young people which would provide meaningful follow-up care and support.

"My friend went to the hospital and all they did was pump out her stomach and send her home ... I think they gave her an appointment with someone but she didn't go as she wasn't sure it would help"

3.5.4. Legislation. The young people were generally scathing about the role of politicians in relation to youth issues. The young people felt politicians did not regard them as important and that this was reflected in the way that young people were treated in the policy arena. As a consequence group participants did not hold much hope of legislation being introduced which would improve the lives of young New Zealanders. They often felt that high expectations were placed on young people to behave and perform in certain ways that were beneficial to the country but that they were kept under-resourced and powerless to express their needs.

"they (politicians) don't try to impress young people. In fact they just try to impress the general New Zealand taxpayer"

All participants endorsed the view that politicians could relieve some of the stresses that young people are coping with by reducing the fees that students have to pay for education, by introducing student allowances for all, and by making it easier for young people to get meaningful jobs once they have finished their education. Some of the participants felt that often young people found themselves in a double bind. On the one hand they were expected to do well at school, pass exams and then get a job, but on the other they were not only expected to pay for a higher education but at the end their job prospects were extremely limited.

"there's a need for more job creation schemes ... there's a real feeling of hopelessness which is a big suicide factor ... what's out there for me, what am I going to do with my future, there's no jobs, there's education costs"

4. SUMMARY AND IMPLICATIONS

Before discussing the implications of the key points identified in this study, it is important to first place them within the context that they were collected. The individuals who participated in these focus groups had volunteered to participate and were aware that the topic to be discussed was youth suicide. They were a small self-selected sample and most of their comments indicated previous involvement with suicide, which may have been their reason for volunteering. For example, they stated that they were aware of the indications of a suicidal friend and were more interested in finding out what to do in times of crisis.

The study identified a number of pressures faced by young people. In general the young people who participated in the focus group discussions felt that suicide was an issue that was a reality for them and their peers. They felt that a build-up of a series of crises rather than one major issue contributed to suicidal ideation and behaviour. They also felt young people would try to cope with a crisis on their own by "toking up' and/or drinking to obliteration point and participating in other risk-taking behaviours. They also found it difficult to cope with the complexities of suicide when the whole area was a taboo subject. One explanation for this is that exposure to suicidal behaviour of others, either personally or through the media, has been identified as a risk factor for suicide (Goldney, 1989; Shafii, Carrigan, Whittinghill, et al, 1985). The three themes which emerged from this study with regard to the perceived warning signs of a suicidal friend (risk-taking behaviours, unusual actions and personality changes) are comparable to those identified in the academic literature (Beautrais, Joyce & Mulder, 1996; Brent, Perper, Moritz, et al, 1993; Shaffer, Garland, Gould, et al, 1988).

This study highlighted a range of strategies that may have implications for the prevention of youth suicide. The finding that young people would turn to their friends or peers if they were feeling suicidal has important implications for the planning of future health promotion strategies. The fact that a lack of knowledge was identified as the major barrier to youth using existing services/resources suggests that health promotion awareness campaigns which provide information on where young people could access help may be worthy of further investigation. Specific suggestions as to how this information should be related, such as through the use of billboards and posters strategically placed, were outlined. Further consultation would be required before proceeding with any such campaign. Participants also stated that life-skills programmes needed to be developed which focused on conflict resolution, overcoming depression, substance abuse and coping with relationship breakups.

In conclusion, this qualitative investigation has highlighted many areas for further investigation: health promotion media campaigns targeted at providing information on how and where to access information; counter-measures to the view that drinking helps to alleviate problems; the development and implementation of ways to improve the identification and referral of "at-risk" young people; and the allocation of resources to ensure that emergency department staff have the skills, time and the availability of specialist referral staff to ensure that appropriate clinical care is provided. Through the use of debriefing sessions, it was also found that the participants endorsed focus groups as a suitable way to discuss the topic of suicide, with the process being reported to be of value to the participants, an overwhelmingly "positive experience."

ACKNOWLEDGMENTS

Our sincere appreciation to all the participants who allowed us to explore their opinions, feelings, attitudes and behaviours on a sensitive topic is acknowledged. This project was funded by the Northern Regional Health Authority, with the research being conducted during the tenure of a Training Fellowship of the Health Research Council of New Zealand.

REFERENCES

Beautrais A. (1994). Publicity and Suicide. Canterbury Suicide Project Bulletin No. 4, Canterbury Suicide Project. Christchurch.

Beautrais AL, Joyce PR and Mulder RT. (1996). Risk factors for serious suicide attempts among youth aged 13 through 24 years. Journal of the American Academy of Child and Adolescent Psychiatry, 30, 741–748.

Brent DA, Perper JA, Moritz G, et al. (1993). Psychiatric risk factors of adolescent suicide: a case-control study. Journal of the American Academy of Child and Adolescent Psychiatry 32(3), 521–9.

Coggan CA, Fanslow JL, Norton RN. (1995). Intentional Injury in New Zealand. Analysis and Monitoring Report No 4. Public Health Commission. Wellington.

Davidson LE, Rosenberg ML, Mercy JA, et al. (1989). An Epidemiological study of risk factors in two teenage suicide clusters. Journal American Medical Association, 262(19), 2687–92.

Diekstra RFW & Gulbinat W. (1993). The epidemiology of suicidal behaviour: A review of three continents. World Health Statistics Quarterly, 46, 52–68.

Disley B & Coggan CA. (1996). Youth Suicide in New Zealand. Journal of Crisis and Suicide Prevention, 17 (3), 116–122.

Goldney R. (1989). Suicide: the Role of the Media. Australian and New Zealand Journal of Psychiatry 23, 30–4.

Kachur SP, Potter LB, Powell KE, Rosenberg ML. (1995). Suicide: Epidemiology, prevention, treatment. In Adolescent Medicine: State of the Art Reviews, Edited by KK Christoffel and CW Runyan, Hanley and Belfus, Philadelphia, 6(2), 171–182.

Morgan DL. (1988). Focus groups as qualitative research. Sage Publications. Beverly Hills.

Morgan DL. (1993). Successful Focus Groups: Advancing the State of the Art. Sage Publications. Newbury Park.

Murphy B, Cockburn J, Murphy M. (1992). Focus Groups in Health Research. Health Promotion Journal of Australia 2(2), 37–40.

Patton, MQ. (1986). Utilization-focused evaluation. Sage Publications. Beverly Hills.

Pope C & Mays N. (1995). Reaching the parts other methods cannot reach: an introduction to qualitative methods in health and health services research. British Medical Journal, 311, 42–5.

Shaffer D, Garland A, Gould M, et al. (1988). Preventing teenage suicide: A critical review, Journal of the American Academy of Child and Adolescent Psychiatry, 27 (6), 675–87.

Shafii M, Carrigan S, Whittinghill R, et al. (1985). Psychological autopsy of completed suicide in children and adolescents. American Journal of Psychiatry, 142(9), 1061–4.

World Health Organisation. (1993). World Health Statistics Annual. World Health Organisation. Geneva.

35

REACHING THE SUICIDAL IN RURAL COMMUNITIES*

Lakshmi Ratnayeke

Sri Lanka, Sumithrayo

The highest rates of suicide in Sri Lanka are amongst the rural farming communities and tea plantation workers. You could attribute this to the free availability of lethal agrochemicals which are widely used in both the farming and estate sectors. The commonest method of suicide in these communities is by the ingestion of these poisons whose potency is such that the victim often dies before being taken to a hospital which may be several miles away in the nearest town.

Remote village areas seldom have access to social services that could offer support in times of crisis, and village traditions discourage the villagers from revealing their difficulties to strangers. There are also strong cultural biases against revealing personal problems and difficulties to others in the village or even to family members. In a village setting, family loyalty, family honour and maintaining face is of great importance. These norms and traditions are barriers to people contacting a crisis intervention centre for help.

In a country where only one in hundred has a telephone and where these telephones are mainly located in the towns, far away from the rural areas, and access to a Befriending Centre in the town by road is not easy and is time consuming as well as unaffordable financially, communication becomes difficult. The situation is further exacerbated by strong cultural biases real or perceived in talking about ones personal problems to a stranger.

Rigid cultural and caste restrictions that ostracize certain communities such as the lower castes, preventing them from mixing with others and completely isolating them and superstitions that defy reason play a major role in village life. For example, if there are three girls and one boy in a family it is considered unlucky and one of the girls would be sent away from home, or should the village astrologer decide that on of the children in a family is unlucky for the parents, it would result in the child suffering a similar fate of being sent away from home to live with an aunt, uncle or grand-parent or whoever would be willing to accept the child.

---

* "Part of this paper was first published as 'Suicide and Crisis Intervention in Rural Communities in Sri Lanka', Crisis, volume 17, number 4, 1996"

Suicide Prevention, edited by Kosky et al.
Plenum Press, New York, 1998

A complete lack of privacy in their lives coupled with the need for maintaining face, curiosity and the total disregard for the privacy of others, extreme poverty, alcoholism, a lack of self esteem and the fatalistic attitude that accepts everything that happens as fate and therefore inevitable, the belief that talking about one's problems does not help, the suspicion of strangers and their difficulty in trusting outsiders are some of the constraints that make traditional befriending in a rural community an uphill task.

The Befrienders have been making efforts to address this situation and the volunteers attached to our rural centres have been trying to adapt traditional befriending to suit the local situation. For example they have been visiting surrounding estates and villages on market days, displaying posters, distributing Sumithrayo brochures and offering open air Befriending.

They have also instituted a regular programme of hospital visits to meet with individuals recovering from suicide attempts. If the patient approves a volunteer visits his or her family at home. The volunteer helps to smooth the Callers return home by helping the family members to come to terms with what has happened and thus to accept the individual when he or she returns home. They also hear other versions of the circumstances leading to the suicidal attempt and this helps them to understand the situation better and respond in a more helpful way. During these visits the volunteer also offers support and befriending to family members, some of whom may also have suicidal feelings. They try and strengthen rapport among the members of the family, and also connect them to institutions that can offer help in areas that the befrienders cannot.

An added benefit of the volunteers visit to a village is that they are able to talk about suicide and suicide prevention with the curious who attach themselves to the volunteers as spectators and also invite the volunteers to hold awareness programmes in the village. They also seem to attract letters from villagers who have hitherto been too shy or apprehensive to visit the Befriending Centre in town.

Although the hospital and home visiting programme is an important outreach effort, it has its limitations. There is little or no privacy in the hospital, nor is there privacy during the home visits, since the arrival of an outsider attracts great attention in the village. Also only male volunteers can make visits to the village due to cultural restrictions and travel difficulties, so individuals who would prefer to speak to a female cannot be accommodated. Moreover the volunteer does not make an advance appointment for fear of arousing alarm and suspicion, so those whom he intends to meet may not be available when he arrives. This is time consuming and expensive. The most important limitation however, is that the hospital and home visits reach only those who have already made a serious suicidal attempt.

The Sumithrayo Befrienders had designed and tested an outreach and prevention programme located in the village and more in keeping with local norms. Based on this the Befrienders are at the moment conducting a fully documented pilot project in a village close to one of our rural Centres, to prove positively the efficacy of the programme. The Befrienders there have organised a series of monthly meetings in the test village, these meetings being open to all in the village.

Each meeting is focussed on common problems and situations faced by villagers such as spouses leaving for employment in the Middle East leaving the family in disarray, alcoholism, failure of crops ad resultant indebtedness, marital disharmony etc. Practical information and common problem solving strategies are discussed, as well as the emotional dimensions of the problems. Interpersonal problem solving communicational skills, recognising and responding to other's feelings are emphasised. Some of the meetings are devoted to knowledge specific to recognising and preventing suicides and to dealing with suicidal emergencies.

As in urban areas, in the village too there are different levels of society which could be broadly divided into three levels; an upper level which is quite small, would consist of the village priests and a few land owners who would be owning most of the village land. The middle level would be a larger group comprised of village shop keepers, school teachers and farmers cultivating their own lands. The lower level which is the largest group would consist of Chena cultivators and other labour class people dependant on the meagre production of their little vegetable plots or a daily wage whenever they are able to find work. This is the level most difficult to reach and who are most vulnerable to suicide.

Over the generations, they have known only privation and penury as realities of life. Their lack of self esteem and self depreciation are not only self destructive but also a hindrance to their growth and liberation. The upper and middle levels attend the meetings and are open to new ideas but the apathy and fatalistic attitude in the lower strata prevent them from attending the meetings or seeking help.

Trying to overcome this obstacle the volunteers have taken to visiting their homes in the village and in an unobtrusive way giving them the opportunity of discussing their problems with the volunteers, gaining trust and acceptance and thereafter encouraging them to seek help when needed.

Two or three volunteers who have built up rapport with the villagers continue to visit the village on a fortnightly basis. During this time they not only visit homes, but also make themselves available in a well publicised location in the village that allows maximum privacy for befriending. It is hoped that one or two of the villagers who attended the initial meetings will have the aptitude and inclination for suicide prevention work. Such individuals may eventually be able to undertake continued befriending in their village or a nearby village, thus providing an on-going source of assistance for those who cannot travel to a Befriending Centre in town.

36

FROM THEORY TO PRACTICE: DO WE REALLY LISTEN

1 — The Clinical-Prevention Position[*]

Alan L. Berman

American Association of Suicidology

The United States is not among those countries with the highest rates of suicide. The latest available data from the World Health Organization places the rate of suicide in America near the median of those countries reporting data.

However, hidden within this moderate ranking are troubling trends. With particular attention to rates of completed suicide among our young, the U.S. documents a dramatic rise in rates since mid-century, such that the U.S. youth suicide rate is currently double the international rate for 15–24 year olds.

Within these statistics are even more disturbing trends. When United States rates for completed suicide are examined in 5-year cohorts over the last four decades, they show youth suicide rates are increasing most rapidly among latency age children and younger adolescents. (See Table 1)

These increases in youth suicide rates have been paralleled by increases in the use of firearms as the means for these suicides. Between 1967 and 1992, the proportion of suicides by firearms relative to suicides by all other methods used by U.S. 15–19 year olds increased from 55 to 68%. Between 1980 and 1992 rates of firearm suicides among 10–14 year olds jumped an alarming 132%. During this same period, overall rates of firearm suicides stayed essentially flat, if not suggesting a slight decline (9.93 to 9.60). Almost three of every four suicides by males between 15 and 19 years old is by firearm. The U. S. Centers for Disease Control and Prevention (CDC) has estimated that among persons 15–19 years old, firearm suicides accounted for 81% of the increase in overall suicide rates.

In 1987 the CDC established among its Year 2000 Health Objectives the goal of reducing youth suicides from a 1987 baseline for 15–19 year olds of 10.2 per 100,000 to a

---

[*] Keynote panel address delivered to XIX Congress of the International Association for Suicide Prevention, Adelaide, Australia, March 27, 1997.

Suicide Prevention, edited by Kosky *et al.*
Plenum Press, New York, 1998

Table 1. Youth suicide rates, United States of America 1952–1992

Age	1952 rate	1992 rate	% increase
10–14	0.3	1.7	567
15–19	2.8	10.8	386
20–24	5.6	14.9	266

target goal of 8.2/100,000. As of 1994, the 15–19 year old rate, however, was 11.1/100,000, an increase of 9%!

The evidence, thus far, appears to suggest that we are either not listening to ourselves or we have yet to master, develop, and propagate effective strategies to stem and prevent these tragic deaths among our young.

Research informs us that among the explanations for the rise in youth suicide rates, two empirically-based findings are of singular importance in informing our preventive intervention efforts:

1. the role of firearms in the home, available and accessible to the adolescent at-risk;
2. the increased prevalence of, and earlier median age of onset of, mental disorders associated with suicide.

I want to briefly describe to you two current approaches to dealing more effectively with our youth suicide problem, one, from a public health prevention model — focusing on our unique issue with firearms; the other from a clinical-intervention model — focusing on adolescents at risk.

1. THE CLINICAL MODEL

First, the clinical-intervention model. This model, established by my colleague David Jobes, is based on an early-detection, targeted treatment paradigm and attempts to alter the pathway to suicide (Jobes, 1995; Jobes and Berman, 1993). It is theory-driven, empirically-based, and, we believe, cost-effective. In the States, this last advantage has become singularly important in an era where clinicians are being increasingly invested in working with the evils of managed care. Most important, this model is built on a foundation of listening to the patient and inviting collaborative problem-solving.

I am not about to present to you any defense of this model from a perspective of its effectiveness. We are only beginning to apply it to a large data-set and to empirically test it. I do, however, wish to briefly share with you why we believe it will be effective and hope, at some later date, to give you evidence of our foresight.

In 1994 the state of Utah, a geographically large but small population state in the Intermountain region of the United States of America, had the 10th highest rate of suicide among all our states. Most alarmingly, among 15–44 year old males, suicide was the *leading* cause of death.

Dr. Jobes and I are working with a large managed behavioral medicine system that operates some 23 hospitals, one-half urban and one-half rural, and 17 outpatient mental health centers throughout Utah that service more than one and one-quarter million people.

We are introducing a model that will be implemented for all suicidal patients. It begins at intake and meshes with an existing screening and triage system modified to assess and track from a patient's initial visit his/her suicide risk and to describe for the clinician a prescriptive treatment model for minimizing and, perhaps, eliminating that risk.

At intake all patients are currently administered a 45-item Likert scaled questionnaire, the OQ-45, as a screening form. This new, well-researched and psychometrically-validated scale screens patients for their "emotional vital signs." Question number 8 asks the patient to rate from "never" to "almost always" whether they have "thoughts of ending their life." Answering anything other than "never" flags the patient who then is triaged to either inpatient or outpatient treatment and the initiation of our "suicide status tracking system."

At the index or first individual therapy session, both the patient and clinician complete the first "Suicide Status Form." The heart of this form lies in the 5-point Likert ratings and rankings given to the seven items and the overall rating of risk noted within a box near the top of the form.

The first five of these ratings refer to empirically-determined risk factors pain, stress, emotional upset, hopelessness and self regard. The astute observer will also note that they are theory-based. Beck's work underlies a further rating of hopelessness and Baumeister's another of self-regard. An earlier version of this measure has shown that these scales function quasi-independently and have good convergent and predictive validity and moderate reliability (Jobes, Jacoby, Cimbolic, and Hustead, in press). Thus, self-perceived impulsiveness and coping ability (items 6 and 7) are rated. The patient also is asked to describe whether their suicidality is motivated by intrapsychic and interpersonal factors and to describe concretely their current ambivalence in the form of reasons for living and reasons for dying. Lastly, a crucial item signals what the patient believes would shift his/her inertia away from suicidality.

Correspondingly, the clinician completes a parallel set of ratings along with a number of other focussed questions regarding risk assessment and treatment disposition and is asked to share his/her observations/ratings with the patient to begin a collaborative, in session discussion and focuses on what the treatment goals will be.

Treatment goals are not dictated, but are left to develop from this alliance between therapist and patient, to be arrived at by whatever means they feel will work. Moreover, they are readily targeted by the Status Form, as intensive therapeutic foci might, for example, be established to change any of the listed risk factors or to accomplish the "one thing" that would help the patient no longer feel suicidal. The therapist is free to work in whatever clinical-theoretical model desired, as long as the focus of treatment is to reduce and eliminate current suicidality. At each subsequent therapy session, the patient completes an OQ-45 to measure their current emotional vital signs. Non-suicidality is documented as reached when responses to the OQ-45's question number 8 are answered "never" over three consecutive sessions. At that point both patient and clinician are asked to complete a "Resolution Session" Status Form, again sharing their ratings and, on the patient's form, attempting to describe what specific impacts the clinical interventions had.

We are cautiously optimistic that we will be able to demonstrate that with this model it will take fewer sessions to reach a goal of no reported suicidality, that satisfaction ratings with treatment will go up, and that overall costs of treatment will go down.

As noted above, this model does not force clinicians into a manual-based, standardized treatment protocol. Instead, as a research-based treatment study, it uniquely allows intuition and personal preference to dictate clinical interventions, simply prescribing that they be targeted to the patient's stated foci. We expect, therefore, a high level of clinician compliance and interest in its implementation.

This model employs a dynamic scaling procedure, in contrast to typical static measures of risk. Note, in particular, that we are not employing an assessment form with some cut-off score defining suicide risk. If the patient is thinking about suicide, there is assumed to be risk.

It focuses on both process and outcome measures. It "listens to the patient," by forging a collaborative alliance between the patient and caregiver and encouraging a consultative role between clinician and supervisor. It ensures that no patient "falls through the cracks," as there is a session by session focus on patient-rated suicidality and a collaborative rating of an absence of suicidality at the resolution session. With the culture of caregiving in the U.S.A. in mind, it promises to be cost-effective, and litigation-defensive (an unfortunate necessity given our overdeveloped legal system). It allows for relatively easy follow-up of patients.

With particular focus on suicidal adolescents, the medical care system in which we are implementing this procedure has a home-based system of assessment and counselling for parents of adolescent patients. Four college-educated counsellors visit the homes of these patients and work with parents on behavioral skills training, providing consultation regarding discipline and support for their children, etc. This system, tends to increase compliance with treatment by developing alliances with parents in the care of their children. The in-home model supports the suicide tracking system for adolescent patients by providing for outpatient clinicians, in-person, intuitive observations of family interactions, environmental cues, etc. that can increase the likelihood of successful outcomes with this sub-sample of at-risk patients. By attempting to increase family stability and functionality, a further layer of protection is built in to support adolescent patients at risk.

Moreover, the in-home model has the potential to dramatically increase attention to the safe storage in and/or removal of firearms from the homes of these at-risk youth. Our concern about firearms as significantly associated mechanisms of risk in the U.S. allows me to shift attention to the second intervention approach I wish to describe to you.

2. THE PREVENTION MODEL

In mid-Novemebr of last year, representatives from the American Association of Suicidology met in conference near Chicago over two days with researchers, public health specialists, social policy experts, and representatives from a number of significant organizations in the States (e.g., the American Academy of Pediatrics, the American Medical Association, the American Academy of Child and Adolescent Psychiatry) including pro-firearms organizations (e.g., the American Shooting Sports Federation) and anti-firearms organizations (e.g., Handgun Control, Inc.) to review and debate the research and epidemiological findings pertaining to youth suicide by firearms in America. Our goal was to attempt to arrive at agreements regarding these research findings and implications and to recommend strategies and, perhaps, policy to reduce the frequency of these tragic occurrences.

Remarkably, we achieved consensus on a number of issues and established a model for future collaboration. A "consensus statement" was issued and is currently in process of being disseminated to hundreds of organizations asking for signatories. That statement currently reads as follows:

Consensus Statement on Youth Suicide by Firearms

Youth suicide is a multidimensional and complex behavior, with many associated risk factors. (Berman & Jobes, 1991; Lewinsohn et al, 1996; Marttunen, et al, 1992; Brent & Perper, 1995)

Youth suicide is a major public health problem in America, with rates now surpassing those for the nation as a whole. (Kachur et al, 1995)

Suicide is the third-leading cause of death among youth (ages 15–24) and second-leading cause of death for 15–19 year olds in the U.S. (Kachur et al, 1995)

Epidemiological surveys indicate dramatic increases in suicidal behaviors particularly among young African American males, Native American males, and younger children, below the age of 14. (Kachur et al, 1995)

Firearms are the most common method of suicide by youth. This is true for both males and females, younger and older adolescents, and for all races (Kachur et al, 1995).

The increase in the rate of youth suicide (and the number of deaths by suicide) over the past four decades is largely related to the use of firearms as a method. (Boyd & Moscicki, 1986; CDC 1986; Kachur et al, 1995)

The most common location for the occurrence of firearm suicides by youth is the home (Brent et al, 1993).

There is a positive association between the accessibility and availability of firearms in the home and the risk for youth suicide (Kellerman et al, 1992; Brent et al, 1993).

The risk conferred by guns in the home is proportional to the accessibility (e.g., loaded and unsecured firearms) and the number of guns in the home (Brent et al, 1993; Kellerman et al, 1992).

Guns in the home, particularly loaded guns, are associated with increased risk for suicide by youth, both with and without identifiable mental health problems or suicidal risk factors (Brent et al, 1993).

If a gun is used to attempt suicide, a fatal outcome will result 78% to 90% of the time (Annest et al, 1995; Card, 1974)

Public policy initiatives that restrict access to guns (especially handguns) are associated with a reduction of firearm suicide and suicide overall, especially among youth (Carrington et al, 1994; Sloan et al, 1990; Loftin et al, 1991).

Therefore, in keeping with a public health preventive approach and the proposed National Academy of Sciences Institute of Medicine's preventive intervention spectrum model, we believe that a significant proportion of suicides by firearms are preventable (Mrazek & Haggerty, 1994). It is vital to try to break the causal chain by separating vulnerable youth from this highly lethal method of suicide, i.e., firearms. To this end, we support the U.S. Public Health Service's *Healthy People 2000* Objectives 7.2 and 7.10 which refer to the safe storage of guns (DHHS, 1994).

2.1. Indicated Interventions

Indicated intervention approaches focus on the education of parents or parental figures who are gun-owners as to:

a. understanding the risk associated with gun ownership with respect to violent death and suicide; and
b. the importance of gun safety, namely making a gun inoperable by and inaccessible to youth.

Professionals who come in contact with at-risk youth and their families must be educated to routinely ask about the presence and method of storage of firearms in the home, and to educate all families about safe storage practice for families who choose to keep guns. This can take place in the context of well-child care by primary care physicians, as well as by any professional who would come into contact with youth at risk for suicidal behavior (e.g., child welfare, juvenile justice, educational professionals, mental health professionals, etc.)

2.2. Selective Interventions

Pursuant to the achievement of firearms-secure homes, we support public health policy initiatives to develop, disseminate, and evaluate technologies that would decrease firearm operability by youth, thereby making it much more difficult for an adolescent to use a gun for a suicide. We support legislative initiatives and efforts to increase market demand for these new technologies.

We endorse training and education with respect to the risks associated with guns in the home; the need for safer storage of guns; and identification of risk factors for youth suicide for all parents, professionals who take care of youth at risk, and all firearms owners.

2.3. Universal Interventions

At the most universal level of intervention, we support models promoting community and parental responsibility for consistent supervision of adolescents; maintenance of alcohol and drug-free homes; and if there is a gun in the home, adherence to safe storage (i.e., inaccessible and inoperable firearms).

We endorse seeking partnerships and collaborations with organizations and agencies that have a shared stake in the issues of youth suicide and violence, e.g., religious organizations, youth service organizations, juvenile justice, child welfare and community service organizations.

3. FUTURE DIRECTIONS

We support epidemiological research that would increase our knowledge about culturally-specific issues associated with youth suicide and firearms, such as those in specific ethnic groups (e.g., African Americans, Native Americans), or in rural areas. Product-based research is needed to develop technologies to increase the safety of firearms. A better understanding of the cognitions, attitudes, and motivations for gun ownership and safe storage behaviors is needed. There is a need to research the gender differences in youth suicide. There is a need to understand the causal sequences leading up to youth suicide by firearms. Studies of the influence of media portrayals of violence and firearms use are urgently needed. There is a need to rigorously evaluate the effectiveness of proposed preventive approaches for youth suicide. There is a need to establish, support, and maintain surveillance and reporting systems of firearm-related suicides and suicidal behaviors.

4. SUMMARY

Given the costs to American society and families wrought by youth suicide, we believe that immediate action needs to be taken. There is clear evidence that intervening in or preventing the immediate accessibility of a lethal weapon can save lives. We have identified the safe storage of guns as one preventive intervention approach that would result in a decrease in the number of youth suicides. We believe that a combination of indicated, selective and universal preventive interventions addressing this objective can successfully lead to a reduction in youth firearm suicides in our homes and communities. The achievement of this goal can only come about through the cooperation, coordination, and collaboration of concerned organizations at all levels of the community.

We currently are actively seeking partnerships and co-signatories to the Consensus Statement from a large number of significant organizations, for example the American Psychological and American Psychiatric Associations. By analogy, if the most important ingredient in our recipe for effective care of the suicidal patient is the therapeutic alliance, then it is through similar collaborative relationships, built upon a solid foundation of theory, research, and our patient's voices, that we feel we can best mount effective suicide prevention programs. I believe that each of the models I have briefly described herein are significant examples of these strategies.

5. CONCLUSION

If suicide might best be conceptualized as a multidemensional problem, its prevention must, as well, require multifaceted approaches. No one domain, e.g., biological or psychiatric, nor no one preventive model will succeed if we think parochially or engage territorial turf wars. The great value to an international conference such as this lies in the forging of collaborative efforts and, at least, our openness to listening to others speak of their successes and failures, their problems, their needs, and those strategic interventions conceptually developed with both universal (i.e., international) translatability and targeted (i.e., indigenous) applicability.

Together our many voices form a chorus of great potential to make a difference…if we only could listen carefully.

REFERENCES

Annest, J. L., Mercy, J. A., Gibson, D. R., & Ryan, G. W. (1995). National estimates of nonfatal firearm-related injury. Beyond the tip of the iceberg. *Journal of the American Medical Association, 273* (22), 1749–54.

Berman, A. L., & Jobes, D. A. (1991). *Adolescent Suicide: Assessment and Intervention*. Washington, DC: American Psychological Association

Boyd, J. H. & Moscicki, E. K. (1986). Firearms and youth suicide. *American Journal of Public Health, 76* (10), 1240–1242.

Brent, D. A., Perper, J. A., Moritz, G., Baugher, M., Schweers, J., & Roth, C. (1993). Firearms and adolescent suicide: A community case-control study. *American Journal of Diseases of Children, 147*, 1066–1071.

Brent, D. A. & Perper, J. A. (1995). Research in adolescent suicide: Implications for training, service delivery, and public policy. *Suicide and Life-Threatening Behavior, 25*, 222–230.

Card, J. J. (1974). Lethality of suicidal methods and suicide risk: Two distinct concepts. *Omega, 5*, 37–45.

Carrington, P. J. & Moyer, S. (1994). Gun control and suicide in Ontario. *American Journal of Psychiatry, 151*, 606–608.

Centers for Disease Control (1986, November). *Youth Suicide in the United States, 1970–1980*. Atlanta, GA: Centers for Disease Control and Prevention..

Department of Health and Human Services (1994). U.S. Public Health Service. *Healthy People 2000: National Health Promotion and Disease Prevention Objectives*. (p. 230). Washington, D.C.: GPO.

Jobes, D. A. (1995) The challenge and promise of clinical suicidology. *Suicide and Life- Threatening Behavior, 25*, 437–449.

Jobes, D. A. & Berman, A. L. (1993). Suicide and malpractice liability: Assessing and improving outpatient policies and procedures. *Professional Psychology: Research and Practice, 24*, 91–99.

Jobes, D. A., Jacoby, A. M., Cimbolic, P. & Hustead, L. A. (in press). The assessment and treatment of suicidal clients in a university counseling center. *Journal of Counseling Psychology*.

Kachur, S. P., Potter, L. B., James, S. P. & Powell, K. E. (1995). Suicide in the United States 1980–1992. Atlanta: Centers for Disease Control and Prevention, National Center for Injury Prevention and Control. Violence Surveillance Summary Series, No.1.

Kellerman, A. L., Rivara, F. P., Rushford, N. B., et al. (1992). Suicide in the home in relationship to gun ownership. *New England Journal of Medicine, 327*, 467–472.

Lewinsohn, P. M., Rohde, P. & Seeley, J. R. (1996). Adolescent suicidal ideation and attempts: Prevalence, risk factors, and clinical implications. *Clinical Psychology: Science and Practice, 3*, 25–46.

Loftin, C., McDowall, D., Wiersema, B. & Cottey, T. J. (1991). Effects of restrictive licensing of handguns on homicide and suicide in the District of Columbia. *New England Journal of Medicine, 325*, 1615–1620.

Marttunen, M. J., Aro, H. M. & Lonnqvist, J. K. (1992). Adolescent Suicide: Endpoint of long-term difficulties. *Journal of the American Academy of Child and Adolescent Psychiatry, 31*, 649–654.

Mrazek P. J. & Haggerty, R. J. (1994). *Reducing Risks for Mental Disorders: Frontiers for Preventive Intervention Research*. Institute of Medicine. National Academy Press: Washington, D.C.

Sloan, J. H., Rivara, F. P., Reay, D. T., Ferris, J. A. J. & Kellermann, A. L. (1990). Firearm regulations and rates of suicide—A comparison of two metropolitan areas. *New England Journal of Medicine, 322*, 369–373.

37

FROM THEORY TO PRACTICE: DO WE REALLY LISTEN

2 — The Voluntary Sector Perspective

Vanda Scott

Befrienders International
23 Elysium Gate
126 New Kings Road
London, SW6 4LZ England

1. INTRODUCTION

Essentially the need for suicide prevention strategies in most societies continues to challenge the mind. Indeed, as we reach the conclusion of this magnificent gathering of the 19th Congress of the International Association for Suicide Prevention we are, I would like to suggest, left with the unanswerable question of why people are prematurely ending their lives in greater numbers today than yesterday.

Or are they? Is it just that the national collection of data on suicide and attempted suicides is more accurate, effective or even more readily available in some countries and communities than others?

As we heard from Professor Srinivasa Murthy earlier this week, suicide rates vary markedly among rich and poor countries reflecting real cultural differences (World Mental Health).

I recently attended a World Health Organisation consultative meeting, with my colleague Professor Diego de Leo, on data collection in which the collection of accurate data on a worldwide basis was reviewed.

The discussions around the table on accurate data clearly showed the difficulty one has in utilising much of the existing data. In Italy, as Professor De Leo pointed out, you will find two official sources from which statistics are collected: the police records and the health authorities. The difference of the Italian national rate on suicide from these sources is 10%, 400 in number. And yet for the scientist and practitioner a 10% differential is not just a matter of numbers or process but to do with actual people — people who kill themselves for a complexity of reasons.

Suicide Prevention, edited by Kosky *et al.*
Plenum Press, New York, 1998

As we struggle with the facts, play with the numbers, as I heard quoted on a number of occasions during this week, are we actually getting any closer to understanding the magnitude of the task that lies ahead of us all ? Do we know if the research, the practice, the strategy and the programme, have any impact on the communities in which we work?

A number of policy statements have evolved at national and regional level based on the World Health Organisation target that:

"By the year 2000 the current rising trends in suicides and attempted suicides should be reversed."

As a policy statement it is not yet clear what impact this specific health target has had, or will have in the next 3 years. By all accounts it is likely that such health targets will not be met.

Each day it is estimated that two and a half thousand people kill themselves. That is almost one million people each year. And are we any closer to understanding why?

This morning Professor Diego de Leo, Doctor Lanny Berman and I, from our respective professional background and experience, will take a look at a number of areas in which our experience has underlined, or emphasised, the need for the close relationship between research and practice.

2. FROM THE VOLUNTARY SECTOR PERSPECTIVE

Cheng, aged about 22, knocked tentatively on the door of The Samaritan centre early one morning in March. He came into the room and sat heavily down, shrouded in depression. He could not talk, had no expression and no life. He was totally dishevelled, tired and without energy. All he had in his world was his sportsbag.

For many hours the volunteer sat with Cheng who, from time to time, closed his eyes and sat in total silence, almost as if sleeping. Occasionally he would take a sip of water but in the main he sat motionless. At other times he would gently sob and say just a few words. Eventually his story evolved: clearly Cheng had decided that this day he was intent on dying.

The distance between Cheng and the volunteer was close but, clearly for a number of reasons, communication was difficult. First, Cheng had been depressed for some time and slowly he had found the doors in his world closed to him. And secondly, when Cheng did choose to say a few words, it was only in Cantonese, his familiar language. Over a period of hours I learnt that the breakdown of his relationship two years ago with his girlfriend had alienated him from her family and their mutual friends; his only work colleagues in the computer company were tired of listening to him and his problems, and his family and friends had supported him for the past two years. By now he had lost his job and sat around day in and day out in darkest gloom. Finally, his uncle, with whom he lived, was getting old and also not coping with Cheng's despair.

He kicked Cheng out on to the street and told him to sort himself. For a number of days and nights Cheng had wandered the streets until he had finally decided that life was no longer an option and that he was going to end the pain by hanging himself. He found himself at a food market where he watched the hustle and bustle of people around him and laughter, children shouting and screaming, dogs barking; everyone communicating, but he had no one to talk to.

He then noticed an old TV set at the edge of the market and watched in silence, hour upon hour, but what he did see was a short advertisement on listening.

"Are you feeling pain — are you alone and want someone to talk to — contact the Samaritans — they listen."

It was almost seven hours since Cheng had walked through the door, although the time had seemingly passed quickly much in silence. Cheng was able to slowly articulate his feelings, his fears and his need for help. He did not want to receive medical attention and yet he knew he was not coping. Eventually he opened his sports bag in which carefully placed was a short rope in the form of a noose. Cheng had been carrying this rope for some weeks and knew exactly how and where he intended to die.

Cheng eventually agreed to see our medical advisor and arrangements were gently made for him to be accompanied by a volunteer to the hospital. On arrival, official procedure in the emergency accident unit was to handcuff Cheng to the bed. The psychiatrist arrived and diagnosed a chronic depression. Cheng was hospitalised and later returned to the community.

In the early '70s there was spate of suicides among young people in Hong Kong. Summer months of intense exhausting heat combined with extreme exam pressures, as experienced in a pyramid educational system where quality senior school education was not guaranteed, caused immense stress. As whole families invested life savings into providing private tuition for their children, so did the fear of failure and shame intensify. In three weeks, seven school children jumped from high rise buildings: two together hand in hand carrying photographs of their family.

It was not unusual for the suicides to occur before the exam results were announced.

The response from the government was to make schooling available for all ages and to block access to high rise buildings.

Families responded by pouring more of their limited funds into private tuition in the hope their child would pass exams.

Accessing extra hotlines for the two month period and increasing awareness programmes went some way towards addressing the problem.

Over the next two decades societal pressure resulted in an anxious government; experts were brought in from the western world to advise on how youth suicide could be combatted. Funds were made readily available for instant solutions but no long term strategy was put into place.

In 1992 a meeting was requested by the secretary of State for Health and Social Welfare to discuss the growing concern of teenage suicides in Hong Kong. At the time Befrienders International local team of volunteers was providing a befriending service, 24 hours a day but clearly not targeting callers in this particular age group and funds were desperately required.

Generous funding and organisational support was offered to provide youth hotlines. International trading companies and banks offered huge sums of money for us to specialise our services for the young — a tempting proposition.

And yet it was evident from the data that suicide over the past 15 years is more serious among the elderly than in any other age group, at a rate of four to five times above the mean rate of the general population. The highest suicide risk groups are the older elderly (above 75 years of age), males and the unmarried elderly.

Funding priorities omitted this group; so therefore did the community carers. They were regarded as the forgotten people. The basic facts were known but society was slow to respond and only recently were we able to commission a study to identify suitable programmes for reaching the elderly.

The study showed that the suicide ratio of economically inactive elderly compared to economically active elderly is 10 to 1. Most deaths occurred either at or near the home of the elderly, and more crowded districts with fewer amenities tend to have higher suicide rates. In 70% of the cases, the elderly person involved had indicated their suicidal feelings to a family member. Most of the suicides studied had suffered from chronic disease; 40% and 27% of these respectively had consulted medical practitioners and psychiatrists shortly before their death.

The plight of the elderly could not be more clearly shown than by this news cutting from the South China Morning Post, Hong Kong, 10 March 1997:

Suicide Bid by Woman, 102, Fails as Rope Snaps

A 102-year-old woman's attempt to hang herself yesterday failed when the rope snapped. Chan Kam told police she wanted to avoid becoming a burden to her family. She lives in Lei Tung Estate, Ap Lei Chau, with her only son and his wife, both 68, and their 40-year-old son. Her daughter-in-law said that earlier this year Mrs Chan was in hospital with a cold and she had not been able to care for herself since returning home. She was seldom able to leave the family's 24th-floor flat in Tung Yat House. Yesterday Mrs Chan's daughter-in-law returned home at about 11.30 am to find her lying on a bed with a 30-centimetre-long rope tied around her neck. She was still conscious. A police spokesman said Mrs Chan had tried to hang herself from a bunk bed but the rope had not been strong enough to support her weight. She was taken to Queen Mary Hospital for treatment and later transferred to Eastern Hospital before being allowed home last night. Mrs Chan has two grandsons and four great-grandchildren.

The study of the science of self destructive behaviour will continue to challenge the mind for years to come. In the meantime there is a need in the voluntary sector for research to be undertaken in which attitudes towards suicide in differing cultures, religions and communities are more clearly understood.

A small two year study is being undertaken by our volunteers in Sri Lanka supervised by a colleague from an American university. As we heard from Lakshmi Ratnayeke earlier this week suicidal behaviour is most common among people who dwell in the remote rural areas where social services are not accessible in times of crisis. An innovative programme is being resourced by volunteers in which:

1. villagers are engaged in a series of meetings at which interpersonal problem solving, coping skills and the need to seek an emotional support are introduced.
2. experienced local volunteers on a fortnightly basis, are available for discussions and to listen.

The traditions of the village discourage the villagers from revealing their difficulties to strangers. There are also strong cultural norms against revealing problems and difficulties to others in the village or even to family members.

The impact of the programme on those who take part in it and others in the village will be documented and an evaluation of the effectiveness in reducing suicide attempts will be conducted.

Comparison with a neighbouring village in which no befriending programme has been introduced will also be key in this project in order for the organisation to find ways in which it can assess priorities and effectiveness in befriending those who are suicidal.

Suicidology is an interdisciplinary science covering the many aspects of human life, whether biological, psychological, medical and psychiatric or psychosocial life events. Comparative studies across age group and across national boundaries address the growing concern amongst many of us that whilst a greater understanding of the complexities of suicide is necessary there is an immediate need to put into practice by clearly interpreting the information that is available and presenting effective strategies to prevent suicide.

Amy was married to a well known medical practitioner in Hong Kong. It was after her third attempt to kill herself that The Samaritans were contacted. When I first met Amy she was still in hospital, heavily medicated, under close supervision and angry that she had failed to kill herself. As she lay in bed, eyes closed in complete silence, all was needed was a quiet presence. It wasn't until the nurse left the room that any connection with Amy could be made. She could only say 'I am not coping' and then started to cry.

Amy finally began to talk of feeling claustrophobic, of being hemmed in and having the role of mother and wife of a highly regarded professional in a highly materialistic society. Her social world was full of meaningless activity and meaningless "contacts and connections." She wanted to "disconnect," "to be heard" for who she was and to have time and space to breathe. She talked of failure and hopelessness: she did not want to live and therefore to have overdosed on her medication was the only answer. Amy, with all the medical support freely available to her in the community, was not coping.

A few weeks later Amy visited The Samaritans. Over the next 6 months Amy's driver would take her twice a week to see the psychiatrist for a fixed time appointment and then on to The Samaritans where she would either cry in deep distress or sit in silence. Volunteers would be along side Amy sitting quietly and providing the emotional support and continuing presence that she required at a time of healing.

Slowly Amy began to live her own life, within the family, within the marriage but with recognition of her own worth. Twenty years on Amy is living and working in Australia having made no further attempts on her life.

There is a continuing role for volunteers in providing emotional support to those who are in despair and in danger of taking their life. There is also a role for the man and woman in the street whether in the black townships of South Africa or the remote rural areas of China.

In an environment of social disintegration the concept of listening, however basic, is an essential component of a strategy to reduce incidence of suicide in a community, an age group or sector of society such as prisons, ethnic minorities, displaced persons and rural areas.

I am going to leave you with someone who can express far more eloquently than me the real need to be heard, which seems to sum up the need to be able to listen to pain, confusion and distress.

A Samaritan (UK) advert of a young girl is shown in which every time the girl opens her mouth to be heard only inaudible noise comes out of her mouth. Increased frustration and distress is evident by her face until she diminishes into a corner, helpless. The words "The Samaritans understand" come up on the screen.

38

THE CAREGIVER'S REACTIONS AFTER SUICIDE OF A PATIENT

Onja T. Grad and Anka Zavasnik

Centre for Mental Health
University Psychiatric Hospital
Zaloska 29, 1000 Ljubljana, Slovenia

1. INTRODUCTION

Suicide is a traumatic event, which has a long-lasting affect on many different people. Most affected people are the relatives, but as a lot of experiences and research have shown, the caregivers are touched by suicide of their patient as well.

The professional role serves as 'a defensive and reparative function to overcome the pain which they (caregivers) feel as human beings' (Litman 1965). The reactions in professionals, most common after suicide of a patient were grief, guilt, depression, personal inadequacy and anger, most of which are very similar to those reported in studies of family survivors of suicide (Ness & Pfeffer, 1990; Farberow, 1992; Watson & Lee, 1993; Valente 1994).

Working with people in crisis, we know, that it is unavoidable to experience patient's suicide — as Brown has put it (1987) 'there are only two types of therapists: the ones who have already experienced a patient's suicide and those who will'.

Should we try to understand why it is so difficult to overcome the patient's suicide, it is necessary to remember that a therapist invests a lot of knowledge, experiences, personal engagement and time on a patient, but if suicide occurs, the caregiver gets back only feelings of failure and devaluation, a lot of doubts and frustration, pain and guilt.

These feelings are not only in the domain of psychotherapists, but are experienced by family doctors as well. Until now, they have been more or less a forgotten group of suicide survivors. How do they get through the suicide of their patient—are they more or less affected by the event than psychotherapists?

While working with the General Medical Practitioners (GPs), on suicide prevention workshops, we realised that death and suicide are their everyday companions. They have to make a home visit regularly when somebody dies or commits suicide. They are the first ones on the scene, serving as the first aid to the person and/or his family. Many times — especially in the small communities, they know the whole family and their circumstances. They might have even seen the patient recently, bud did not ask about his suicidal thoughts.

Suicide Prevention, edited by Kosky *et al.*
Plenum Press, New York, 1998

Compared to the GPs, psychotherapists have some advantages in coping with death and dying of their patients arising out of:

a. postgraduate education and specialised training
b. experiences (reducing omnipotence, being aware of the limitations of therapy)
c. work setting (more team work, supervision)
d. psychiatrists' awareness that suicide is something which awaits them in their practice

2. METHOD

A special questionnaire was constructed, containing 15 yes-no items and three open-ended questions, asking about the emotional reactions of the caregiver after suicide of their patient. The questionnaire was mailed to psychiatrists and clinical psychologists (further referred to as psychotherapists) who work in psychiatric hospitals and clinics throughout Slovenia (Group 1) and to general practitioners (GPs), who have experienced their patient's suicide (Group 2) and GPs who have experienced the death of their patient (Group 3).

The data were compared and chi-square test of independence was used as the statistical method to determine significance.

2.1. Samples

Three groups of caregivers answered the questionnaire:

a. psychiatrists and psychologists experiencing suicide of a patient: a response rate of 72% (n=87).
b. general practitioners experiencing suicide of a patient: a response rate of 68% (n=75)
c. general practitioners experiencing death of a patient: a response rate of 84% (n=75)

3. RESULTS

When comparing the three groups, the data are similar. More than 80% of the caregivers in all three groups became more cautious and spoke to the colleagues after the event, while in Groups 2 and 3 the majority of the respondents spoke to their partner as well (68% and 82%).

Table 1. Respondents by vocation and gender (age and working years)

| | Gender | | | | |
| | Male | | Female | | |
Vocation	Mean	Standard deviation	Mean	Standard deviation	Total
GP (suicide)					
Age	45	9	39	6	**51**
Work (years)	16	7	13	7	
Psychotherapist					
Age	48	11	41	6	**63**
Work (years)	18	11	15	8	
GP (death, not by suicide)					
Age	43	8	37	4	**63**
Work (years)	16	8	12	4	

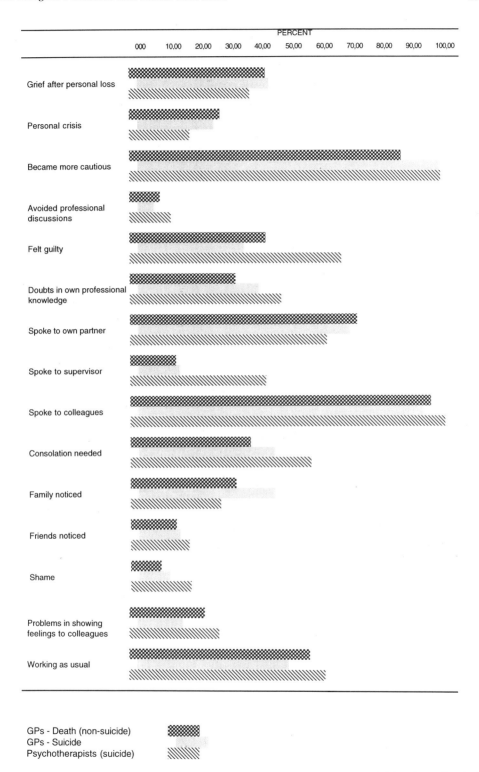

Figure 1. Percent of 'yes' answers comparing psychotherapists after suicide, gps after suicide and gps after death (non-suicide) of a patient.

When calculating the significant differences between the two groups who lost a patient by suicide, we have found three differences (Fig. 1): psychotherapists were more likely to have felt guilty (<0.001), spoken to supervisor (p<0.01) and had experienced problems in showing feelings to colleagues (p<0.05).

Comparing the Groups 1 and 2 for men only, we found significant differences between the groups in one item: psychotherapists felt significantly more guilty than GPs (p<0.05).

In women there were three items that differentiated the two groups: female psychotherapists felt significantly more guilty (p<0.001), spoke to their supervisor more (p<0.01) and had more doubts in their own professional knowledge (p<0.05) than did female GPs.

Comparing groups 2 and 3 we found no significant differences, comparing male GPs after experiencing suicide and GPs experiencing death of their patient, nor comparing these two groups in women.

4. DISCUSSION

Suicide and death of a patient affects any caregiver. The authors have experienced it with their own patients; they have observed the effects of the event while supervising younger colleagues, and when working with GPs on suicide prevention workshops. All of these experiences have triggered the present study which confirmed the impact on the caregivers and added some new conclusions.

The results of the questionnaire showed similarities between the experiences of the psychotherapists and family doctors losing their patient by suicide. As a result of the event the caregivers became more cautious with other patients, were preoccupied with the loss, even to the extent that they have brought their feelings about it to their own families. More than 40% of caregivers experienced the event as a personal loss. All these results confirm the hypothesis that not only the relatives, but the caregiver is emotionally affected by the loss of his/her patient (Grad, 1996)

However, the training and professional discipline make the majority of the caregivers work as usual after the event. When we compared the group of psychotherapists and the group of GPs after their patient's suicide, psychotherapists significantly more often responded that they had felt guilty. The reasons might be various:

1. Psychotherapists are the last in the chain of professional caregivers — they have nowhere to refer the patient, so everybody expects them to solve the problem, therefore they feel more responsibility, which provokes more guilt, when unsuccessful. Obviously it doesn't help to know that the incidence of suicide amongst the mental health patients is much higher than in general population.
2. Fear that a therapist overlooked something or did something wrong, which can both be connected to guilt.
3. GPs felt less guilty because their role is more defined: they don't feel they are the experts for psychological problems and can refer the patients to the psychiatrist.

The second significant difference between psychotherapists and GPs was that the psychotherapists more often spoke to a supervisor than did GPs. This could be explained by the established practice in psychotherapeutic work to have one's work supervised. Also, the system is that GPs are mostly working alone and have no team and no supervisor to consult with.

The third significant difference found between the two groups was that psychotherapists stated that they have had problems in showing feelings to the colleagues more often than GPs have. This difference might again be connected to the guilt feelings and responsibility that psychotherapists feel more intensely. Even though they speak with colleagues, it might mean that they speak more about 'technical' problems — case study, what was done, what wasn't done, how should the patient be treated otherwise, etc. One of the explanations for this difference between both groups could also be that psychotherapists perceive it is within their professional role that they have to cope with every emotional stress.

Female psychotherapists more often had doubts in their own professional knowledge ($p < 0.05$) after suicide. This is probably connected to the fact that women psychotherapists reported feelings of guilt more often than their male colleagues.

All three groups showed a lot of similarity. This means that psychotherapists and GPs are affected by the suicides and by the death of their patients. It also means that they all need a support system to cope with the aftermath of these losses.

A programme to provide help to the bereaved caregivers should be partly structured and partly individualised. The structured part could be in the hospital wards and include a team meeting with all participants present, lead by a neutral external supervisor with the aim to diminish the guilt feelings of all staff members, make new plans how to support patient's relatives, what to do about the funeral, and how to cope with feelings of grief and with grief of the other patients on the ward.

When caregivers are working alone, the structured debriefing should also include an external supervisor to let the professional consider their own feelings.

The individualised support system should respect the person's own needs, which could include: gender differences, level of education, personality traits of the caregiver and working years, etc.

Our study has proved that it does not help if a caregiver denies his own feelings or emotional involvement when losing a patient, but it helps to talk to somebody, to accept support if needed, and help the caregiver find his or her way through the grief.

REFERENCES

Brown, H (1987). Patient suicide during residency training. *Journal of Psychiatric Education,* 11, 201–216

Farberow, N L (1992). The Los Angeles survivors-after-suicide program. An Evaluation. *Crisis,* 13, 23–34.

Grad O T (1996). Suicide: How to survive as a survivor? *Crisis* 17/3. 136–140.

Grad O T, Zavasnik A, Groleger U (1997). Suicide of a patient: Gender differences in bereavement reactions of therapists. *Suicide and Life Threatening Behaviour* 27(4), 379–386.

Litman, R E (1965). When patients commit suicide. *American Journal of Psychotherapy,* 4, 570–576

Ness, D E & Pfeffer C R (1990). Sequelae of bereavement resulting from suicide. *American Journal of Psychiatry* 147, 279–285.

Valente, S M (1994). Psychotherapist reactions to the suicide of a patient. *American Journal of Orthopsychiatry* 64, 614–621.

Watson, W L & Lee, D (1993). Is there life after suicide? The systemic belief approach for 'survivors' of suicide. *Archives of Psychiatric Nursing,* 7, 37–43.

39

SUICIDE SURVIVOR PROGRAMS IN IASP MEMBER COUNTRIES*

A Survey

Norman L. Farberow

Los Angeles, California

Programs to help survivors in their bereavement after a suicide has been a comparatively new development in the field of suicide and its prevention. Early activity in suicide prevention was focused almost entirely on the suicidal person, with efforts at identification, assessment, and intervention or treatment. Significant others such as family, lovers, friends were involved but they were only regarded as part of the context; the concern was on the person who was thinking, talking about or had already started to kill himself. We knew that the family was important, but at that time it was primarily as a source of information about, or as the necessary support for the suicidal person. Also, when we started conducting psychological autopsies, we had noticed how beneficial the interviews with the families had been, how helpful it had been for the family members when given the opportunity to talk about the death to someone who was interested and non-judgmental. Still, it took a long time for any activity in the field to develop It seemed to develop primarily as the result of the demands for help that came from those survivors who attended the early conferences of the professional associations, who were looking for answers to their pressing questions and for some help for their feelings, and finding it mostly only from each other.

The movement has grown considerably over the past two decades — but unevenly, more in some parts of the world than in others. Now, with the recognition of the suicide bereavement field, through the establishment of an award to recognise contributions in the area, a significant step forward has been taken toward completing the round of services that suicide prevention practitioners first undertook almost a half a century ago.

In order to gain a more comprehensive picture of the extent and kind of services currently being offered in this area, a survey was undertaken of all the 52 countries listed as

* Appreciation is expressed to all the National Representatives who completed and returned the survey questionnaire.

Suicide Prevention, edited by Kosky *et al.*
Plenum Press, New York, 1998

Table 1. Respondent countries with no formal
programs for survivors of suicide (N=16, 1997)

Europe	Near/Middle East	Far East	Central America
Iceland	Iran	South Korea	Cuba
Portugal	India	Japan	
Yugoslavia		People's Republic of China	
Greece			
Lichenstein			
Romania			
Bulgaria			
Lithuania			
Spain			
Russia			

members of the IASP. A short questionnaire was sent to all National Representatives in the IASP, along with a cover letter asking for information about the programs, if any, in their countries, and for some descriptive details of their operation. Responses were received from 31 or 60%, or at least more than half, and actually not too bad for a request of this kind (Table 1).

COUNTRIES WITH NO SURVIVOR PROGRAMS

The first question asked of the National Representatives (NRs) whether programs for survivors existed in their country — 14 answered yes, and 17 no. Of the European countries answering 'no' most were in eastern Europe (Russia, Lithuania, Romania, Bulgaria, Greece, Yugoslavia); the others (Iceland, Portugal, Spain, Lichtenstein) could be considered in the western region. The rest of the countries, except for Cuba, were in the eastern part of the world (Iran, India, South Korea, Japan, and Peoples Republic of China).

The second question asked of the NR was—'If no, what were the reasons why not?' Five of the countries (Iceland, Lithuania, India, Russia and China) felt their programs in suicide prevention were just beginning, some with a struggle, and that it was not yet possible to turn to helping the survivors. India's national representative, Dr Vijayakumar, for example, said that India's suicide prevention program has barely started, with only five crisis centres serving in a population of 530 million. Six of the countries (Portugal, Spain, Yugoslavia, Iran, South Korea and Japan) felt the problem was that suicide itself was considered too great a religious sin or was culturally unacceptable behaviour. Japan is in this category, contrary to common opinion that suicide is viewed more acceptably there. Reverend Saito, Japan's national representative, wrote, 'Although there are some circumstances where suicide is acceptable, in modern times suicide evokes a stigma on the individual and the family survivors, leaving a sense of shame which is experienced as deeply painful. This is complicated by feelings of guilt. Given these feelings, it is thought that survivors of suicide will not be able to talk to others. They will be inhibited by their shame in sharing their experience with others.'

Romania and Bulgaria were described by their national representatives, Dr Scripcaru and Dr Marinow respectively, as being concerned more with just surviving in these difficult transitional times. The national representative for Cuba, Dr Perez report that there was no regular program for survivors, but he was working with general practitioners who have had survivors as patients. Lichtenstein's national representative, Dr Nagele, reported that there were just not enough requests to form a special service, so people used individual therapy if and when needed; and in Greece, authorities simply had not felt that suicide was such a big problem, according to its national representative Dr Botsis.

COUNTRIES WITH SURVIVOR PROGRAMS

Fourteen (27%) of our 52 IASP member countries report having suicide survivor programs in place. Eight (28%) of our 29 member countries in Europe reported there were programs; the rest were scattered throughout the world. A glance at the numbers indicates that the greatest numbers were reported by the English speaking countries, England (16+), Ireland (5), Australia (6+), Canada (50), the United States (363), and the Scandinavian countries, Sweden (10), Denmark (5) and Norway (3).

Several of the national representatives stated that there were ad hoc groups and groups that were formed in private clinics that were difficult to count. The survivor movement in most of the above countries seemed to derive its impetus from non-professionals, from survivors who chanced to meet, found shared needs and decided to continue to meet. Word got around, others joined, regular meeting dates were established, advertisements of availability appeared, and before long, branches were formed. In some countries there were already established bereavement organizations that organized special groups for suicide survivors, such as CRUSE in England (often a resource for Samaritans), Compassionate Friends in a number of countries, SPES in Sweden and 'Verwaiste Eltern' (abandoned or deserted parents) in Germany (for parents who had lost a child by suicide).

In some countries, the survivors program was affiliated with, or a part of the IASP, as in England, Ireland, Norway, France, Canada and USA. In Israel, suicide emergency teams from the Ministry of Education and Army provided immediate intervention for survivors who where students and soldiers respectively. In most of the countries survivor programs were also offered by individual suicide prevention centers, sometimes ad hoc, and at other times on a regularly scheduled basis when the number of requests was large enough.

Information was requested on the operational details of the programs, where available. Table 2 shows the sources of support for the programs in the various countries.

Practically all show more than one source. Government support rarely provides full support for a clinical program, but more often will take the form of funds for training, conferences, publishing of material and incorporation into national programs for suicide

Table 2. Sources of support for survivor programs

Government	Church	Participant fees	Donations	Professional association/self help/ volunteer/non profit	University hospital/ hospice	No information
Ireland	Norway	Sweden	Ireland	England	Turkey	France
England	Slovenia	Australia	England	Denmark	Slovenia	
Denmark	USA	Argentina	Australia	Germany	Argentina	
Sweden		USA	Canada	Canada	USA	
Slovenia			USA	USA		
Turkey						
Israel						
Canada						
USA						

prevention. Norway (listed as church supported only) might also have been shown as multi-sourced inasmuch as a National Plan for Suicide Prevention, which will include bereavement activity support, is about to be initiated, according to national representative Prof Retterstol. It is apparent that many of the non-institutional programs depend on fees, donations and dedicated self or volunteer help to function. Israel, Turkey and Slovenia were the only countries that did not indicate these as sources of support.

Professionals or paraprofessionals were conducting survivor groups by themselves in 9 of the 14 countries. Three countries, Australia, Canada and USA also reported groups in which the professional works with a survivor. Denmark and Turkey were the only countries in which the support groups were led only by professionals. Often the survivor leads the group by him/herself or with other survivors, as reported in eight countries (Ireland, England, Sweden, Norway, France, Germany, Canada and the USA). Each of the formats have their proponents. Most of the time, the leader seems to be determined by how the programs got started and by whom (on a personal note, I remember meeting with a group in Honolulu that was adamant that no professionals be involved. They felt they would be taken over and they would lose their focus on their own emotional needs).

Information was sought about research activity on survivors, and whether or not there were any formal programs for schools. Five countries (Slovenia, Turkey, Australia, Canada and USA) reported that research was being conducted on various aspects, such as comparing survivors of automobile and suicide deaths (Turkey, USA) therapists who are survivors of a suicide of a patient (Slovenia), attitudes toward suicide (Australia, USA, Canada and others). Eight countries (England, Denmark, Norway, France, Turkey, Israel, Canada and USA) indicated that there were programs for schools when a suicide occurred among their students. Denmark, Norway and France stated their programs for responding to the event in schools were in the planning stages. In Israel, a team from the Ministry of Education was sent to the school to handle the impact on the school and on the other students and staff (a similar team is located in their armed forces). Some programs in England and Canada viewed the death as a critical incident and applied the Critical Incident Stress Briefing (CISD) process when they were called to schools. The Los Angeles School District had its own crisis team, this was sent out when the suicide (or other deaths) occurred on the school grounds, otherwise, the individual school called the Suicide Prevention Centre when a suicide death occurred, whether at home or elsewhere, and distressed reactions occurred among classmates and teachers. From one to six meetings might to be arranged depending on need. A related question that is currently being hotly discussed in Australia and the United States is whether suicide prevention should be taught in schools.

SURVIVOR SUPPORT GROUPS IN THE USA

The American Foundation for Suicide Prevention has, with considerable effort, tried to locate all the survivor groups currently functioning in the US and has put out a directory of suicide survivor groups in the US, listing 363 groups. The list supersedes that put out by the Survivors Division of the American Association of Suicidology in 1992–92, which listed 258 groups.

There is an average of 7 programs per state and a range of 1 to 32. California has the greatest number of programs, 32, followed by New York with 30 and Michigan with 21. Six states have only one survivors group. Most of the groups (135) are led by a professional with a peer (survivor) facilitator (135). A similar number (131) are run by survivors alone. Most of the programs (85%) do not charge a fee. The rest depend on fees based on sliding scales and on donations. Many publish newsletters which are distributed to present and past participants in the program.

The names adopted by the groups are of interest. In Los Angeles there was a deliberate effort to distinguish between those persons who attempted suicide and survived and those persons who experienced the suicide of a loved one. The result was Survivors After Suicide rather than '...of Suicide.' However, Survivors Of Suicide was used quite often by other groups. The words identifying the purpose 'survivor' or 'suicide' was retained in the title by groups such as 'Suicide Survivors Bereavement Support,' 'Friends for Survival,' 'Hope after Suicide' , 'Healing after Suicide,' 'The Suicide of a Loved One' and 'Loving Outreach for Survivors (LOSS).' Others offered encouragement in the title itself, as with 'Day by Day,' 'Take Heart,' 'Ray of Hope,' and 'Transitions.' Others promised support and security with names like 'Safe Place,' 'Listening, Sharing, Caring (LSC)' and the 'Caring Network.'

CONCLUSIONS

A number of countries are not represented, so a lot of information is missing. Yet it is possible to draw some conclusions from the data received. Survivor help is a growing field. At the IASP Congress in Montreal four years ago there were only a few people who expressed interest in the field. There seems little doubt that it will eventually be as big and as formalized as the field of suicide prevention has become. Like that field, the process of growth will not only provide help to the individual through an intensely painful experience of loss and transition, but will aim to reduce prejudice, facilitate research, develop standards through investigations of effectiveness and initiate studies on overcoming cultural hurdles and restrictions.

All of these will contribute to our basic goal of helping grieving suicide survivors.

CONTENTS OF ABSTRACTS

Oral Papers

Plenary Sessions

Posters

ORAL PAPERS

STUDENT'S ASSESSMENTS OF THEIR RISK OF REPETITION FOR SUICIDAL BEHAVIOUR

Stephen Allison, Graham Martin, Leigh Roeger, and Colby Pearce — CAMHS, Flinders Medical Centre, Australia

The objective is to investigate the relationship between adolescent's self-assessments of their risk of repetition and a range of psychological risk factors for suicidal behaviour.

As part of a suicide prevention project in South Australian high schools (Early Detection of Emotional Disorders; EDED) 1813 students from 17 schools completed standardised questionnaires for depression, hopelessness, delinquency, family dysfunction and previous suicidal behaviour. Self-assessment of the risk of suicidal behaviour was measured using a series of questions about the self-rated probability of suicidal thoughts, plans, threats, deliberate self-harm and attempts occurring in the following 6 month.

Of 1813 students, 111 (6.1%) reported previously having tried to kill themselves. Among these students, 27% rated themselves as likely or very likely to repeat their attempt, 26% were uncertain and 47% indicated that a further attempt was unlikely or very unlikely. These self-assessments of suicide risk were significantly related to the recency of the previous attempt and self-reported hopelessness, delinquency and family dysfunction ($p<0.01$ to $p<0.0001$).

Suicide attempters' estimate of their risk of repetition were significantly related to established risk factors for future suicidal behaviour. Further analysis of the self-assessment questions will include their predictive validity for suicidal behaviour reported in the second year of the study (1995–96).

SUICIDE AND CYBERSPACE

Simon Armson — The Samaritans, United Kingdom

The increase in the suicide rate of young men in the Western World has been well documented. The extent to which the Internet is used as a means of uninhibited communication by those who may find it difficult to converse using more conventional means is also well known. This presentation will describe the way in which the means of providing emotional support to the suicidal, given by Samaritans volunteers, has been extended to include "befriending by E-mail" using the Internet. This appears to have been a successful initiative in providing support to some of those who fall within this high risk group.

Against a background of a brief description of the Samaritan movement, the presentation will focus on the work that has been done during the past three years in developing this service which now operates within twelve Branches of The Samaritans in the UK. It will be demonstrated that this new means of providing the traditional Samaritan service has been able to reach callers who otherwise may not have been able to make contact face to face, via the telephone or through correspondence. It will also be demonstrated, in overall terms, that the suicide risk of callers using the E-mail befriending service, who are predominantly male, is consistently higher than that of callers using the other forms of contract.

The effectiveness of the emotional support provided in this way will be discussed, together with the ways that this can be integrated with other forms of support or intervention. Consideration will be given to the way in which this initiative can be developed further, so as to increase the availability of the service to meet an apparent growing demand.

ADDRESSING CHANGES IN CRISIS CENTRES SERVICES

Nada Barraclough and Neville Twine — Distress Centres Ontario, Canada

The objective is to examine Critical Success Factors (CSF) as one useful way to ensure a viable link between a Crisis Centre's vision and client need in a changing and turbulent environment.

CSF method was applied to a crisis intervention organisation serving 30 Crisis Centres in Ontario, Canada. The C.F.S. method entailed the examining of the environments macro and micro, the resources people-formal & informal, and the internal functioning of the organisation including the history, mental health reform, accessibility & organisational change efforts. Materials used were literature searches, marketing initiatives and results of the organisations planning strategies.

"Social psychologists have concluded that to change behaviour you must unfreeze basic beliefs". Our need was to get at the "unfreezing", knowing the degree of possible entrenchment. It is evident that efforts related to changing key parts of Crisis Centres work are becoming circumvented in an environment thick with history and embedded in the seductive connection between ear and voice through the telephone, CSF's focussed on the components most important to the success of the organisation and least threatening to the existing structures. CSF language focussed thinking on vision and client need and was easily adaptable to the 'cognitive' thinking of the organisations planners.

CSF were determined to be readily adaptable to organisational planning because of the amoeba-like ability to accommodate and to influence the existing and sometime entrenched and obsolete planning process.

SOCIAL SUPPORT AMONG EUROPEAN SUICIDE ATTEMPTERS

U. Bille-Brahe, P. Crepet, H. Egebo, A. Kerkhof, D. De Leo, J. Lönnqvist, K. Michel, E. Slander-Renberg, A. Schmidtke, T.C. Stiles, and D. Wasserman — Centre for Suicidological Research, Denmark

The aim of the study has been to develop a model, where social support could be studied as an outcome of personal *interactions*, to examine this outcome from the individual's point of view, and to try and see whether various cultural settings influence on this view.

The model comprises four elements, namely needing support/receiving support and being needed for support/giving support, referring to emotional and practical support as well as for family and friends, respectively.

The analyses are based on information on 773 suicide attempters interviewed at 10 European research centres participating in the Repetition-Prediction

Study, which is part of the WHO/Euro Multicentre Study on Parasuicide carried out in cooperation with the EU Concerted Action on Attempted Suicide.

Preliminary results indicate unexpectedly marked differences between the various European areas both with regard to the individual elements of the model and as far as balances between the various elements are concerned.

Knowledge of common traits, experiences and learned coping strategies in this group may facilitate and shorten the time needed in psychiatric care.

COMORBIDITY OF SUICIDE ATTEMPTS IN ADOLESCENTS AND YOUNG ADULTS

Thomas Bronisch, U. Wunderlich, and H.U. Wittchen — Max-Planck-Institute of Psychiartry, Germany

The data presented came from the first wave of the Early Stages of Psychopathology (EDSP) study, designed to collect data on the prevalence, risk factors, comorbidity and course of mental disorders with specific emphasis on substance use disorders. The sample was drawn from 1994 government registries of all residents in metropolitan Munich expected to be 14–24 year old at the time of interview during the first half of 1995. Psychopathological as well as diagnostic assessment were based on the Munich version of the Composite International Diagnostic Interview (M-CIDI, Wittchen et al. 1995). From the total of 4809 sampled individuals 3021 could be interviewed (response rate 71%). Seventy individuals reported on suicide attempts. Data about comorbidity of suicide attempters as compared to non-suicide attempters will be presented.

TOWARDS ALTERNATIVE SUICIDE INTERVENTION STRATEGIES

Peter Carstairs and Graham Lane — Wyong Community Health Centre, Australia

To develop an appropriate means of consulting with people who had attempted suicide, to improve practices in responding to these people and to establish networks for this group.

"Co-research" was developed from the ideas of Michael White and David Epston and utilised in this project to privilege the expert knowledge of people who had attempted suicide. It culminated in a two day phone-in, the results of which have been published in the report, *Armstrong, S., Towards Alternative Suicide Intervention Strategies: Central Coast May Day Phone-in May 1995, ITRAC/CCAHS, 1996, ISBN 0 646 27135 0.*

One hundred and seventeen people who had attempted suicide contacted the service and responded to the questionnaire. Parametric statistical treatment of the data was not undertaken.

Discussion: The majority of respondents were female (70%). 67% had attempted suicide more than twice in their lives. More than 60% cited relationship difficulties as contributory to their suicide attempt(s). 56% of respondents' comments indicated preferences to turn to formal services, such as psychiatric intervention, for support in suicidal crises, but 69% of the comments about formal services were that they were unhelpful.

CHANGES IN RATES OF DIFFERENT METHODS OF SUICIDE IN THE BRITISH ISLES 1978–1994

John F. Connolly,[1] Orfhlaith McTigue,[2] and Anne Cullen[3] — [1]St. Marys Hospital, Ireland, [2]University College Hospital, Ireland, and [3]Tyrone + Fermanagh Hospital, Ireland

Official suicide, accident and undetermined mortality data was obtained from the appropriate departments of the Republic of Ireland, Northern Ireland, Scotland, England and Wales for the years 1978–1994 inclusive. Overall rates of suicide are considered for each jurisdiction as are changes in the rates for different methods of suicide.

Possible sources of error in the under-reporting of suicide are discussed in the light of the current literature. Likewise, choice of method of suicide is discussed as is the literature pertaining thereto.

It is noted that of the four countries studied, the Republic of Ireland is the only country in which drowning as a choice of method of suicide, has remained stable as a proportion of total suicides. In all other jurisdictions, drowning as a choice of method, has decreased.

The increasing accuracy of suicide mortality data in the Republic of Ireland is noted and commented on.

THE DEVELOPMENT OF A NATIONAL YOUTH SUICIDE PREVENTION STRATEGY FOR NEW ZEALAND

Maria Cotter — Ministry of Health, New Zealand

Like many countries New Zealand has seen the suicide rate of young people escalate dramatically over the past decade. New Zealand now boasts the unenviable position of having one of the highest youth suicide rates in the world.

This paper will outline the previous governmental strategies to address youth suicide in New Zealand and will detail the processes and components of the National Youth Suicide Prevention Strategy which is currently under development.

The multiplicity of factors which lead to poor mental health and the risk of youth suicide makes the coordinating of agencies whose activities impact on the mental health of young people an especially complex task. Ensuring that such strategy is widely accepted, recognised, credible, implemented and monitored is crucial to the success of a national prevention effort.

The challenges involved in formulating a National Strategy will be detailed, such as the importance of acknowledging the political environment and of inter-governmental agency support, the difficulties of addressing polarised approaches regarding risk factors for suicide and the importance of having a conceptual framework on the prevention of youth suicide to guide the implementation process.

YOUTH SUICIDE PREVENTION, A STATE-WIDE SCHOOLS STRATEGY

Jenny Cugley and Vera MacKenzie — Student Support Branch, Education Department, Western Australia

State initiatives for a youth suicide prevention schools strategy in Western Australia began in December 1988 within the framework established by the state Youth Suicide Steering Committee. The strategy initially targeted government schools.

This paper considers why and how the strategy evolved within the context of the state strategy. Development has been via a clear, common framework for identification, intervention, postvention and primary prevention. Strengths and weaknesses of the approach are considered.

YOUTH SUICIDE PREVENTION, A STATE-WIDE SCHOOLS STRATEGY INCORPORATING NON-GOVERNMENT SCHOOLS

Jenny Cugley and Vera MacKenzie — Student Support Branch, Education Department, Western Australia

Subsequent to the agreement for a state wide schools strategy through the Western Australia Youth Suicide Steering Committee efforts began in the non government sector to determine how this might be achieved within a highly devolved system. This paper examines the process by which a structure was established across the non-government schools sector of Western Australia.

In an endeavour to achieve a comprehensive strategy issues of management and maintenance emerged as crucial components. Both the non-government schools system and individual school perspective's of these issues are examined.

GATEKEEPING IN YOUTH SUICIDE PREVENTION: REPORT ON A STUDY ANALYSING GATEKEEPER TRAINING

M. Frederica and Cathy Davis — Australian Catholic University, Australia

The aim of this study was to identify needs of gatekeepers in youth suicide prevention.

Literature review and interviews with key informants were undertaken to determine differing perspective on training for youth suicide prevention gatekeepers. In addition, training programs designed for youth suicide prevention training were analysed.

A major component of this study was to define gatekeepers in youth suicide prevention. The findings suggested that there are three levels of gatekeeping and that training should address the needs of each level. The range of gatekeeping activities included referral, assessment, networking, linkage, caregiving and triage functions. There was disagreement amongst key informants as to what the desired role should be. The findings indicated that context was important in exploring and defining the gatekeeper's role and that the functions of the gatekeeper were strongly influenced by the context. The researchers made a number of recommendations in relation to gatekeeper training. These covered the areas of access, implementation, content of youth suicide prevention gatekeeper's training programs, gatekeeper's training delivery and development of best practice principles and guidelines.

A COMPARISON OF THE PSYCHOPHYSIOLOGY OF SELF-POISONING AND SELF-MUTILATION

Carolyn Driscoll, Kerryn Brain, Janet Haines, and Chris Williams — University of Tasmania, Australia

To compare the strength of the tension reduction experienced during self-mutilation with the reduction in arousal experienced during intentional self-poisoning.

Eighteen individuals who had intentionally taken an overdose of tablets and 18 self-mutilators participated in the study. Personalised guided imagery scripts (Haines, Williams, Brain, & Wilson, 1995) of the act of self-harm and a neutral event were presented in four stages (scene setting, approach, incident, consequence) and psychophysiological measures recorded.

Results indicated a reduction in arousal during the act of self-harm and immediately afterwards for both groups of participants. However, self-mutilation participants experienced a larger reduction in arousal during and after the act of self-harm.

Both groups experienced a distinctive tension reduction pattern of arousal. This reduction may serve to negatively reinforce the behaviours. The stronger pattern of tension reduction for the self-mutilation group may be due to the greater frequency of engaging in the behaviour. It is proposed that the reduced tension reduction response to the self-poisoning group may be due to the wider range of motives ascribed to the behaviour.

It can be concluded that both behaviours are used as a method of coping with an aversive psychological state. These results have clinical implications for management of these self-destructive behaviours.

SUICIDAL THOUGHTS AMONG NORWEGIAN MEDICAL DOCTORS

Oivind Ekeberg,[1] Torgeir Finjord,[1] Erlend Hem,[1] and Olaf G. Aasland[2] — [1]The Research Institute, the Norwegian Medical Association and
[2]Department of Behavioural Sciences in Medicine, University of Oslo, Norway

The aims of the present study are to study how common suicidal thoughts are among Norwegian MD's and relate such thoughts to psychological factors.

In 1993, an extensive study on the living and working conditions of the Norwegian MD's was conducted. In a sub-study, a questionnaire on suicidal thoughts was competed by 1041 subjects (response rate 72%).

There were 10% (females 14%, Males 8%) of the MD's who had seriously considered to commit suicide, and 1.5% had actually made a suicidal attempt.

Serious suicidal thoughts were more common among psychiatrists (17%), non-specialists (13%) and surgeons (12%) in contrast to doctors working in laboratory (2%) and social medicine (2%). Serious suicidal thoughts were associated with depression (OR=12.2), anxiety (OR=2.2), unmarried status (OR=2.6) and somatic problems (Ursin Health Index) (OR=2.6).

In conclusion, suicidal thoughts among MD's are higher in speciaists, those who are unmaried, and have depression or somatic problems.

IF YOU CAN HEAR ME WHY WON'T YOU LISTEN?

Kelli Farrow — Australia

Secondary school students attitudes to what needs to be done with suicide prevention. A survey of 4000 students was conducted around Tasmania showing that young people are attempting suicide at a much higher rate than people think.

PREVENTING CONTAGION: CLINICAL INTERVENTIONS FOLLOWING A SUICIDE

Karen Dunne-Maxim, Frank Jones, Edward Dunne, and Kjell Rudestam — UMDNJ–UBHC, Office of Prevention, USA

Following a completed suicide, contagion in the community is of prime concern to postvention consultants. Specific settings such as schools and mental health facilities, pose additional risks because of the vulnerability of their populations. Consultants need to be informed about interventions which target these settings and to be able to implement them in the most expeditious manner. The authors present their experiences in developing a number of specific strategies including working with key personnel such as school administrators, families, police, clergy, and the media. These interventions are included in the United States Center for Disease Control's recommendations for preventing contagion following a suicide.

SOCIOCULTURAL ATTITUDES TOWARDS SUICIDE IN LITHUANIA

Danute Gailiene — Vilnius University, Lithuania

One of the major among numerous factors determinating suicide, is the sociocultural factor. Some tendencies of sociocultural attitudes influencing suicidal behaviour in Lithuania were discerned on the basis of historical chronicles, archaeological data, mythology and folklore, and the newspapers reports on suicide. At least three active tendencies, influencing suicidal behaviour in Lithuania nowadays, can be discerned.

1. The tendency of romanticising and glorifying suicides that manifests more prominently during historical periods of struggles against various occupations;

2. A reserved and negative attitude to suicide becomes notable already in pagan times, and is reinforced with the establishment of Catholicism;

3. The state of anomie in the present society, conditioned by the later 50 years of Soviet occupation and by difficult transition into a democratic state which is still in progress.

SUICIDE IN SAXONY-ANHALT IN THE DECADE 1985–1994

Axel Genz — Fachkreankenhoas für Psychiatrie, Germany

Description of the development of the suicide risk in East Germany in relation to political and economic changes following the unification of Germany.

Age and sex-specific rates in the 10 year interval have been calculated using official statistics and evaluated using regression methods; the correlations to age and sex-specific unemployment rates and the general availability of suicide methods were determined.

With an average suicide rate of more than 40/100,000/year in men and half of this rate in women East Germany suffered one of the highest suicide rates in Europe; following the fundamental socioeconomic changes accompanying the unification in general the suicide rates of men as well as those of women declined significantly; there was, however, in men a contradictory trend in the age group of the 50 - 65 year old. The decline of the suicide rate in women outnumbered that in men; while in the '80s domestic gas was used to commit suicide by 14% of men, but 28% of women, the use of this method had nearly vanished due to the detoxification of domestic gas.

In general the fundamental political and economic changes in East Germany had a positive effect on the suicide risk of the population. It is assumed that 2 factors mainly contributed to the decline of the suicide risk: The experience of a 'general charge' also resulting in a parallel decline of the birth rate exceeding that in World War ll and the detoxification of domestic gas. A contradictory trend in men aged 50–65 is attributed to a third detectable factor — unemployment — enhancing the suicidal drive in the age group mostly struck with it.

Economic and sociological factors once again proved very important as determinants of suicide; the concept of primary suicide prevention should take this into account.

NARCISSISTIC DISORDER AND MOTIVATION FOR SUICIDE

Paul Götze and Georg Fiedler — University Hospital of Hamburg, Germany

The importance of the theory of narcissism to the understanding of the psychodynamics of suicidal behaviour has not yet been empirically-statistically examined, for a suitable questionnaire has been lacking up to now. The Narcissmus Inventory developed by Denecke and Hilgenstock (1989) appeared to us to be very suitable; it contains systematically differentiated, theoretically relevant aspects of the organisation and regulation of the narcissistic personality system, as far as these aspects are accessible to self-observation.

The sample: of 240 patients consecutively interviewed following their suicide attempt, 100 patients could be surveyed with the narcissmus questionnaire.

The results of the evaluation of the narcissmus questionnaire, supplemented by an evaluation of the clinical interviews, were correlated with the motivation for the suicide attempt.

SELF CUTTING: FACTORS ASSOCIATED WITH TENSION REDUCTION

Janet Haines, Kerryn Brain, and Christopher Williams — University of Tasmania, Australia

To investigate the behavioural and cognitive factors associated with increased psychophysiological tension reduction to self-cutting.

A series of experiments were conducted investigating a range of behavioural and cognitive factors that are associated with an increased strength of psychophysiological tension reduction, namely, frequency of behaviour, premeditation, covert conditioning of the behaviour, cognitive control and impulsivity. Personalised guided imagery scripts of the act of self-harm and a neutral event were presented in four stages (scene setting, approach, incident, consequence) (Haines et al., 1995) and were used to assess heart rate changes as they developed over the course of behaviour.

Results indicated that strong tension reduction responses to self-cutting were evident in relation to increased frequency of the behaviour, no premeditation, high levels of covert conditioning of self-cutting, little cognitive control of thoughts and images associated with self-cutting, and higher levels of impulsivity.

Previous research has demonstrated a strong tension reduction mechanism is in operation that negatively reinforces the act of self-cutting. It has been determined that a range of behavioural and cognitive factors are associated with an increased strength of tension reduction. This information has provided the basis for a model for repetitive, impulsive self-mutilative behaviour by examining the covert processes associated with the psychophysiological response to the behaviour.

The results of these investigations further the understanding of a behaviour that has proven difficult to control.

EVIDENCE OF COGNITIVE DISTORTION IN THE CONTENT OF SUICIDE NOTES

Janet Haines and Christopher Williams — University of Tasmania, Australia

To determine if the dysfunctional attitudes, as described by Beck, of suicidal individuals can be determined from the content of suicide notes.

A sample of 50 suicide notes were selected on the basis that they contained reasons for suiciding rather than instructions only. Two independent clinician raters assessed the content of these notes for evidence of each of Beck's categories of cognitive distortion.

Evidence of cognitive distortion from each category was apparent. A range of demographic variables and suicide factors were associated with increased cognitive distortion.

Cognitive distortion has been reported to be evident in samples of suicide attempters. This investigation has provided a means of assessing similar information from a sample of completed suicides. Given the debate about the extent to which suicide attempters and completers represent the same population, it is important to determine the extent to which factors such as cognitive distortion are apparent for both groups.

The present study has provided a means of assessing the psychological state of individuals who subsequently complete suicide with the aim of increasing the understanding of risk factors for completed suicide.

INFORMATION SHARING — THE TRULY GLOBAL REALITY

Gerry Harrington — Suicidal Information and Education Centre, Canada

To review and demonstrate some of the current technology available for sharing suicide prevention information on a global basis, and to encourage the exchange and distribution of research results, curriculum development, national and regional policy and innovative strategies.

If there is one truly global aspect of suicide prevention which we can all benefit from it is in the field of *Information Sharing*. Suicide prevention services which may prove effective in some cultures may not be transferable to another culture, but information, knowledge and research which arises from efforts in one area may very well include significant components which are transferable to other cultures.

With current readily available technology such as the World Wide Web on the Internet, CD-ROM's, fax machines and satellite telecommunications it is possible to instantly access existing information databases which have been developed on suicidal behaviours. The accumulated knowledge from the suicide prevention field is already available to personnel worldwide.

This presentation will review the current leading technology in information transmission and dissemination and will demonstrate the use of the Internet and CD-ROM technology as they can be related to information sharing in the suicide prevention field. Participants will have the opportunity to add their expertise and experience and share knowledge.

FRIENDS OF ADOLESCENT SUICIDE ATTEMPTERS: A DETAILED PILOT STUDY

Philip Hazell, Terry Lewin, and Natalia Turnbull — University of New Castle, Australia

To pilot a methodology for examining the longitudinal effect of exposure to peer attempted suicide.

Immediate and remote friends of five known suicide attempters (n=11), three previously non-disclosing suicde attempters (n=10), and four non-suicidal psychiatric controls (n=12) were examined at 0, 3 and 6 months on measures of relationship to the focal adolescent, emotional and behavioural symptoms, and suicidality.

Control adolescents nominated more friends, and their friendship groups overlapped to a significantly greater extent (p<.05) than the suicide groups. There was an increase in depressive symptoms in the suicide groups, while depressive symptoms decreased in the controls (differences significant at the level of p<.05). There were similar differences in suicidal ideation, but only at 3 months. There were no significant group differences in behaviour problems.

Friendship groups of suicide attempters are less cohesive than those of psychiatric controls. The relative increase in depression and suicidal ideation in the suicide groups compared with controls over time suggests some pathogenic influence over and above assortive friendships. Further analyses will examine the association between the intensity of the relationship with the focal adolescent and outcome.

An understanding of the social ecology of adolescent friendships is essential to the investigation of the transmission of suicidality in such groups, and the planning of preventive strategies.

FOOTPRINTS IN TIME

Trish Hill-Keddie — Ministry of Justice/Aboriginal Visitors Scheme, Australia

"Mum remembers being dragged away kicking and screaming, Nanna was collecting the eggs when the welfare car came up and a policeman grabbed them. They were trying to get out of the car window and Nanna was trying to grab their hands and get them out". *(abridged from an article in "The Bulletin" June 27, 1995. Used with permission).*

This scenario is one to which I can relate. I am a 'stolen child', this extract is from an article written by my sister about a social experiment which went wrong. I am a survivor of this genocide, but there are many Aboriginal people who have past and present, mutilated, self harmed, and attempted suicide in an effort to erase the pain they endured from this experiment. The successful suicide attempts are at present growing, and are exacerbated by present government, ill health, unemployment and dislocation of family breakdown. The majority of these attempts are youth. Most attempts are made within the communities, they are hidden from the public.

"To take the most damaging example, the 99 deaths in custody investigated by the Royal Commission, 43 of the deceased had been separated from their families as children". *(Royal Commission Final Report April 1991).*

Suicide in Aboriginal communities is "taboo" it becomes a shame issue. Family of the victim is either shunned, or the actual event never occurred. Life goes on. No intervention takes place, no loss and grief, no questions asked, it is accepted, why? Suicide is ever increasing with our young Aboriginal youth, as early as 12 years of age — what can be so traumatising as to push a young person to neck themselves. This is the reality of living with a minority group that has been imprisoned with white ideologies, alcoholism, ill health, imprisonment and an inconsolable sense of loss.

This paper will endeavour to provide reasons why adolescent suicide is so prevalent in the Aboriginal community, and propose some solutions to reducing and educating those persons who are directly involved with suicide intervention within the Aboriginal Communities.

PARASUICIDE: PREDICTION OF REPETITION

Heidi Hjelmeland — Dept. of Psychology, Norwegian University of Science and Technology, Norway

The objective is to identify factors predicting non fatal repetition of a suicidal act.

Repetition was studied both retrospectively and prospectively. In the prospective analyses, patients with and without a previous history of suicidal behaviour were analysed separately. The data were analysed by hierarchical logistic regression analyses. To partial out their effect, sex and age were entered in the first step of the analyses, and the potential discriminators were entered in the second step. 1220 parasuicide patients registered in a Norwegian county during a period of six years were included in the study. In the retrospective analyses 11 variables were found to discriminate between repeaters and non-repeaters. In the prospective analyses of the patients with no prior history of suicidal behaviour (first-evers), only two of the variables were significant predictors of repetition of the suicidal act within 12 months following the index parasuicide, namely a lifetime history of sexual abuse and report of own psychiatric problems as their main concern at the time of the parasuicide. In the prospective analyses of the patients *with* previous suicidal behaviour, the only variables predicting repetition within 12 months were alcohol abuse and experience of suicide among relatives or friends.

In retrospective analyses of repetition there is no way of knowing which factors found to discriminate between repeaters and non-repeaters are actual predictors of repetition. Moreover, when studied prospectively, predictors of repetition are dependent upon which stage of the suicidal career the patients are in. Implications for secondary prevention will be discussed.

YOUNG PEOPLE AND PSYCHIATRIC ILLNESS — INTERVENTION AND ASSESSMENT (YPPI–IA)

Deborah Howe, Kim Braasch, Catherine Mackson, Martin Gallagher, and Kim Vukelich — Central Coast Area Health Service, Australia

The project will develop, pilot and evaluate an acute, home-based assessment service for young people experiencing significant mental health issues and at risk of suicide to promote better access and improved interventions.

This project has been successful in obtaining $325,000 over 2 years and 4 months, from the Commonwealth Department of Health and Family Services, Youth Suicide Initiative. This is one of three national projects funded for this specific client group.

Young people with a mental illness have been identified as being at high risk of suicide, homelessness, substance abuse and engaging in risk taking behaviour. The Young People and Psychiatric Illness (YPPI) Programme was initiated on the Central Coast of New South Wales (NSW) in response to the needs of these young people. YPPI is an innovative partnership programme between the Youth Health and Mental Health Services and has direct service and consultative components which has been in operation for the past two years. The YPPI–IA. Project will extend this model further to one which is complete with protocols and is measurable against specific indicators and transferable to other health areas. Attention will be given to addressing the impact of drug and alcohol comorbidity on suicide in this target population.

The literature identifies gaps in current modes of service delivery to the target group and points to early intervention strategies to address these services. In addition, local Central Coast data emphasizes a need to examine and implement programmes aimed at suicide prevention.

THE INFLUENCE OF CANNABIS, HOMOSEXUALITY, CHILD ABUSE, AND SEXUAL ABUSE ON THE INCIDENCE OF SUICIDE: A CONSUMER PERSPECTIVE

Tony Humphrey — Australian Mental Health Suicide, Consumer-Alliance Inc, Club Speranza, Australia

Suicide in Australia is now beginning to get political recognition as well as consumer power. Its capacity to threaten public health, immobilise and traumatise individuals and even government in its wake cannot be underestimated. The high incidence of youth suicide has attracted considerable attention and has generated considerable emotion.

What are some of the influences among young people? The use of cannabis is on the increase, again in the younger population. Figures also show a relationship with the number of admissions with symptoms of schizophrenia and a high incidence of suicide and suicide attempts among schizophrenia sufferers.

Often parents and parental users take the view that the occasional use of cannabis does no harm. Research is now showing that the effects of even low doses are considerable and result in impaired cognitive functioning, loss of self esteem, diminished responsibility, mood changes, auditory and visual hallucinations etc.

Suicide threatens young people in two other areas. Adolescent homosexuality and child sexual abuse are significant precursors to suicide and the evidence can be withheld from the consciousness to re-emerge as a threat to health and indeed to life.

Consumer involvement awareness and education are important mechanisms in addressing suicide among young people.

CONSUMERS IN PARTNERSHIP: A GLOBAL OBJECTIVE — THE SPERANZA CONCEPT

Tony Humphrey — Australian Mental Health Suicide, Consumer-Alliance Inc, Club Speranza, Australia

This paper looks at the raison d'etre, beginnings, and progress to date in developing and marketing a practical 'global' consumer driven concept to minimise suicide, moderate mental illness, and promote mental health and vital living in Australasia. SPERANZA the concept, is based on research, personal identification, long experience, empirical judgement and evaluated practice. It holds a set of national policies, objectives, and marketing strategy encapsulated in its name, and a working community approach of self-help support and recovery in partnership with service providers, agencies, other NGOs and government. 'Club SPERANZA' is the working model. It believes that like women and pregnancy, only from personal suicide experience can you relate to the grieving and the hopeless. With 90% of suicides suffering from a diagnosable mental illness and 70% from treatable depression and 10% of suicides occurring as known clients of the system or in protective care, new connections must be found.

SPERANZA promotes mental health and prevention, therefore it must also provide outreach and support to those who are actively or intermittently or chronically suicidal as well as those left behind. Its business/marketing plan is based on standardising services to conserve resources while creating personal interaction, establishing interrelated support groups of people on both sides of the event and facilitating the advancement of other agencies and health services' suicide prevention endeavours.

Among other things it advocates: a national *'HIGHLIGHT'* easy 3 or 4 digit telephone number adjunct to 000, for immediate access to universal and/or local services; and 'Friendship Houses' (time-out healing centres) for suicidal people pre or post hospital and for respite for bereaved family members.

EMPIRICALLY DERIVED RISK GROUPS IN ADOLESCENT SUICIDAL BEHAVIOUR: A REVIEW AND A NEW APPROACH

Erik Jan de Wilde, Ineke Kienhorst, and René Diekstra — Leiden University, The Netherlands

To present a state of the art in the field of adolescent risk groups for suicidal behaviour and to formulate a new approach towards it.

A review of the literature is combined with the results derived in a survey of approximately 2500 depressed adolescents, who were followed up one year after the first measurement. Data were gathered on various socio-demographic characteristics, suicidal behaviour, attitude towards suicidal behaviour, self esteem, hopelessness, depreciation and symptomatology. Data were analysed using the Chi-Square Automatic Interaction Detection (CHAD) program for segmentation modelling.

Risk groups were identified using the CHAD-algorithm. One group of 60 adolescents even gave a retrospective suicide attempt rate of 75%.

This sub-risk group approach, finding specific risk groups within a group of adolescents already identified as being at risk at a higher level than the general population, may provide better insights in the prediction of suicidal attempts at a group level.

"LIVING WITH SUICIDE": A MOTHER'S STORY

Carol C. Jefferson — Australian Mental Health Suicide Consumer-Alliance Inc., Australia

This paper is to be presented from a mother's perspective and gives an insight into what it is like to live with a son who is intermittently suicidal and eventually succeeds in completing the act after numerous attempts. It shows the frustration of being a nurse and a mother and not being able to cope adequately to prevent an eventual suicide. The paper covers a period of the son's life of 32 years and shows how the mother has dealt with the loss and how she feels ten years after the event. It points out the ongoing need for care of the son but also the need for attention of those close to him. This is often not taken into account when treating a patient and it is important for the academic and the service providers to be aware of this need. The story illustrates the two grieving processes ie. the loss of the complete interactive person to the family before the event as a long term life pattern disruption as well as the massive dislocating loss after the suicide itself. How the parent deals with the grieving during the life of her son has an effect on the son and the grieving after the event should be of importance to the understanding of those service providers endeavouring to meet the needs of their clients.

The paper shows the difficulty the mother has in sharing her feelings until she meets someone who has also experienced the loss of a child through suicide. It demonstrates the need for support groups for both those who have lost someone from suicide and those who have attempted and illustrates how beneficial it is to combine the two groups. The loss of her son through suicide enables the mother to empathise with those who have suffered that loss and, having lived with a suicidal son, enables her to give support to those who have attempted. In helping develop the Suicide Consumer-Alliance and its support groups the mother feels that, however devastating that loss was, something good has come as a result of losing her son.

SUICIDAL IDEATION AND SUICIDE ATTEMPTS AMONG 15–24 YEAR OLDS IN THE DANISH EDUCATIONAL SYSTEM

Gert Jessen, Karin Andersen, and Unni Bille-Brahe — Centre for Suicidological Research, Denmark

To evaluate background factors for suicidal ideation and suicide attempts among young people.

The instrument used was an anonymous and voluntary questionnaire study with 15–24 year olds in the Danish educational system. Beyond suicidal behaviour, focus has been placed on the well-being of the individual in every day life in relation to school, family, friends, leisure time, and the future. 3042 young people participated in the study.

About 40% of those interviewed had at least once had suicidal ideation and almost one in every twenty confirmed that they had attempted suicide. Furthermore, the study showed that almost one in every ten had experienced suicide in the family.

The study showed that frequent or chronicle suicidal ideation and self destructive behaviour can be considered risk factors of suicide attempts and possible predictors of future suicidal behaviour.

It appeared that the students who had experienced suicide in the family had a risk of committing suicide that was three times as high as that of the students who had *not* experienced suicide in the family.

It is probably only the tip of the iceberg which is detected or registered by the treatment system. To all appearances, close to 75% of these suicidal attempts by young people are *not* registered officially. This bears witness to the fact that many of these 15–24 year olds apparently received no help after their suicidal attempt.

PARASUICIDE IN PAKISTAN: ROLE OF SOCIO-CULTURAL FACTORS

Murad Moosa Khan and Hashim Reza — Department of Psychiatry: The Aga Khan University, Pakistan

To study the pattern of parasuicide in Pakistan, a Muslim country where due to a variety of social, legal and religious reasons data on suicidal behaviour is difficult to obtain.

A retrospective case note analysis of all index parasuicide admissions to a university hospital in Karachi was carried out between January 1989 and July 1995.

Of the 447 cases (262 females & 185 males) majority were under the age of 30 years. Compared to males females were younger (mean age 25.6 years, sd 8.81), more often married and their act was precipated by conflicts with their husbands or in-laws. Housewives were the predominant group. Males were more likely to be single and students. Medication self-poisoning was the most common method employed in 74% of cases of which 85% used benzodiazepines. 39% subjects bought the drug 'over the counter'. Organophosphate insecticides used by 21% subjects were responsible for 5 of the 7 fatalities. The gender was significantly associated with marital status ($p < 0.05$), age ($p < 0.001$), occupation ($p < 0.0001$) and reason for parasuicide ($p < 0.0001$).

Our findings suggest that marriage is a significant source of distress for females in Pakistan. The easy availability of benzodiazepines and access to organophosphate insecticides contributes to their high incidence in this series.

A change in law, greater public awareness and continued research into this important but neglected subject in Pakistan is recommended from our findings.

ABOUT THE DIFFERENTIATION OF THE CONSTRUCTION 'SUICIDALITY'

Manfred Kuda — University of Göttingen, Germany

For persons committing or attempting suicide, typologies with different criteria have been propounded and partly empirically verified. Suicidal intentions are less frequently investigated this way. But concerning the valid diagnostic of suicidality, the prophylaxis and an effective psychotherapy it is very necessary to register and differentiate this pre-phase of suicidal actions.

- What kind of prevelances (basis-rates) of suicidal intentions are present amongst clinical and non-clinical treated persons (here: university students)?;
- What kind of conformities exist between self-estimations and expert-ratings about suicidal tendencies?
- Which subgroups–typologies can be differed amongst individuals with suicidal tendencies?
- Are there differences between clients and non-clients?

Criteria of suicidality:

- Self-estimation and extension of acute suicidality by SCL-90;
- additional estimation for clients by prediction of suicidality in future;
- naming of symptoms by therapists after the first consultation.

Sample-tests:

a. students without previous psychological care, and
b. student clients of a psychotherapeutical welfare centre.

Accordances/divergencies between self-estimation and estimation by others were examined for the clients and likewise personality features for the two sample-test. We also examined correlative reciprocal effects between "suicidality" and the social biography. To differentiate the heterogenity of the construction "suicide intentions" cluster-analyses for the typology are calculated seperated by clients and non-clients.

THE PREVALENCE OF SUICIDAL FEELINGS

John Lawrie — The Samaritans, United Kingdom

Attempts to identify factors which predispose people to suicide are often not conclusive and no certain distinction between those who might be at risk and those who are not can easily be achieved.

The Samaritans in Britain and Ireland record approximately 21% of their callers as admitting to suicidal impulses, but this figure is understated due to the difficulty of establishing the state of mind of some callers, particularly those who end their call prematurely. A study which was undertaken on a limited scale will be described, with the tentative conclusion that suicidal impulses are much more prevalent among Samaritan callers than was previously recognised, even among those who initially deny such feelings.

A further exercise, designed to elicit the history of suicidal impulses among groups of Samaritan volunteers, will also be described. Though the nature and scale of the exercise were insufficient to produce data which could be relied upon to support firm conclusions, it will be postulated that the proportion of the population susceptible, in certain circumstances, to suicidal impulses may be large, with the consequence that a random element among suicides in the population at large may be inevitable.

TRENDS IN SUICIDAL SELF-POISONING
IN TALLINN, ESTONIA
(1980–1994)

Boris Loogna — Estonia–Swedish Institute of Suicidiology, Estonia

The objective of this paper is to determine trends in attempted suicide by poisoning during social revolutionary events (from socialism and stagnation through Gorbatchev's perestroika to independence and capitalism) in Tallinn, Estonia.

Data form patients being treated after suicidal self-poisoning in Tallinn Mustamäe Hospital have been analysed and compared in several different years through 15 years periods.

Besides a moderate increase in the number of suicidal poisoning's, there were found most significant changes in toxic agents used for attempted suicide.

Social instability is usually followed by dramatic increase in suicide rates. This has also happened in Estonia in the last few years. As suicide and parasuicide reasons are different, the motion of both rates does not straightly follow each other. Year by year the number of self-poisonings with psychotropic drugs has increased. This is in direct way connected with prescription of these drugs by doctors and with their preference. Life threatening poisoning's with strong acetic acid and organophosphate insecticides, very common in the beginning of eighties are rarely met after the open sale of these chemicals in shops was prohibited.

Among other social factors legislation and availability of chemicals and drugs seem to have the most strong and straight influence on the selection of toxic agent used for attempted suicide by poisoning.

SUICIDAL IDEATION AND PICTORIAL EXPRESSION

Alexanda Marinow — Clinical Psychiatric Hospital, Bulgaria

Plastic works done by depressive patients show sometimes important signs of the patients' suicidal ideation, represented in a symbolic and abstract way. Our study comprises a series of spontaneous drawings and paintings done by schizophrenic and drug-addicted patients during depressive episodes. The analysis exemplify how crisis and life-events as well as suicidal ideation could be visualized in these art works.

Thus, these pictorial art works could be helpful for:

- The *diagnosis*, as nonverbal communication in depressed patients with suicidal thoughts.
- The *prevention of suicide*, by means of interpreting the pictorial self-expressions as a symbolic sign of present suicidal ideation.
- The *therapy*, by facilitating the verbal communication during Art-therapy and Art-psychotherapy.

SUICIDE INTO THE 21ST CENTURY — A MULTI-FACETED PANDEMIC

Joan C. McVay — USA

This abstract is a preview of a book in progress which began the day I found my 28 year old son dead from a self inflicted knife wound in the heart. It holistically presents a unique blend of the cultural, environmental, economic, psychological, and physiological facets of suicide, citing current research in each area.

Particular emphasis is placed upon the newest research areas related to biochemistry and depression/suicidal mind-body processes: photochemistry, photobiology, photosensory biology, photomorphogenisis, and others. The interconnectedness between perceptions of environment and human biochemical responses is emphasized. The author proposes in the "Searching for Solutions" section that modern technology should be used to gather and report greater data world-wide on the biochemical evidence of those who suicide via more extensive forensics by coroners and laboratories.

The paper also includes cultural aspects, related to survivors experiences coping with loved ones' suicidal behaviour in an American society which keeps suicide stigmatized and "in the closet". At the conclusion of this presentation, the participants should be able to discuss from a multidimensional perspective the variables related to suicide, their trends into the 21st century, and an advanced insight into prevention, using 21st century research and technology. They will also understand that the end result of suicide is the result of a long continuum of interactions of perception and emotion and the human biochemical response system to the environment.

SUICIDE AS GOAL-DIRECTED ACTION: THE SUICIDAL PERSON'S NARRATIVE

Konrad Michel and Ladislav Valach — Psychiatrische Poliklinik, Universitätsspital, Switzerland

This is a theoretical paper, outlining an action theoretical concept of suicide. Suicidal behaviour has traditionally been seen in the frame of a biomedical causal illness-model. An action theoretical approach is proposed as an alternative basis for understanding suicidal patients and for establishing a meaningful communication with people at risk of suicide.

This model is based on the view that human behaviour is goal directed, intentional and planned, socially and cognitively steered and regulated. It is a developmental model that can be applied to long term projects such as life careers as well as to short term projects such as suicide. An action theoretical model of suicidal behaviour is compatible with a large number of empirical facts as well as with everyday practice.

Action theoretical concepts are based on social conventions, and it can be assumed that such concepts are naturally used in patient's narratives of the reasons why they attempted or considered suicide. We believe that in order to achieve a better mutual understanding between patient and helper, it is important to develop models of suicidal behaviour that are meaningful for patients.

Examples of patients' narratives (in the form of letters and oral accounts) will be used to illustrate the concept of suicide as goal-directed action. First experiences from the pilot phase of a research project based on systematic observation of video recorded interviews with individuals who recently attempted suicide, and self-confrontation discourse using video-playback will be discussed. We hope that the results of this study will answer the question if action theory is a useful approach to improve communication with attempters, and if, as a further step, an evaluation of its potential in prevention will be feasible.

EDUCATIONAL MOBILITY AND SUICIDE IN HUNGARY

Ferenc Mokosony — Budapest University of Economic Sciences, Hungary

Department of Sociology, Budapest University of Economic Sciences, Hungary. The aim of the study was to test two competing explanations of the effect of social mobility on suicide. The first regards t he *direction* of change as the decisive factor and expects loss of status to increase the risk of self-destruction. The second, in contrast, maintains that what really matters is change *per se*, not its direction, and, accordingly, mobile people are, regardless of whether they move up or down, more vulnerable to suicide than those keeping their social position.

To check the validity of these two explanations, I performed a case-control study, comparing people who lived in Budapest and committed suicide in 1994 with a random sample of non-suicidal individuals residing in the same city. Data on suicides came from interviews with relatives and other survivors, whereas information on the control sample was collected in 1994 as part of a large nation-wide longitudinal survey. Social mobility was measured as the difference in education level between the person in the sample and his or her father. The method of analysis was logistic regression.

The results indicate that, in keeping with the first explanation, downward social mobility greatly increases the risk of suicide. The second explanation, in contrast, received no support, since with the direction of change disregarded, suicide declined, rather than grew, with rising levels of educational mobility. It thus seems that the causal mechanism underlying the effect of mobility is not so much the anomie produced by the change, but rather the loss of status induced by moving down in the social hierarchy.

LAW AND SUICIDE PREVENTION — THE INDIAN EXPERIENCE

R. Srinivasa Murthy — National Institute of Mental Health & Neurosciences, India

Suicide prevention requires efforts from many sectors and professionals. The legal status of attempted suicide clearly describes the larger society attitude and response to the issue of suicide. In India, till 1994, attempted suicide was a punishable offence, punishment including imprisonment and fine. In 1994 this was reversed as 'inhuman' by the Supreme Court.

The reaction of the different groups to this historic judgement was conflicting. The issue was again examined by the larger constitutional bench of the Supreme Court and in April 1996 the punishability of attempted suicide was upheld as constitutional. The reasons for this were the issues of right to live and right to die, euthanasia, fear of misuse in dowry deaths, insurance etc.

It was also significant that professionals and non-governmental organisations did not use the 1994–1996 period to organise community level programmes and public education. In India, as in other developing countries, law plays an important role in the development of policies and programmes. The broader aim of suicide prevention has to include the legal status of attempted suicide. The 'criminalisation' of attempted suicide can lead stigma, avoidance of seeking help and lack of involvement of professionals and limitations in developing innovative programs of suicide prevention.

The paper presents the background to the legal status of attempted suicide till 1994, the 1994 judgement and the 1996 judgement and the implications of these developments for suicide prevention in India.

SUICIDAL IDEATION AND ATTEMPTS IN EARLY ADULTHOOD IN A COMMUNITY SAMPLE: PREVALENCE AND RISK FACTORS

Shyamala Nada-Raja, Rob McGee, Michael Feeham, John Langley, and Sheila Williams — University of Ontago Medical School, Injury Prevention Research Unit, New Zealand

The objective is to determine the prevalence and risk factors for suicidal ideation and attempts in a community sample of young adults in New Zealand.

A modified version of the Diagnostic Interview Schedule was used to assess the one year prevalence of mental disorder, including suicidal ideation and attempts in a birth cohort of 903 New Zealand young adults when they were aged 18 and 21 years. Self- and parent- report data gathered when the participants were aged 15 years were included in a logistic regression model to examine risk factors for suicidal ideation and attempts in early adulthood.

At ages 18 or 21, 17% of the sample (significantly more women than men) reported that they had thought about committing suicide (suicidal ideation) in the previous 12 months. At least one suicide attempt was reported by 33 study members. Overdose was the most common method used, and few had sought any help following their suicide attempt. A low perceived attachment to parents and peers at age 15 (OR=3.5) was the most significant risk factor associated with suicidal ideation in early adulthood for both women and men. Conduct problems and an external locus of control at age 15 significantly differentiated study members who had attempted suicide from those who had not attempted suicide.

A low perceived attachment to family and friends in adolescence was associated with the highest odds of suicidal behaviours. These findings are similar to those found by Kosky and colleagues who suggested that further research is required to identify the mechanisms underlying the relationship between family discord and suicidal behaviours in adolescents and young adults.

STAFF'S ATTITUDES TOWARD SUICIDAL PATIENTS

Ludvig Olsson, Inga-Lill Ramberg, Bo Runeson, and Danuta Wasserman —
Centre for Suicide Research and Prevention, Sweden

The objective is to investigate how suicidal behaviour and work condition of mental health personnel influence their attitudes toward suicidal patients.

A questionnaire of validated questions about social climate and supportive factors in work with suicidal patients, attitudes toward suicidal patients, and personal suicidal behaviour has been distributed to a random sample of mental health care workers in Stockholm county. Response rate was 60% (n=1025).

Seven percent report suicidal thoughts during the last year and 5% report that they have made a suicidal attempt during their lifetime. But they did not report difficulties in caring for suicidal patients. Those who report a bad relationship with superiors (p=0,01), conflicts in working environment (p=0,06), or getting unclear and unsatisfactory instructions about how to deal with suicidal patients (p=0,02) to a larger extent also report that they feel mentally exhausted in their work with suicidal patients. Compared to women, men seem to be more vulnerable to their work environment as men who report less supportive factors to a larger extent also report that they feel mentally exhausted in their work with suicidal patients.

Social climate and supportive factors in the working place has an impact on ones attitudes toward suicidal patients. Men especially seem to be vulnerable to conflicts and unsupportive social relationships. Staff's own previous or current suicidal behaviour does not influence their attitudes toward suicidal patients. Contrary to previous Swedish investigations with smaller materials the prevalence of suicidal thoughts or suicide attempts is not exceedingly high in mentally health personnel compared to the general population (7% suicidal thougths during last year and 3.5% lifetime suicide attempt, n=8800).

The results of this investigation shows the importance of a satisfactory social climate and supportive factors in work with suicidal patients.

ROLE OF THE BODY EXPERIENCE IN SUICIDE

Israel Orbach — Bar-llan University, Israel

The objective is to deal with the role of the body experience in suicide.

It is postulated that early caretaking processes have a powerful impact on self-destruction through the formation of alterations in the experience of the body and negative attitudes toward the body. Relevant theoretical and empirical literature in this area is reviewed.

The hypothesis that emerges is that the internalization of early negative caretaking processes and negative attachment may lead to a distorted experience of the body, as well as to a basic negative attitude and feelings toward one's body. Such body experience and attitudes are believed to interact with anguish, hopelessness, and mounting stress and culminate in self-destruction.

Some of the destructive processes intervening between distorted caretaking, experiences of and attitudes toward the body are described. These include lack of taming of self-aggression, lack of attunement to bodily needs, lack of representational learning to care for the body, symbolized hate toward the body, twisted perception of pain and pleasure, and dissociation. It is suggested that the role of the body in suicide may turn out as a most important avenue for future research in suicide.

ATTEMPTED SUICIDE AND UNEMPLOYMENT IN HELSINKI: 1989–1992

Aini Ostamo, Sari Valjakka, and Jouko Lonnqvist — National Public Health Institute, Finland

The objective is to analyse the relationship between attempted suicide and unemployment.

The individual data consist 2101 attempted suicide persons aged 15 years and over with some clinical and socioeconomic variables. The WHO/Euro Multicentre Study on Parasuicide monitoring data have been completed with official individual unemployment information. Attempted suicide rates among subgroups, characteristics of unemployed and the sequence of unemployment periods and suicidal behaviour are analysed.

The unemployed were highly overrepresented among suicide attempters and their relative rate rose sharply from 1989 to 1992. The attempted suicide rates of unemployed fell markedly from 1989 to 1992. The sociodemographic characteristics of suicide attempters remained rather constant at the same time when the proportion of the unemployed persons increased among attempters. In 1992 every second of the subjects who attempted suicide in 1989 had had unemployment periods whereas in 1989 every fifth of the same subjects had been unemployed.

Unemployment seems not to be so much the cause of attempted suicide as it is a marker of dysfunctional persons in relative employed society. The connection between unemployment and attempted suicide seems to be more due to a selection process.

The risk of becoming and staying unemployed is highest among those worst off, who also demonstrate higher risk of attempted suicide whether they are unemployed or not.

ADELESCENT SUICIDAL BEHAVIOURS: AN AUSTRALIAN POPULATION BASED STUDY OF RISK

George Patton, Ros Harris, Carolyn Coffey, John Carlin, and Glenn Bowes — Centre for Adolescent Health, Australia

The objective is to examine the characteristics and preditors of non-fatal suicidal behaviours in a representative adolescent sample.

Information has been gathered over a period of three years involving Australian secondary school students in year 10 (15 to 16 year olds) at 44 schools in the state of Victoria, Australia.

Self report of episodes of deliberate self harm were characterised using subject description and a modified Beck Suicide Intent Scale. Psychiatric morbidity was assessed using the Clinical Interview Schedule (CIS). Alcohol and marijuana use were evaluted using diary and self-reported frequency of use measures.

The twelve month weighted prevalence estimates for deliberate self harm was 5.1% with a significantly higher rate reported by females (6.4%) than males (4.0%). The commonest forms of self harm were self-laceration (1.7%), self poisoning (1.5%) and deliberate recklessness (1.8%). Gender differences in pattern of self harm were evident in higher rates of both self-poisoning and self-laceration in girls. The prevalence of true suicidal self harm, where the episode was reported as definite attempt to kill was 0.2%. The majority of self-harmers did not perceive death as likely, plan self-harming episodes at length nor inform others of the episodes. Psychiatric morbidity had the strongest association with deliberate self-harm in both boys and girls, an association which held for all subtypes of self-harm. Antisocial behaviour and substance abuse were associated with self-harm in girls but not boys. Sexual activity was independently associated with higher rates of self-harm in both genders. Further analysis will examine predictors of adolescent self-harm.

SUICIDAL IDEA: KEYSTONE IN THE SUICIDE PREVENTION

Sergio Perez Barrero — SCM: Dpto Psia Hosp "Carles M. Cespedes" Bayamo, Cuba

The suicidal idea is one step in the suicidal behaviour which include also the wish of death; the suicide image, the suicide threat, the suicide gesture, the suicide attempted, the failed suicide and the completed suicide. The suicidal idea is classified according to its internal evolution till the suicidal plan and some interview techniques are given as well as others semiological aspects (verbal and non verbal) of the suicidal idea.

THE ROLE OF GENERAL PRACTITIONERS IN YOUTH PARASUICIDE: A WESTERN AUSTRALIA PERSPECTIVE

Jon Pfaff, Melanie Wilson, and John Acres — Perth Central Coastal Division of General Practice, Australia

The objective of the present study was to determine the role of general practice in 194 patients presenting to a Perth public hospital, accident & emergency department, due to parasuicidal behaviour. The method consisted of a survey of 194 general practitioners (GP), identified by hospital records as the patient's family doctor. Each GP was contacted to determine the date of the patient's last visit prior to the parasuicidal act, nature of the consultation (somatic/psychological), and the source of medication for those patients engaging in overdosing behaviour. This data was compared across gender and age ranges, and represented 75% of all parasuicidal patients presenting to hospital during the study period.

Results from this sample of parasuicidal patients indicate that 67.6% were seen by their GP in the month prior to their presentation to hospital, 35% in the week before. The nature of these GP consultations were for psychological reasons in 42.8% of the cases, while 57.2% of the visits were for somatic complaints. Youth aged less than 25 years comprised 23.7% of the sample and tended to have a shorter duration between their parasuicidal act and their last GP visit (p<.01). In general, males tended to be older (p<.01), with a shorter duration to the parasuicidal act following GP consultation than females (p<.01).

Overdose was the predominant parasuicidal method, employed by 82% of the sample, where 31% of the subjects obtained the drug of overdose on prescription from their GP. A further 49.6% of the drugs used were over-the-counter medications. Conclusions; the present study expands previous research, demonstrating that young people in particular consult primary health care physicians within the month prior to engaging in suicidal behaviour. An under-recognition of psychiatric symptomatology, however, may occur in general practice settings. This emphasises the importance of training for general practitioners in recognising and responding to underlying psychosocial factors that place patients at an increased risk for psychological distress and suicide.

EVALUATION OF A "TRAIN THE TRAINER" MODEL OF YOUTH SUICIDE PREVENTION

Robert McKelvey, Jon Pfaff, Stephen Edwards, John Acres, and Geoff Riley —
National General Practice Youth Suicide Prevention Project

The objective of the present study is to determine the effectiveness of a training program for general practitioners in recognising and responding to psychological distress and suicidal ideation in young people ages 15–24. The method consists of a pre-post experimental design in which three randomly selected groups of general practitioners in Western Australia, Tasmania and Victoria are compared in terms of their ability to recognise psychological distress and suicidal ideation among young people presenting to their surgeries. The control group receives no training in the recognition of psychological distress and suicidal ideation. A second group receives training by means of a handbook addressing the recognition of suicidal ideation and suicide risk. The third group receives training in a four-and-a-half hours seminar based on the handbook.

The two educational groups (handbook/workshop) will evaluate the presence of psychological distress and suicidal ideation among their 15–24 year old patients six months after the training period. The control group will conduct identical patient evaluations prior to the educational period, to provide a baseline measurement, while a second randomly selected control group will complete patient evaluations during the six month post-training period.

Results of previous studies suggest that general practitioners can be taught to recognise psychological distress and suicidal ideation in their patients, and that such training may lead to a reduction in overall rates of suicide.

Conclusions; the present study seeks to expand previous research on youth suicide prevention by utilising an experimental model and applying it to a wide-spread geographical area.

UNEQUAL REGIONAL DISTRIBUTION OF THE INCREASE OF SUICIDAL BEHAVIOUR IN ITALY

Anotnio Preti — CMG Psychiatry Branch, Italy

CMG, Psychiatry branch, via Costantinopoli 42, 09129 Cagliari, ITALY. For about twenty years in Italy, as in other Western Nations, there has been a progressive rise in suicidal acts. Different factors have been invoked to explain this rising trend: the rise in existential stress, caused by the changes in the Western World after the Second World War, and the rise in incidence and prevalence of medical and psychiatric disorders which imply a suicidal ideation, are both considered to be very important. Since many factors with a well-known impact on suicidal behaviour are unevenly distributed across the National territory, regional differences in the distribution of suicidal acts were investigated in Italy.

The data were taken from the ISTAT Year Books, from 1980 to 1994. The yearly variation of suicide and attempted suicide rates have been analyzed in Italy from 1980 to 1994 according to their regional distribution. Furthermore, the Italian regional distribution of suicide and attempted suicide rates have been put in relation with some social and economical indicators according to their regional distribution.

Analyses shown an unequal distribution of self-inflicted acts according to their regional distribution. The unequal regional distribution of suicides and attempted suicides associate with the unequal regional distribution of wealth, as can be measured from Gross Domestic Product or from internal consumers rates per inhabitant, with greater changing in suicide and parasuicide rates in richer areas. Wealth, in effects, influences the microenvironment in which an individual expresses him or her self. The distribution of wealth also influences the regional distribution of marriages, separations and divorces, which show a strong relationship with suicide rates. A larger presence in wealthy area of people who are biologically predisposed to develop a disorder which imply suicidal ideation could be the condition that links suicidal acts to these social indicators. If the hypothesis outlined above is correct, a further increase of suicidal acts in the near future can be expected.

Efficient strategies of prevention should include an accurate evaluation of the class of individuals at risk, according to the demographic composition of the area. These strategies should also include accurate evaluation of the medical and psychiatric diseases with suicidal ideation, particularly when other risk factor concur, like a separation or the loss of employment. The setting up of crisis intervention centers become an important instrument for controlling suicidal behaviour in the region with greater risk.

POST-VENTION: A STUDY FROM MADURAI, INDIA

A. Venkoba Rao — President, Indian Association of Suicidology, India

The study comprised 250 consecutive suicide attempters (first attempt -234; M:128, F:106) from the Medical, surgical wards, intensive care unit and those attending the Institute of Psychiatry, Govt Rajaji Hospital, Madurai, India between 1 November 1986 to 15 March 1987. Of these, 16 proved fatal (M:11, F:5). One of the objectives of the project (Indian Council of Medical Research funded) was to examine the psychiatric morbidity in the members of bereaved families of the completers and their felt-need for intervention and offering post-vention measures to them. The follow-up lasted up to 31 August 1988.

Psychological autopsy was carried out in 13 out of 16 completers.

The clinical diagnoses (DSMIII) were: Depression (N=2) and Adjustment problems (N=2). Family history of psychiatric illness was elicited in 3. The impact of suicide on family was classified under three categories: Financial (n=2) Social (n=13) and Emotional (n=11). In 2 cases relatives felt a 'relief' from burden. Coping mechanism and supportive measures were: employment, turning to religion, psychiatric consultations and 'acceptance' as 'Karma'. Eight survivors (61.5%) felt the need for intervention and 2 (15.4%) for a need for employment while 4 felt intervention unnecessary. The interviewers found 11 needed counselling, 2 employment and 2 psychiatric consultation. Counselling was offered to 11 survivors at their door steps, while others were referred to psychiatric department. Two subjects were confident enough to cope with situation. Many survivors, though stigmatised, were surprised and felt consoled that such measures were available.

Post-vention is a neglected area and generally not sought due to stigma. Nevertheless the study has indicated the need for such measures.

SUICIDE BEHAVIOUR AND PHYSICAL ILLNESS — A SCREENING QUESTIONNAIRE FOR RISK DETECTION

A. Venkoba Rao — President, Indian Association of suicidology: Madurai Medical College, India

The material consisted of 250 cases of consecutive suicide attempters admitted into medical, surgical wards and intensive care units of Institute of Psychiatry of Govt Rajaji Hospital, Madurai. Sixteen of them ended fatally. Schedules used were: Intentionality - Lethality Scale (Beck); Beck's Depression Inventory (BDI); Beck's Scale of Hopelessness (BHS); Presumptive Life Events Scale. The DSM III criteria were used for diagnosis.

Among the objectives of the project (Indian Council of Medical Research funded) were (a) diagnostic categorisation of the cases of suicide behaviour and (b) to evolve a screening schedule for detection of suicide tendency in those with physical illnesses.

The Group 1: Seventy four (31.6%) subjects were psychiatrically ill; major depression (N=24); Adjustment disorders with depression (19); Dysthymia (9); Schizophrenia (6); Drug dependence (12); Atypical psychosis (3); Mental retardation (2); Grief reaction (1). The Group II: 104 cases had physical illness (44.4%): Peptic ulcer (N=26); Premenstrual syndrome with abdominal pain (N=6); Dysmenorrhoea (N=4); DUB (N=5) and unclassifiable abdominal pain (N=33). The Group III (N=145): Conflicts in various spheres; domestic, occupational, social or sexual. Overlap was observed between this and the first 2 groups.

Ninety subjects (33.5) were in contact with health care agencies: Sixteen of them under psychiatric care and 74 for physical illness. Twenty eight were in contact with medical personnel, one month, 75 within three months and 90 within six months before the attempt. However, the risk of suicide behaviour in them escaped detection. Hence a simple screening questionnaire was prepared for use by non-psychiatric medical personnel to elicit suicidal risk in the physically ill especially those with 'pain'.

Subjects with physical disorders comprise a large proportion of suicidal attempters. Assessment of suicide risk in them is essential. A screening device has been evolved for this purpose. This will enable institution of appropriate preventive measures.

MOTOR VEHICLE EXHAUST GASSING SUICIDES IN AUSTRALIA

Virginia Routley — Monash University, Australia

The objective is to investigate the epidemiology of motor vehicle exhaust gassing (mveg) suicides and the impact of catalytic on suicides by this method.

Australian data on completed mveg suicides and Victorian mveg hospital suicide admissions was collected. A sample of 1994 and 1995 Victorian Coroner's files of mveg suicide victims was investigated for vehicle details. Additional information on year and model was obtained by checking against a vehicle registration database. Inclusion of catalytic converter in the vehicle (post 1986 models) was noted. A literature search was undertaken for articles on mveg and other means of suicide. Discussion and correspondence were undertaken with personnel from relevant bodies.

In 1994 mvegs were the third major means of suicide. Victims were predominantly middle-aged males. Since at least 1970 mveg suicides have been increasing in both total numbers and as a proportion of all suicides despite the introduction of stricter CO emission standards and catalytic converters in 1986. Coroner's files revealed suicides to be occurring in vehicles fitted with catalytic converters. Victorian hospital admissions for mveg suicides have increased considerably since 1989/90.

There is evidence that reducing access to the means of suicide can reduce the overall suicide rate, especially if any transfer is to a less lethal means. The anticipated decline predicted from the introduction of catalytic converters has not yet occurred. Suicides are occurring in vehicles fitted with catalytic converters possibly because the device does not operate efficiently until warmed up. The increase in hospital admissions suggests the revised standards may be preventing some deaths. Allowable limits of CO emission have been reduced from 24gm/km to 9.4gm/km in 1986 to 2.1gm/km in 1997. The impact of the 1997 limit will be of interest.

Recommendations to reduce suicides by this method are — continued monitoring of mveg suicide data both in Australia and internationally, modification of catalytic converters to operate more immediately, modification of exhaust pipes to impede the attachment of hoses and installation of sensing devices.

REVISITING THE ACUTE-CHRONIC DISTINCTION IN SUICIDE PREVENTION

Kjell Rudestam — The Fielding Institute, USA

Suicide prevention efforts during the past several decades have been particularly helpful in responding to individuals with acute psychological crises. In this context the crisis intervention model works well, and basic principles of stress management and brief psychotherapy are generally effective. However, the crisis intervention model is not well-adapted to dealing with chronically suicidal individuals.

The purpose of this presentation is to clarify the nature of chronic suicide by taking a social constructivist perspective and placing the problem within the context of profound social and psychological changes in contemporary society. I will argue that the predominating values of American culture - rampant individualism, self-liberation, and consumerism - directly contribute to the experience of what Cushman refers to as the "empty self," and that this syndrome is related to high rates of depression, hopelessness, substance abuse, and suicide. What is particularly discouraging is that most models of traditional psychotherapy are poorly suited for dealing with such individuals, who more often than not carry Axis II diagnoses.

I will conclude this presentation by recommending interventions which are most likely to instil hope and optimism and which makes major use of social networks and communities.

MODELS FOR SUICIDAL BEHAVIOUR IN YOUNG SUICIDE VICTIMS

Bo S. Runeson — Centre for Suicide Research & Prevention, Sweden

Previous exposure to suicidal behaviour by next-of-kins was investigated in a sample of 58 consecutive suicides in 15 to 29 year olds. The method was a modification of the psychological autopsy.

22/58 (38%) of the subjects had at least one family member who had attempted suicide, but in only three families someone had actually committed suicide. Role models were more common in suicide victims with a diagnosis of Schizophrenia (63%) or Borderline personality disorder (56%) than in subjects with Adjustment disorder (13%, p=0.06 and 0.05 respectively) or Major depression (31%). Models were also more common in Substance abusers than in non-abusers (56 vs 23%, p=0.01). The suicide victim rarely used the same method as the family member. Plausible mechanisms for the family clustering were:

- heredity for depression among parent and victim;
- common personality traits of impulsivity in both generations;
- disturbed psychological development caused by exposure to parent's (repeated) suicide attempts;
- destructive coping patterns in the families.

Death of a close family member was more frequently found in male than female suicide victims (19% vs 0, p=0.06).Including models for the suicide among other relatives or close friends, any model was described by the informants in altogether 36/58 (62%) cases. Five subjects had been inpatients at the same psychiatric unit and revealed contagious elements such as:

- identification with a previous victim's problem;
- introduction to a certain method used by the model and later by the victim.

In a majority of the young suicides, interviewer identified models of suicide or contagious factors.

THE PATTERN OF SUICIDE IN JAPAN

Yukio Saito — Tokyo Inochi No Denwa

In the field of suicidology, the situation in Japan is obscured by many myths. It seems to be generally thought that hara-kiri is still common practice in Japan, together with other feudalistic practices. Another myth is that we have a very high suicide rate among children. Yet another is that we have a lot of cases of parent-child suicide, whereas in the West such suicides do not exist. In fact, 2% of Japanese suicides involve parent and child, while in the West figure is more like 1%. The Japanese rate may be double but the actual incidence is very low. As regards to child suicide, the pattern of high rates among the young peaked in 1979 and since then the Japanese curve has come to be very similar to that of Europe, where suicides increase with age. This is a sign of the times, as is the reduction in suicides among women, from 3:2 in the 1950s to 2:1 in the 1990s when women have easier lives. This paper will examine the myths and realities of suicide in contemporary Japan.

SUICIDE IN THE MILITARY: ITS RELATION TO PEACEKEEPING STRESS

Isaac Sakinofsky, Michael Escobar, Alain Lesage, Albert Wong, Michael Loyer, and Claude Vanier — Clarke Institute, Canada

The objective is to investigate causes of suicide in the Canadian Forces (CF) with particular reference to the possible role of UN peacekeeping stress.

Between January 1990 - June 1995, 66 suicides occurred among CF personnel. CF commissioned a study to investigate the problem. The study was tripartite: an electronic personnel database study comparing the suicides with a random sample of 4042 CF personnel, a matched case control of records, and a psychological autopsy investigation of a small sample and controls.

Peacekeeping did not emerge as a risk factor overall or for the land and sea forces; there was an increased risk for (non-combatant) air personnel which increased (O.R. 5.3) when single status and low rank were added. A higher proportion of psychiatric diagnoses including adjustment, mood and personality disorders and substance abuse but not PTSD was found among the suicides.

Air personnel are currently not deployed in formed units as are land forces; hence may feel isolated and without comrade support. Francophone suicides (higher than overall) may be due to more frequent single status with economic duress causing them to enlist. Contrary to expectation post-peacekeeping PTSD does not seem to contribute to suicide in the military but suicide preventive recommendations can be made.

COLLEGE SUICIDE: A FEMALE PAGLIACCI ALL-AMERICAN THREE SPORT ATHLETE

Charlotte J. Sanborn — Dartmouth College, USA

The suicide of a female, all-American, three sports, senior athlete in an Ivy League college had a profound effect upon classmates and coaches at a college that had not experienced any suicide for several years. The level of anxiety among student survivors was intense. The tendency to identify with the victim was felt most by fellow team members and assistant coaches closer in age to the team athletes.

The campus response to the suicides via community meetings, candlelight marches and open forums affected the study body in different ways. Age, class year, team sport, and the individual student's value system all played a part in the meaningfulness and rationality of life while the media attention "ad nauseum" added to the inability to allow the healing process to take place.

At Convocation one year later, we are dealing with the students' internalized sorrow surfacing once again. In his speech to the freshman, the Student Assembly President requests that they "Please ask an upperclassman about Sarah." The all-star female athlete, role model, and friend who could not sustain the cost leaves the survivors to wonder about themselves. How apt the Dartmouth motto, "Vox Clamantis in Deserto" — (a voice crying in the wilderness). A brief vignette will be presented.

COGNITION, FEELING, AND WELL-BEING IN THE ELDERLY

Sylvia Schaller — Otto-Selz-Institut fur Psychologie und Erziehungswissenchaft, Univesitat Mannheim, Germany

Because life of the elderly is often characterized by a loss of social roles and status, standards for successful aging are not provided by our western society. The purpose of this study is to investigate whether a state of subjective anomia influences feelings of hopelessness and depressive-suicidal tendencies in elderly persons (>65yrs), who are not in psychiatric or psychotherapeutic treatment. The cross-section study revealed a significantly higher subjective feeling of anomia in the group of the "old-old" as compared with the group of the "young-old", females, and the group with a low socioeconomic status.

The older age-group as well as the females and the group with low SES also had higher ratings on the scales designed to measure depressive symptoms. The group of elderly who experience subjectively high anomia reported more suicidal-depressive behavior and suicide ideas than people with a low grade of anomia. The longitudinal study shows that anomia was also a good predictor for future cognitions of hopelessness and loss of control as well as depressive feelings and suicidal ideas.

PUBLIC HEALTH NURSE AS OMBUD FOR
SUICIDE ATTEMPTERS

G. Schjelderup — National Institute of Health, Norway

The objective is to evaluate the post-suicide-attempt intervention performed by public health nurse in a community based "ombud-team" -designed for providing adequate treatment and support to suicide attempters. Factors such as motivation, strategies for clarifying patient-problems and planning interventions, theoretical understanding of suicidal behaviours, team-organisation, co-operation with other professionals and supervision were studied. Among the evaluated factors, *motivation* and *supervision* will be presented here.

A utilization-focused evaluation, where team-members were invited to formulate strategies and goals for the evaluation, was chosen. Semi-structured interviews were conducted with present and earlier team-members concerning motivational factors for working with suicidal people. Observation of team-members during formal and informal supervision sessions was carried out to categorise different elements of the supervision.

A desire to extend their professional experience and competence, a wish to care for suicidal patients, and of professionalism and supporting friendship woven through supervision, seem to be basic motivational factors associated with the ability to deal with suicidal patients. The availability of supervisor both in weekly sessions and whenever needed is the <<team glue>>. At the same time most team-members additionally also share their strongest emotions with their spouses when coming home after crisis interventions. Prior to the establishment of routine supervision a suicide resulted in one team member leaving the team.

Continuous professional supervision and informal support is necessary to maintain motivation for dealing with suicidal crises over a long period of time. Motivational factors influence on continuity and development of professional skills in the community-team as a unit.

Ombud-teams for suicidal patients should not be operated without suitable and continuously professional supervision for team-members.

TWO DETERMINANTS OF THE SUICIDAL BEHAVIOUR OF ADOLESCENTS — THEIR CONCEPTS OF DEATH AND ATTITUDES OF THEIR SOCIAL SURROUNDINGS

Gunter Schmitz — University Kiel, Child and Youth Psych., Germany

The summerarized results of two series of examinations:

The motives (aims of the action) for the suicidal dynamics of a person are firstly closely connected to his concept of death, secondly to the attitude of his social surroundings, the addressee of the suicidal acts. The concept of death (in fantasy) of adolescents demonstrates dimensions of mystic-paradisiacal, occult illusions and correspond with the stability of their feelings of self-esteem.

The attitude of teachers, social workers, adolescent therapists towards adolescent suicidal acts is hardly determined by age, occupation and sex. the decisive determinants of the evaluation are their own experiences with suicidal occurrences and the experience and full development of their own suicidal dynamics.

SUICIDAL FEELINGS IN A SAMPLE OF COGNITIVELY UNIMPAIRED OVER-SIXTY-FIVE-YEAR-OLDS INTERVIEWED AT HOME

P. Scocco, M. Dello Buono, O. Urciuoli, P. Marietta, G. Meneghel, and D. De Leo — University of Padua, Italy

The Authors undertook to survey the frequency of suicidal feelings, ideation and any suicidal behaviour over the preceding month in a sample of elderly subjects interviewed at home. An initial sample 100 subjects tested as part of a more extensive population study currently in progress in Padua, Italy, were interviewed on the basis of the Paykel et al system. The subjects were also assessed through administration of the Brief Symptom Inventory by Derogatis & Melisaratos to evaluate psychological status. At the time of the interview, and the Mini Metal State Examination by Folstein et al, in order to exclude cognitive impairment. In this respect, only subjects who scored 24 or over out of 30 on this test were included.

The paper presents and discusses the findings relating to those subjects who in the preceding month had considered that life was not worth living or had desired death, or actually planned or attempted to take their own life. A comparison is then made between subjects for whom psychiatric symptoms emerge on the Brief Symptom Inventory and had a psychiatric record, and those subjects with no psychiatric disorders. In view of the high suicide rates in the elderly population, awareness and assessment of suicidal ideation and behaviour in this age group may help provide answers to needed intervention, also considering the ever increasing number of individuals who reach old age.

STANDARDS OF CARE FOR SUICIDAL PATIENTS

Morton Silverman — University of Chicago, USA

The most common legal cause of action involving psychiatric care is the failure to reasonably protect patients from harming themselves. Independent of malpractice and tort law considerations, the suicidal death of a patient has significant ramifications for the therapist and the surviving family members and friends. The standard of care dictates that the clinician make a reasonable attempt to detect elevated risk for suicide. Where the risk is elevated, the standard requires that the clinician exhibit reasonable clinical management efforts based on the detection of elevated risk.

One approach to limit the risk of suicidal behaviours in psychiatric patients is to develop and operationalize minimum standards of care for the inpatients.

This presentation will provide a framework for developing such standards of care and offer a set of standards for both outpatient and inpatient settings. These standards will include those actions appropriate for the practicing clinician, hospital staff, and hospital administrators.

PSYCHOLOGICAL AUTOPSY OF 100 SUICIDES: COMPARISON OF PRE AND POST-WAR PERIOD

Slavica Selakovic-Bursic, Lidija Culibrk, and Olivera Sekulic — Institute of Neurol. and Psychiatry, Yugoslavia

The objective is to determine whether the rise in suicide rates in Vojvodina was influenced by dramatic events in former Yugoslavia.

Psychological autopsy was conducted over suicides committed in 1993, 1994 and beginning of 1995 on Vojvodina territory. The results were then compared to those of a similar study carried out in 1980. Comparison comprised 3 areas of data: socio-demographic (18 items), psychopathological (27 items) and suicidological (9 items).

In the post-war period there was significant increase in the number of retired persons, aged over 60 suffering from physical illnesses. The use of firearms also increased from 4 to 20 per cent. War experience and combat participation contributed to suicide in only 10 per cent. Economic situation worsened significantly and was barely adequate in 48 per cent and totally inadequate in 21 per cent. Among psychiatric cases there were significant increase of alcoholism and depressive reactions.

Contrary to our expectation, actual war experience contributes little to the genesis of suicide, but socio-economic factors appear to be dominant in generating suicide in post war period.

MENTAL DISORDERS AND CRISIS INTERVENTION

Zhai Shutao — Nanjing Neuropsychiatric Research, China

Aside from common causes of crisis, there are some special reasons responsible for crisis formation for mental patients. The susceptibility and vulnerability to life event is also higher in patients with mental disorders.

The peculiar origin of crisis for recovery of mental patients include some bias against the patients by the surrounding and hence affect their schooling, employment and marital life. In order to prevent relapse, crisis intervention must be provided to these patients and their families.

Seventy cases were reported, 36 males and 34 females . Most of the invalids had affective disorders and schizophrenia. After crisis intervention, the situation of the patients improved.

ELDERLY SUICIDE IN HONG KONG

Ewan Simpson — Befrienders International, Hong Kong

The objective is to determine the cause of the disproportionately high levels of suicide amongst the elderly population in Hong Kong.

Research was commissioned by Befrienders International and carried out by the University of Hong Kong, using data made available by the Census & Statistics Dept of Hong Kong and the police files of all suicides in a specific year.

The results, which will be published in February 1997, will enable Befrienders International to address the issue of elderly suicide with the most appropriate prevention methods.

PROGRAM EVALUATION OF THE NORWEGIAN NATIONAL PROGRAM OF SUICIDE PREVENTION

Irene Soeraas — Agenda Utredning and Utvikling AS, Norway

The objective is to evaluate the implementation and the results of the National Program for Suicide Prevention in Norway during the program period of five years.

The evaluation design is encompassed a formative and a summative evaluation. The focus of summative evaluation is the results of the program at pre-defined decision points. The formative evaluation is designed to contribute to the success of the program by giving feedback during the program implementation concerning implementation, strategies, organisational factors, and allocation of resources. The program will undergo five series of data gathering followed up by recommendations.

The evaluation is monitoring the National Program in Norway, and the first data gathering has been completed. Our recommendations so far is to adjust the program on some key issues.

A successful implementation will be more likely with an appropriate and professional evaluation design.

STRUCTURED DISPOSITION PLANNING FOR ADOLESCENT SUICIDE ATTEMPTERS IN A GENERAL HOSPITAL: PRELIMINARY FINDINGS ON SHORT TERM OUTCOME

Anthony Spirito, Deidre Donaldson, Jennifer Aspel, and Mark Arrigan —
Child and Family Psychiatry: Rhode Island Hospital, USA

The purpose of this project was to determine if a brief intervention specifically designed to enhance treatment compliance would improve the rates of outpatient psychotherapy in this high-risk group. Twenty -three adolescents (19 females and 4 males) who received medical treatment in an emergency department following a suicide attempt received a psychotherapy compliance enhancement intervention which included the following: expectations for and information about outpatient psychotherapy, discussion of the factors that may impede psychotherapy attendance, and a verbal agreement between the adolescent and parent/guardian to attend at least 4 psychotherapy sessions. After discharge from the hospital, each participant received 3 phone interventions over an 8 week period. The telephone intervention utilised a problem-solving format around 2 key areas: suicidal ideation and psychotherapy.

Compared to a 3-month follow up of 78 subjects who did not receive an experimental intervention, the experimental group had fewer outpatient psychotherapy "no-shows" (9% vs 18%) and a trend toward more sessions attended (5.5 vs 3.9). The effect size of the intervention was substantial (.47). There were no repeated suicidal attempts in the experimental group whereas the comparison group had a 9% re-attempt rate. The results of the intervention appear promising.

An intervention designed specifically to enhance compliance with outpatient treatment was effective despite the fact that the adolescents were referred to 16 different sites for outpatients care.

A randomised intervention trial to experimentally test the efficacy of this approach is planned.

YOUNG MEN'S DISCOURSE ON COPING — TELLING OTHERS HOW THEY SURVIVE

Matt Stewart — Australia

This paper attempts to address the effect of gender in suicide with particular reference to the social construction of masculinity. A related concern is the increasing high level of young male suicide in spite of the amount of suicide prevention research conducted in this country. The study was based on a radical theoretical approach which insightful suicide prevention research demands, but which is sadly lacking in much of it to date. The three theoretical components of the study are poststructuralist discourse analysis as used by Bronwyn Davies, Aaron Antonovsky's concepts of Salutogenesis and the Sense of Coherence and Edward Sampson's idea of the dialogic nature of the Self.

Qualitative methodology of the study featured unstructured interviews with a group of young men aged between 17 and 22. I analysed and discussed selected transcripts of the young men's discourses on coping techniques in four broad and related areas ie: The Hard

Masculine Culture of Drugs and Crime; Support After Sexual Abuse; Coping, Suicide and Guns; and Concerns about Sexuality.

Analysis and discussion lead to the conclusion that formation of small, confidential, and supportive discussion groups for marginalised young men is useful for sharing and developing coping skills and improving their management of stressors which are ever-present in the social (gendered) environment. The supportive group can be a place where more caring, nurturing and communicative discourses of masculinity can be developed. Such groups could have long term benefits in reducing the numbers of young male suicides if they are conducted by youth support agencies throughout the community.

ALL ABOARD? WORKING INTERSECTORALLY IN THE PREVENTION OF YOUTH SUICIDE

Barry Taylor — Centre for Social Health–NEHCN, Australia

Intersectorally collaboration has become the new buzz word in health promotion and health service delivery. But what does it really mean and how can this model be effectively applied to youth suicide prevention? It is just a new word to describe multidiscilinary or is about networking.

As part of the two year Statewide Youth Suicide Prevention Project in Victoria, Australia, intersectoral collaboration pilot projects were undertaken in two communities, one rural and one urban. A brief description of each project will be given as an introduction to the paper. Using the experiences learnt from this project, this theoretical paper will critically examine intersectoral collaboration and its application in the prevention of youth suicide.

It will outline the principles of intersectoral collaboration and describe the strengths as well as the weakness of the model. It will assess the impact of differing theoretical and professional paradigms on how collaboration can occur. Using the qualitive data from the projects evaluation, the paper will explore the issues of intersectoral collaboration can be sustained in a community post an intervention such as a project. The model of the Community Resource Team will be presented as a means of sustainbility.

The paper will conclude that intersectoral collaboration has a variety of meanings and that it is a new way for some sectors to relate with others. Collaboration often occurs in informal means at the worker's level but is never formalised at the agency or sector level. Collaboration requires a great deal of goodwill from all sectors and requires the development of common goals and a common language to work together. Overall, intersectoral collaboration is a useful strategy of the many strategies required to address the complex social phenomenon of youth suicide prevention in the late 1990's.

CHOICES: INTRODUCING A ONE HOUR YOUTH SUICIDE AWARENESS SEMINAR

Darien Thira — Vancouver Crisis Centre, Canada

CHOICES is a one hour *youth suicide awareness seminar* which is currently being used by over 150 suicide prevention programs in Canada, the USA, and Australia. Sensitive to demographics and diversity, the international-award winning 16-minute *video* invites the viewers to identify with young adults who have overcome their suicidal feelings as teenagers, and family that lost their 14 year old boy to suicide as they speak candidly of their personal experiences and insights. Woven throughout the interviews is a dramatised example of how a youth (or adult) can help a peer in crisis. The *facilitator's manual* includes: necessary background information on youth suicide, some essential pointers for teaching suicide education; video transcript, a suggested seminar outline; and an optional facilitator's "script" with all visuals and references to the video included. Designed for youth and those who work with them, the seminar can be facilitated by suicide prevention professionals, trained crisis centre volunteers, teachers, counsellors, or other committed persons. The video, manual and seminar itself will be explored in this interactive workshop.

PROTECTIVE FACTORS IN ADOLESCENT SUICIDE PROBLEM

Martina Tomori — Chair of Psychiatry, Slovenia

The objective of the study was to identify and assess the main protective factors in adolescent suicidal ideation and behaviour.

A comprehensive questionnaire including depression and self-respect measuring validated scales was applied in the sample of 4706 high-school students in Slovenia. The data on various patterns of self-destructive behaviour as well as suicidal attempts and ideation were collected and their correlation to family, social behaviour, attitudes towards health, sport and some other issues were studied. Depression and self-esteem were assessed and their role in suicidal behaviour and ideation was evaluated.

The study identified several protective factors in the adolescents' family peer-group, school and social environment. Some of the characteristics of low risk group of adolescence were found as well.

Prevention of suicide in children and adolescents is a complex task. It should take into account all the relevant factors specific fro the developmental period. Suicidal behaviour in adolescence is often connected to high depression and low self-esteem.

Suicidal risk in adolescence is high. All the relevant protective factors should be identified and promoted by preventive programs specially adapted to the specific needs of the population of this age group.

SUICIDE HELP!! PROMOTING FIRST RESPONSE SKILLS

Eric Trezise and Rodney Lynn — Teakl Education Pty Ltd, Australia

The objective is to provide each person in the community with an easy to use resource for responding to situations of suicide. A Quick Look Handbook and associated training programme were developed to provide suicide awareness training and response skills.

The Handbook provides thumb indexed, concise, instant, reference materials to the reader.

The associated training programme provides:

1. Awareness of actions to take in situations of suicide;
2. A take away copy of the Quick Look Handbook;
3. Interaction and Discussion;
4. A self development and personal preparation project, to affirm questionnaire, SCID, FH-RDC and SAP (Standardised Assessment of Personality).

5. Appraisal / assessment of the project with a certificate of participation issued upon successful completion;

6. Provision of a *Suicide Counselling Available Here* symbol for use by participants.

Reception of the Handbook by community leaders and service providers has been impressive.

The handbook recently published, and is being eagerly accepted by Lifeline around Australia, Educational Institutions (Schools and TAFE), Juvenile Justice Centres, Community Services Departments, Area Health Services, The Salvation Army, Wesley Mission and its Lifeforce Suicide Prevention Programme, Medical Practioners etc.

The Handbook has been immediately recognised as a uniquely easy to use, and "friendly" resource.

The training programme has been well accepted, but is yet to be more extensively tested over time, before definitive results can be claimed.

Provision of this programme has met a community need and is being acclaimed by those who have come in contact with it. Further positive and practical developments are expected.

GROUP WORK AS A WAY TO PREVENT SUICIDAL BEHAVIOUR OF PUPILS

Olga Vasilyeva and Sergey Ulanitsky — Rostov University, Dept. of Psychology, Russia

According to our idea, the main cause of suicidal behaviour of teenagers is a non self-acceptance, the inability to understand self-value and as a result , a tendency to give more significance to the attitude of other people to them (especially relatives and friends). To prevent suicidal behaviour of teenagers we invented special programms of group work (training). The main aim of these programms is a rising of self-understanding and self-acceptance (it's possible only as a result of high appreciation of oneself from the other members of the group). We also work with life values and life aims, especially we emphasise the value of life.

In these groups we use special exercises which give us an opportunity to find out the actual values and understanding of life and mark the persons in risk zone (we work with them in special groups). Besides, during these exercises and after them, while discussing their results (the feed-back) the pupils change their attitude to their life.

During the studies we model different stress situations that provoked the aggressive behaviour. We analysed the different forms of aggressive behaviour, especially the suicidal behaviour as an extreme form of autoaggressivness.

The main result of the group work- the strengthening of mental health of pupils and reducing the risk of suicidal behaviour.

RISK FACTORS FOR COMPLETED SUICIDE IN SOUTH INDIA

L. Vijayakumar and S. Rajkumar — India

Around 90,000 people commit suicide in a year in India, but there is a paucity of studies on completed suicide. So it is essential to find the risk factors to plan for effective suicide prevention strategies.

We tried to determine the role of psychiatric illness, life events and family psychopathology as risk factors for suicide.

Population based case control study design was chosen. 100 suicides which occurred in a defined geographical area in Madras and 100 neighbourhood controls matched for age, sex and socio economic status were studied using the psychological autopsy technique. The instruments used were a predesigned detailed questionnaire, SCID, FH-RDC and SAP (Standardised Assessment of Personality).

The odds ratio for the presence of Axis 1 disorder as a risk factor was 19.5 (CL 7.32 < OR < 73.35), for family history of psychopathology was 12.75 (CL 4.69<OR<48.59) and for lack of faith in God was 6.83 (CL 2.88<OR <19.69). The other risk factors identified were recent life events, personality disorder, early parental loss and previous suicide attempt.

Presence of DSM-III-R Axis I diagnoses, family history of psychopathology and recent life events were found to be significant risk factors for completed suicide. Individual strategies like effective treatment of psychiatric illnesses, social strategies like restriction of alcohol consumption and preservation of religious faith may reduce suicides in India.

FINLAND'S NATIONAL SUICIDE PREVENTION PROJECT: IMPLEMENTATION, EXPERIENCE, AND EVALUATION

Maila Upanne, Jari Hakanen, and Marie Rautava — National Research and Development Centre for Welfare and Health, Finland

Finland was among the first countries to create and implement a national strategy for suicide prevention. The strategy was based on Suicides in Finland -87 research programme. The internal evaluation shows that the aim of comprehensive nationwide implementation has been largely achieved.

Survey data (1996, sample N=1693) reveal that practical activities have emerged all over the country and in many professional fields. 37% of the respondents reported that a project had been initiated at their workplace during the implementation phase. Some dozen sectors, from health care to police and rescue service, have been involved. Multisectoral cooperation has been chosen as an approach by 50% of working units. The broad strategy developed for the national project, including suicide-specific, nonspecific and promotive targets seems to have been generally approved

and applied. Two thirds of those running activities estimated that they would continue for at least a few years after the project. Over one third of the respondents estimated the project to have somewhat or greatly stimulated suicide prevention in practices.

Apart from activating by networking, another strategy has been to collaborate with key sectors in order to develop practical models in the nationwide context. Examples of these are cohort-orientated training programmes for the army and church, and "good practices" - programs for schools (crisis model) and health care (suicide attempters). Our cooperative process model has proven a promising strategy in the evolution and implementation of new challenges and practices.

GENDER-SPECIFIC PSYCHOBIOLOGICAL ASPECTS OF SUICIDAL BEHAVIOUR: A STUDY OF TEMPERAMENT, CHARACTER AND BIOLOGICAL MARKERS

Kees van Heeringen, Lieve Van de Wiele, Alain Verstraete, and Stijn Jannes —
Depts. of Psychiatry & Clinical Biology, University Hospital, Belgium

Recent research indicates important gender-specific differences in the efficacy of treatment and in the outcome of suicidal behaviour. This study aimed at investigating the contribution of Cloninger's recent psychobiological personality model to an explanation of these differences.

Measurements included Cloninger's TCI, and the levels of HVA, MHPG, 5-HT, and MAO-activity in venous blood, and urinary cortisol(HVA not yet available). Personality dimensions and biological characteristics were compared to deliberate self-poisoning (DSP) patients and patients without a history of DSP, stratified by gender.

When compared to females without a history of DSP, female DSP patients showed lower scores on reward dependence (RD3), cooperativeness (C2), and MHPG. RD3 and MHPG correlated negatively ($r=-.50, p<.05$). Among males, DSP patients showed comparatively higher scores on novelty seeking (NS2 & NS3), and cooperativeness (C1), and lower 5-HT levels. 5-HT correlated negatively with HA scores ($r=-.50, p<.05$).

The results indicate important differences in the psychobiology of DSP between females (reward dependence/noradrenaline) and males (impulsivity/serotonin).

Application of Cloninger's psychobiological personality model reveals important gender-specific differences in the mechanisms underlying deliberate self-poisoning. Further study is needed to replicate these findings, and to evaluate psycho- pharmacotherapeutical implications.

SUICIDE PREVENTION IN SECONDARY SCHOOLS: AN EDUCATIONAL AND CONCERTED ACTION PROGRAM IN BELGIAN SCHOOLS

Kathleen De Rycke and Kees van Heeringen — Dept. of Psychiatry, University Hospital, Belgium

During the past three decades there has been an alarming increase in suicidal behaviour among young people. Although a substantial number of actions towards a solution of this problem have taken place, suicide rates do not decrease.This lack of effect can be attributed to the complexity of the problem. Preliminary investigations, however, indicate that a lack of co-operation between health care organisations is another important contributory factor. Therefore,there is a great need for a concerted action program for suicide prevention among young people including all institutions involved in the care for young people.

Previous suicide prevention programs have focused on raising awareness of the problem of adolescent suicide among secondary school students. Evaluative studies have, however, not found any beneficial effect of these interventions. Therefore, the goal of the current prevention project is to train teachers to identify adolescents at risk of suicide, and to educate them about community mental health resources and referral techniques. More-over, feed-back from these resources to the schools is included in the program.

The prevention program aims at the implementation of a concerted action including the teachers, schools and mental health care providers, primarily in a well-defined pilot-region. Before the program is extended to other regions, it will be evaluated. Implementation will occur if indications for the efficacy of the program are found.

MALE AND FEMALE SUICIDES IN THE FORMER USSR

Danuta Wasserman and Airi Varnik — Estonian-Swedish Institute of Suicidology, Estonia

In 1988, secret information held by the Sate Statistical Committee of the USSR in Moscow became accessible.

Data were collected from primary documents in Moscow for the whole of the USSR and its constituent republics.

Suicide rates in 1990, the last year of the Soviet Union's existence, were 34.4 per 100, 000 males and 9.1 per 100,000 females. Regional differences within the USSR were studied according to groups of republics: Baltic (Estonia, Latvia, Lithuania), Slavic (Russia, Belarus, Ukraine), Central Asian (Kasakhstan, Uzbekistan, Tajikistan, Turkmenistan, Kirgizstan), and Caucasian (Gergia, Azerbaijan, Armenia). Male suicide rates varied between republics, from 2.6 in Azerbaijan to 44.3 in Lithuania in 1990. Suicide rates of women were lower and less variable than those of men, ranging between 0.7 in Azerbaijan and 14.1 in Estonia in 1990.

The former Soviet Union is a vast conglomeration of diverse languages, cultures, traditions and lifestyles. Cultural background appears to be a factor related to suicide attitudes and behaviour. Regions with a historically Christian background- the Slavic and Baltic countries had the highest suicide rates. Central Asia, with its prevalence of Islam among native people who strongly disapprove of suicidal behaviour, had suicide rates one-third to half of Christian people, as well as smaller ratios of male to female suicide. Cultural background also influences alcohol consumption, which is strongly associated with suicidility. Alcohol consumption in Central Asia and the Caucasus is between one-fifth and half that in the Slavic and Baltic republics.

EXPERIENCES RELATED TO A CONSCIOUS WISH TO END ONES LIFE — ATTEMPTED SUICIDE

Kari Vevatne — Rogaland Psychiatric Hospital, Norway

The study was carried out in 1995. It consisted of 16 interviews with Norvegian persons, between 20 and 64 years old, who had attempted suicide. Each person was interviewed twice, the day after the attempt and two weeks later.

The intention of the study was to understand experiences after the attempted suicide and it was used a qualitative, hermeneutic method. The theories of Melanie Klein and Julia Kristeva were used as the most important theoretical framework.

The interpretation of the interviews showed 5 central consepts, integrating each other. The concepts are: empty, shameful, lonly, envy, hopeless. An abstraction of these 5 concepts, make the consept: *Powerless*.

In the involvement with suicidal persons it will be important to have knowledge about powerlessness as a deep feeling in a person's mind.

SUICIDAL THOUGHTS IN WOMEN —
A GENERAL POPULATION SURVEY

M. Waern,[1] J. Beskow,[1] P. Allebeck,[2] and F. Spak[2] — [1]Dept. of Clinical Neuroscience, Section of Psychiatry, Sahlgrenska Hospital and [2]Dept of Social Medicine, Vasa Hospital, Sweden

The objective is to test the association between suicidal thoughts and depression, anxiety disorder, alcohol dependence or abuse (ADA), and low social functioning according to GAF in women in a community setting. Personality characteristics will also be examined.

Face to face interviews were administered to a stratified selection of 25–65 years old women (N=316) in the second phase of a general population survey. The women completed the Karolinska Scales of Personality, a self-report personality inventory. Suicidal ideation was rated according to Paykel. Diagnoses were made according to DSM-III-R.

The prevalence of suicidal thoughts during the past year was 6.6%. A stepwise logistic regression showed that independent contributions were made by last year diagnoses of depression and anxiety disorder but not by ADA or low social functioning according to GAF. A third of the women who had suicidal thoughts during the last year had no mental disorder during this period of time. Women with suicidal thoughts had significantly higher scores on somatic anxiety ($p<0.01$), psychic anxiety ($p<0.001$), muscle tension ($p<0.01$), psychastenia ($p<0.01$), indirect aggression ($p<0.05$), irritability ($p<0.05$), suspicion ($p<0.01$), guilt ($p<0.01$), and low socialization ($p<0.05$) than women without such thoughts.

The last year prevalence of suicidal thoughts in this female sample was only half that found in a previous Swedish study using the Paykel questions in an anonymous questionnaire. This highlights a methodogical problem in the assessment of suicidal ideation. The finding that ADA is not associated with a higher frequency of suicidal thoughts is unexpected and supports the notion that concommitent mental illness plays an important role in the suicidal process in female alchohol abusers. Further study on the interactions between personality, mental disorder and suicidal ideation is called for.

SALUTOGENETIC ASPECTS OF SUICIDOLOGY

Wedler Hans — Burgerhospital, Germany

The concept of Salutogenesis (Antonovsky, 1971), developed for better comprehension of the course of chronic illness supposed to be in line with stress, has been influential in the field of psychosomatic, but not in suicidology. This study tries to find out traces of this concept in actual suicidology and crisis intervention practice.

Sociological and epidemiological data support the interpretation of suicidal behaviour to be an inherent element of human life, usually prevented by salutogenetic factors.

Crisis intervention techniques are more directed on the chance of longer life, than on the elimination of "suicidogenetic" factors.

External organisation, in spite of attracting a lot of people, mostly do not elevate suicide rates. The chance to commit suicide is known to minimise special human fears.

The actual debate on medical assisted suicide seems to involve even as an "salutogenetic" element of a widely individualised and disintegrated society.

PREVENTING SUICIDE IN RURAL AUSTRALIA: DEVELOPING STANDARDS OF BEST PRACTICE IN COUNTY HOSPITALS

Bronwyn Williams, Katrina Hithersay, and Anthony Collier — Community Mental Health Services, Australia

During 1994/95 surveillance was conducted in the Great Southern Region of Western Australia, which aimed to detail the incidence, clinical management and follow-up arrangements for people at risk of self-harm.

From the information collected during this study, and according to the guidelines provided by the state's Youth Suicide Advisory Committee, the next phase has commenced to develop best-practice protocols for the main regional hospital.

Currently, the project consults with key hospital and community stakeholders. It is anticipated the development of these procedures will act as a pilot for the remaining hospitals and nursing posts in the region, and other rural areas.

This paper details the outcomes and obstacles to the development of best-practice protocols in a regional hospital in Western Australia.

COMMUNITY ATTITUDES TO SUICIDAL BEHAVIOUR: A 20 YEARS FOLLOW-UP

Lisa Thomson, Janet Haines, and Christopher Williams — Depatment of Psychology: University of Tasmania, Australia

The objective is to examine the relationship between attitudes and suicidal behaviour by surveying the beliefs and knowledge of high risk cohort members (16–26 yrs; 55+ yrs) of suicidal behaviour.

400 members (200 x cohort) of the Hobart community completed a questionnaire (Sale, Williams et al., 1975). Attitudes and knowledge regarding motives for suicide, lethality of methods, personal contact with victims, and the contribution of the media to knowledge and beliefs concerning suicidal behaviour were examined. Results were contrasted with those of a study conducted 20 years ago in Hobart with the two samples matched for age, sex and social class.

Sex differences in attitudes to suicidal behaviour were evident. Unlike the previous study, no difference was identified between cohort groups' attitudes with the development of less sympathetic attitudes among the young over the 20 years period. Differences in the sources of information influencing attitudes between the young and the older groups were noted; the young had a wider range of sources of information.

The reduction in reported sympathetic attitudes to suicidal behaviour over the past 20 years coincides with increases in rates for the behaviour over that time period. The results provide support for the proposition that unsympathetic community attitudes may be related to the occurrence of the behaviour. Increased sources of knowledge, including the media, may promote less sympathetic attitudes.

Further understanding of community attitudes toward the behaviour may provide information relevant to the targeting of prevention programmes.

POST-SUICIDE-ATTEMPT INTERVENTION — A NATIONAL PERSPECTIVE

M. Ystgaard, L. Mehlum, and E. Major — Suicide Research Unit, University of Oslo, Norway

In 1996 the Norwegian Ministry of Health established the National Suicide Research Unit as part of the Ministry's Program of Suicide Prevention. This paper will describe and discuss one of the main research areas of the research unit: the treatment chain for suicide attempters, which comprises 1) the hospital evaluation and care, 2) the community based «ombud-team» and 3) the collaboration between the hospital and the local team.

Since the municipality of Bearum established an «ombud-team» in 1983, several other communities have formed similar teams giving help to the suicide attempter immediately after the hospital discharge and thus representing a link between the hospital and further counselling.

In Norway all somatic and mental health services are sectorised and cover all subgroups and classes of patients. In this way it's possible to organise collaboration between the hospital and the community health service for all suicide attempters within a certain sector, and to do follow-up studies on representative samples. The clinical evaluation of this ombud model are promising, but more systematic evaluation of the effect of this intervention, and information about adaption to local conditions are needed.

STUDY ON ATTITUDE TOWARD SUICIDE AMONG MEDICAL STUDENTS IN CHINA

Xiao Ming Yu — Institute of Child & Adolescent Health: Beijing Medical University, China

The objective is to understand the attitude toward suicide among medical students, and to provide the suggestions in preventing suicide.

The study used self-reported questionnaire that includes 45 items made up of 38 items on suicide opinion questions (SOQ) and 7 items requesting demographic information. The SOQ was scored by five levels, namely "strong agree", "agree", "undecided", "disagree", "strong disagree". The subjects were selected randomly from a medical university in Beijing, total number were 231, in which males were 74 and females were 157.

The attitudes toward suicide among the medical students investigated were shown very complex and interesting inclination with different questions.

When the medical students begin their medical career after graduation, they will be likely to have many opportunities to contact the suicide attempters, so their attitudes toward suicide can have effect on their behaviours and services toward attempters. Through our study, we found that medical students could not accept general suicide caused by some reasons such as failure in learning or loving, but the suicide committed by individual who suffers from incurable disease, which reflect the multiple influences of Chinese traditional culture and primary experience of medicine.

The study will provide medical students with the education for prevention of suicide in the framework of the whole medical education so as to help them deal with the problems related to suicide confidently in the future career and to improve services in preventing suicide.

STUDY OF SUICIDE AS AN AUTOAGGRESSION ON THE OEDIPAL STAGE OF PERSONS DEVELOPMENT

Elena Zolotilova — Russia Institute of Family Social Care Centre, Russia

The Psychoanalysis considers suicide as manifestation of autoaggression, destructive action aimed at the introjection.

Let us suppose aggression to be primary and autoaggression secondary, then sense's ambivalence about significant objects determines ambivalent attitude to himself, or rather to those sides of person's structure, which results of internalisation. As a rule one of the ambivalent sides is repressed, usually this hate or other negative emotional experiences, contain destructive effect. The aggressive image of rival mother or rejecting father is internalised, forming person's aggressive energetic potential. If energy release via libido is frustrated it comes out through destructive actions.

The conditionally three suicide risk degrees may be defined:

1. A low risk with energetic potential release via libido cathexis;
2. Risk increases when libido mediated energy release is frustrated, but they are in social environment object to whom the aggression may be projected (outward aggression);
3. A real danger of suicide. An unrealised, repressed aggression turns against the self. Thus, it manifests as somatic diseases, accident liability, asocial behaviour and finally suicidal attempts.

Oedipal stage problems study on the group of patients with suicidal attempts or thoughts allow projection onto social objects, causing intensive negative emotional experiences, transference and reveal aggressive introjection.

PLENARY SESSIONS

ABORIGINAL SUICIDE IN TAIWAN

Andrew T.A. Cheng — Institute of Biomedical Sciences, Taiwan

To examine the psychiatric and sociocultural risk factors of suicide and their implications for suicide prevention among two major aboriginal groups (Atayal and Ami) in Taiwan. A matched (1:2) case-control study with biographical reconstructive intervention was conducted for 60 consecutive aboriginal suicides in East Taiwan.

The incidence of suicide was significantly higher in Atayal (64.8/105) than in Ami (16.1/105). In both groups, 97% of suicides suffered from mental illness before committing suicide. The most prevalent psychiatric disorders significantly associated with the risk of suicide were severe depressive disorder, substance use disorder and emotionally unstable personality disorder (EUPD) (F60.3 in ICD-10-DCR). While the prevalences of severe depression were similarly high in both groups (83.3% and 86.7%), that of substance use disorder and EUPD were much higher in Atayal (70.0% and 56.7%) than in Ami (53.3% and 26.7%). A higher risk of suicide was significantly associated with a lower degree of acculturation in Atayal. Although 43%-53% of suicides had consulted medical professionals in the last six months, the medication was insufficient for the treatment of depression.

The higher incidence of suicide in the Atayal was speculated to have come from their higher prevalences of alcoholism and emotionally unstable personality disorder, a lower degree of acculturation, and a weaker family support and kinship tie. It is suggested that early detection and proper treatment of depression might be a feasible and effective measure for suicide prevention in these two Taiwanese aboriginal groups.

AUSTRALIAN STUDIES

Jennifer Chipps, Gavin Stewart, and Geoffrey Sayer — NSW Centre for Mental Health, Australia

Using existing data sets such as the Australian Bureau of Statistics Death Data, The NSW Inpatient Statistics Collection and the Department of Health's Suicide Surveillance System of Clients of Mental Health Services in NSW, the Centre for Mental Health produced a series of articles on suicide statistics in NSW at an Area and LGA level, an evaluation of the risk of suicide in clients of mental health services and an analysis of the flow of suicide related events and the associated morbidity and morality. This presentation will discuss the insights gained from this work relevant to the prevention of suicide.

REACH OUT: SUICIDE PREVENTION AND THE INTERNET

Jack Heath — Executive Director, New Australia Foundation, Australia

The Australian-based Reach Out service will be the world's first fully interactive youth suicide prevention service on the Internet. Reach Out! consists of three distinct areas: Chill Out! for young people; Family and Friends for older people; and the Professional Forum for those working directly with young people. All the information provided will be of benefit to older people as well.

Reach Out! will provide advice, information, referrals, forums for discussions, networking and a national database which will allow anyone in Australia to find out the relevant suicide prevention services in their immediate vicinity. For professionals here will be specific areas for professional groups dealing with youth suicide. It is expected that once fully developed the service will be replicated in other States and countries around the world.

YOUNG PEOPLE AND PSYCHIATRIC ILNESS — INTERVENTION AND ASSESSMENT (YYPI–IA)

Deborah Howe, Kurt Braasch, Catherine Mackson, Martin Gallagher, and Kim Vukelick — YYPI–IA Programme Central Coast Area Health Services, Australia

The project will develop, pilot and evaluate an acute, home-based assessment service for young people experiencing significant mental health issues and at risk of suicide to promote better access and improved interventions.

This project has been successful in obtaining $325,000, over 2 years and 4 month, from the Commonwealth Department of Health and Family Services, Youth Suicide Initiative. This is one of three national projects funded for this specific client group.

Young people with a mental illness have been identified as being at high risk of suicide, homelessness, substance abuse and engaging in risk taking behaviour. The Young People and Psychiatric Illness (YYPI) Programme was initiated on the Central Coast of New South Wales (NSW) in response to the need of these young people. YPPI is an innovative partnership programme between the components which has been in operation for the past two years. The YPPI–IA Project will extend this model further to one which is complete with protocols and is measurable against specific indicators and transferable to other health areas. Attention will be given to addressing the impact of drug and alcohol comorbidity on suicide in this target population.

The literature identifies gaps in current modes of service delivery to the target group and points to early intervention strategies to address these. In addition, local Central Coast data emphasises a need to examine and implement programmes aimed at suicide prevention.

THE CANTEBURY SUICIDE PROJECT

Peter Joyce, Annette Beautrais, and Roger Mulder — Christchurch School of
Medicine, New Zealand

New Zealand, like most Western countries, has a rising rate of suicide in young people. This is a new phenomenon and has not previously been an issue in New Zealand's history. Over the last six years in Christchurch, New Zealand, we have undertaken a large case control study which has collected data on 200 people who died by suicide, 300 who have made medically serious suicide attempts and over 1000 control subjects. Initial analyses have been completed and we confirm high rates of mental disorder in both suicides and attempted suicides.

THE NATIONAL CORONIAL INFORMATION SYSTEM — AND THE REDUCTION OF SUICIDE

Graeme Johnstone — State Coroner, Australia

Australian coroners from 8 States and Territories are working with a number of Federal and State agencies to establish a National Coronial Information System. the system is designed to provide key data and detailed information on areas such as deaths at work, in fire, deaths in custody, drownings, on the roads, from drugs, from products and in the home and recreational areas, etc. The system is intended to assist coroners in the investigation/identification of problem areas and in making recommendations.

In Australia, all States and Territories are moving towards a uniform system of data collection and investigation in the violent and unnatural death area. Coroner's files are a rich source of information for early hazard identification, trend analysis, and detail on a variety of factors and potential systems failures. At the present time data is difficult and costly to access. The value of coroner's investigations and data to injury prevention is only just being fully appreciated.

The proposed system is also designed to alleviate the access problem for researchers and those concerned with prevention of injury/death and provide some degree of uniformality in the data collected in each investigation. Once established the information system will provide timely data on causative factors and means used in suicide and self-harm.

SUICIDE IN SWEDEN: THE IMPORTANCE OF TREATMENT OF DEPRESSION

Göran Isacsson — Karolinska Institute, Department of Psychiatry, Huddinge
University Hospital, Sweden

Suicide occurs seldom (if ever) in the absence of depressive disorder. In spite of the availability of effective antidepressant medication for several decades, however, it has not been shown that such medication has any impact on suicide rates or lowers the risk for suicide in depressed patients. In a series of pharmacoepiemiological studies, we have shown that this might be due to the fact that depressed patients who have committed suicide seldomly were treated with antidepressants in the population, we could estimate to which extent the use of antidepressants in Sweden in 1990–91 prevented suicides. The risk for suicide among depressed patients who were *treated* with antidepressants was found to be 141 per 100000 persons per year and, among those who were *untreated*, 259 per 100000 person per year (ie. 100 suicides annually were prevented in Sweden, which practically equals the actual decline in Swedish suicide rates 1970–1990). During 1990–91 probably only 1-in-5 of persons with major depression were treated with antidepressants. It was therefore predicted that 500 more lives could be saved if all depressives were to be treated. In the years 1991–94 the use of antidepressants trebled in Sweden and this was parallelled by a 15% decrease in suicide rates (300 fewer suicides in 1994 compared to 1991). We cannot claim a casual relationship. Our clinical conclusion is, however, that strong evidence exists supporting increased detection of depression and treatment with antidepressant medications as basic strategies for suicide prevention.

EARLY DETECTION OF YOUTH SUICIDE

Graham Martin, Leigh Roeger, Vikki Dadds, and Stephen Allison — Southern CAMHS, Flinders Medical Centre

This presentation will launch a report on the first two years of a longitudinal study of suicidal behaviours in young people in South Australia, funded under the National Mental Health Strategy.

Seventeen high schools in the southern region have taken part allowing study of some 1,800 students. A composite questionnaire — the Youth Assessment Checklist — was developed to examine demographic factors, family issues, recent life experience, current psychological functioning and in particular reports of suicidal behaviour.

We will discuss the complexities of the program, preliminary descriptive statistics of the first two years of the program and the risk indicators from the first year which relate to suicidal behaviours in the second year. Plans for the third year of the study are well under way. Issues to do with data collection from young adults will be examined.

ARE WESTERN MODELS OF SUICIDE APPROPRIATE FOR OTHER COUNTRIES

Srinivasa Murthy — National Institute of Mental Health and Neuro Sciences, Bangalore

Suicide is a global tragedy. Suicide and attempted suicide represent a public health challenge in all countries of the world. A striking aspect of the rates of suicide and attempted suicide is the wide variation across countries, communities and at different points of time. The most striking is the consistently low rates in Islamic Countries and the rising trends in societies experiencing rapid social change (e.g., urban places).

Life and death are viewed differently in different religions and communities. The predominant western model of suicide is the focus on the individual experience and individual pathology preceding suicidal behaviour. This is reflected in the theories of crisis intervention and befriending, as a method of suicide prevention.

The non-western countries currently have (I) differing legal status regarding attempted suicide, (ii) differing levels of care programmes.

A striking illustration of the differing approaches of countries is the way India continues to consider attempted suicide and is punishable when Euthanasia is 'legal' in Australia. At the levels of service there is still major emphasis on primary group rather than professions and organised service. At a philosophical level there are differences across different religions. It is well recognised that suicide prevention should be rooted in cultural, social, political and historical realities of communities and countries. There is not enough innovative thinking and action programmes reflecting this awareness.

In conclusion, suicide is a global phenomenon and to that extent is universal. The forces working at the individual, family, community and the national vary widely across countries. This is especially so in the non-western countries. This facet needs to be considered in understanding suicidal behaviour and planning suicide prevention programs.

JESUIT SOCIAL SERVICES CONNEXIONS PROGRAM

Father Peter Norden — Jesuit Social Services, Melbourne

Psychiatric disturbance during adolescence is not uncommon, but the effective delivery of mental health services to adolescents themselves has its difficulties.

Those who find themselves with the dual disability of mental illness and substance abuse are doubly disadvantaged. As the seriousness of their needs increase, they become less likely to receive assistance from either mental health services or drug and alcohol services. Connexions, a program of Jesuit Social Services in Melbourne is directed towards young people aged 16–25 who have this dual disability.

Through development of a model of professional intervention which overcomes the barriers of youth culture and dual disability 'Connexions' employs a project worker whose task it is to bring about a policy change towards inclusion rather than exclusion, within the mainstream mental health and drug and alcohol services.

AUSTRALIAN STUDIES

Beverley Raphael, Jonine Penrose-Wall, and Judy Jones — NSW Centre for Mental Health, Australia

Programs in NSW drawing together suicide prevention initiatives will be reviewed. How these programs sit in the context of mental health service enhancement will be considered and specific programs to address this will be reviewed. This will include the implementation and evaluation of the guidelines concerning depression in young people.

AUSTRALIAN STUDIES

Sven Silburn, Stephen Zubrick, and John Acres — Western Australia

Evaluation of the feasibility and efficacy of a public health intervention to enhance the hospital management and community follow-up care of teenagers presenting to Perth hospital emergency departments following deliberate self harm.

A non-randomised, cohort design was used to evaluate the phased introduction of 'better' practice protocols for the management of deliberate self-harm at three Perth hospitals. A total of 654 teenagers were ascertained in three differing treatment conditions with clinical and demographic information on admission being recorded by the attending clinician. Prospective follow-up of 640 of these cases (97%) was achieved by record linkage with the Western Australian epidemiological registers of deaths, hospital admissions and use of public mental health services.

The limitations of the study design are discussed together with the some of the clinical and systemic issues which arise in the implementation and evaluation of 'better' pracitce in hospital settings. The findings provide general support for the value of efforts to improve hospital practice and the awareness, knowledge and skills of clinicians and other caregivers who assist suicidal young people and their families.

WORKSHOPS/SYMPOSIA

SUICIDE AND VIOLENCE:
A COMMON BIOLOGICAL SUBSTRATE?

Alexander Botsis — Director, Department of Psychiatry, Athens

At present, the only compelling evidence of neuro-transmitter related to suicide and violence stems from the data on serotonin. Decreased levels of 5-hydroxy-indoleacetic acid (5-HIAA) in the CSF have consistently been found in patients with suicide attempts, particularly in those using violent means across a wide variety of diagnostic categories. Further, CSF studies have reported the same finding in patients who engage in different kinds of violent behaviour such as assaults, firesetting and criminal acts. In order to obtain information about the functional state of specific 5-HT neurons, neuroendocrine challenge studies using direct or indirect 5-HT agonists have been conducted.

In conclusion, it seems that impulsivity, not premeditated aggression suggests an underlying psychopathological entity more likely to associated with the 5-HT dysfunction. Although aggression is far from being a simple unidimensional psychological concept, the interpretation that a low-output or a low-stability serotonin system may render an individual more vulnerable to act impulsively in a suicidal or violent way could be made.

COMMUNITY BASED TRAINING IN YOUTH SUICIDE PREVENTION: STRATEGIES FOR IMPLEMENTATION AND EVALUATION

Kerry Bidwell, Christine Petrie, and Eleesa Johnstone — Ipswich Health Plaza, Young People at Risk Program, Australia

The objective is to present practical strategies for developing, implementing and evaluating training programs in youth suicide prevention within a community development framework.

The facilitators will provide an overview of core content areas included in the training and will identify factors which have enhanced training outcomes for service providers and community members - including the invaluable role of consumers in training delivery.

Strategies specifically developed for evaluating the training programs will be presented in conjunction with samples of preliminary evaluation results which indicate that training is an effective tool for increasing helpers' knowledge about youth suicide prevention.

Participants will have the opportunity to investigate a community development process for creating and maintaining networks of trainers and/or resource personnel. A resource manual produced by the Program will be available outlining strategies for developing, implementing and evaluating training programs within a community context.

Training can be an effective tool for prevention of suicide in young people. However, a number of factors have been found to influence the effectiveness of training, including community "readiness" and participant cohesiveness. In order to be effective, training programs need to incorporate sound evaluation methods and be cognisant of core competencies for workers.

WOMEN AND SUICIDAL BEHAVIOUR

Silvia Sara Canetto — Colorado State University, USA

This workshop focuses on advances in the understanding and treatment of non-fatal suicidal behaviour in women. Participants will learn the latest research on risk factors for non-fatal suicidal behaviour (including social, economic and cultural factors), and the limitations of traditional theories of etiology.

The psychotherapy outcome research will be reviewed so that participants can understand why traditional psychotherapies have not been effective for suicidal women. Finally, participants will learn new ideas for intervention and prevention, based upon knowledge of risk factors, new treatment outcome studies of suicidal behaviour, and insights from the literature on women and depression.

THE MEDIA AND MASS HOMICIDE

Chris Cantor — Australian Institute for Suicide Research and Prevention, Australia

In August 1987 in Melbourne a gunman killed six people and injured 18 others. Ten days later in England a gunman similarly killed 14 people and injured 16 others before killing himself. Analysis of British newspaper reports of the former incident compared with Australian reports of the latter revealed many similarities.

The recent Port Arthur massacre, although not subjected to formal media analysis, closely followed that in Dunblane (Scotland). A further assault of school children in Britain was reported as being associated with the stories of both Dunblane and Port Arthur.

Suggestions are invited regarding media responsibilities.

DEVELOPMENTAL MODELS OF SUICIDE

Robert Kosky, David Clark, and Patrick O'Carroll

David Clark will present a unique study where adolescents are randomly assigned to different forms of suicide prevention management. This is a very intriguing attempt to work out best practice models. Patrick O'Carroll and Robert Kosky will comment on

David Clark's experiment and in particular, we want to work out some of the issues which might be challenges or obstacles for suicide prevention programs involving young people. We will be looking especially at the developmental process of adolescence and how they might impact on public health programs for suicide prevention, eg; their sense of invincibility, their different levels of maturation, their struggles with autonomy and independence and so on.

We want this workshop to be interactive and would hope that the participants will contribute and address some of these issues from their own experience. Perhaps at the end we will have 2 or 3 points that we would like included in the final report of the Congress.

BEREAVEMENT THROUGH SUICIDE

Sheila Clark, Norman Farberow, Onja Grad, Jon Stebbins, and Sue Stebbins

Professor Norman Faberow will workshop an international survey of the status of bereavement services for suicide survivors. He will discuss bereavement services.

Mr. Jon and Mrs. Sue Stebbins will workshop, from crisis control; a model of community support for those bereaved by suicide. They will discuss issues for the community.

Dr. Onja Grad will workshop, postvention for caregivers after suicide or death of their patient. This will also discuss issues of the therapist.

Dr. Sheila Clark will workshop models of grieving, discussing issues of therapy.

As knowledge about suicide bereavement and postvention expands, there follows a need to share these advances amongst therapists and care givers. Presenters will focus on various important issues which will then be workshopped in small groups. This workshop will provide a forum for discussion and exchange for participants form different countries working in various fields of postvention.

EVALUATING A COMMUNITY DEVELOPMENT PROGRAM TO PREVENT SUICIDE AND SELF-HARMING BEHAVIOUR AMONG YOUNG PEOPLE

Jo Dower, Maria Donald, and Tim Windsor — Department of Psychiatry, University of Queensland, Australia

This workshop will highlight important issues in the development and implementation of the comprehensive research and evaluation program of the Young People At Risk Program (YPAR). YPAR is an intervention program funded by Queensland Health. It uses a community development model to improve the community and health system response to young people at risk of suicide and self-harming behaviour. Pilot programs are in progress in four regions of Queensland.

The workshop will feature discussion of the lessons learned from the development and implementation of the Program and recommendations for future program evaluations. It will include:

- A brief outline of the YPAR Program;
- The development of the Program Goal, Objectives, and Evaluation Plan;

- Formative evaluation provided to program staff to inform ongoing planning and implementation of the program. Components include interviews with young people, service providers, and program staff;
- The process evaluation;
- The impact evaluation which includes two cross-sectional surveys of over 500 key services for young people;
- Preparation for future outcome evaluation which includes a statewide survey of young people's mental health and access to services.

This workshop will provide practical information which will assist in the collaborative planning and evaluation of intervention programs

SUICIDE IN OLD AGE

Brian Draper and John Snowdon — Prince Henry Hospital

The theme of the workshop will be "Is suicidal behaviour in old age understandable, rational and untreatable?"

Invited international and local speakers will talk to each of the three aspects of the theme during the first half of the 3 hour workshop. In short we will ask the speakers to consider:

- "understandable" What are the stresses that contribute to suicidal behaviour in old age?
- "rational" What are the mental health correlates of suicidal behaviour in old age?
- "untreatable" How can we prevent suicidal behaviour in old age and treat the survivors?

The second half of the workshop will be a panel discussion, possibly based around a "hypothetical" case with invited participation from the audience.

COMMUNITY DEVELOPMENT IN SUICIDE PREVENTION — BEAUTY OR THE BEAST?

S. Drew, J. Ward, T. McGuire, E. Johnstone, and A. Nathan — Queensland Health, Australia

This workshop will examine the role of community development in the development and implementation of the 'Young People at Risk: Access, Prevention and Action' (YPAR) program to improve the community and health system response to young people at risk of suicidal and self harming behaviour. Using as a working model the YPAR program, this workshop will examine the strengths and weaknesses of community development as a working model in suicide prevention. YPAR is aimed at the prevention of suicide and self harming behaviour amongst young people between 10–24 years of age and funded by Queensland Health.

The workshop will feature discussion of the issues which impact on the development and implementation of a community development based program within the constraints of the bureaucracy and the opportunities to achieve systemic change which ensures health system equity for young people.

The workshop will include:

- an outline on the initial development of the program, including the framework and underpinning principles;
- presentation of individual pilot regions participating in the program with discussion on local program developments;
- common issues and differences between pilots and what this means for evaluation;
- relationships with key stakeholders, local, statewide and national;
- consideration of the quality (community development) versus quantity (clinical intervention/research) debate;
- future directions.

There will be the opportunity for participants to question, share experiences and discuss the principles of community development.

RURAL YOUTH SUICIDE

Michael Dudley — University of New South Wales, Adolescent Service, War Memorial Hospital, Australia

This workshop will aim to illuminate the phenomenon of suicide in rural areas.

It will consist of three papers: one by Michael Dudley (University of New South Wales) on rural youth suicide trends and possible explanations in Australia: one by Peter Dunn and colleagues (Australian Rural Health Research Institute) on the Australian rural youth suicide prevention project; and one by Lakshmi Ratnayeke (Sri Lanka–Sumithrayo) on the prevention of rural suicide in Sri Lanka. Presenters will speak for 20 minutes each, and a half-hour discussion will follow.

Suicide Among Young Rural Australians: 1964–1993

The study tested hypotheses that from 1964 to 1993, suicide and firearm suicide rates among 15–24 year old males rose more sharply in rural than metropolitan areas, and corresponding rates among 15–24 year old females did not change. Suicide rates among 15–24 year old males rose by a factor of 2.2 in metropolitan locations, by 4-fold in towns with populations between 4000 and 25000, and by 12-fold in town with populations less than 4000. Male firearm suicide rates continued to rise in rural locations, and the greatest proportion of deaths in those locations were by firearms, though male hanging rates increased most in recent years in all locations. Female youth suicide rates did not change overall, but in towns with populations less than 4000 they increased 4.5 fold. Possible explanations for this epidemic, which are mostly speculative and require confirmation, are discussed.

FIREARMS AND SUICIDE

Michael Dudley — Adolescent Services, War Memorial Hospital, Australia

This workshop will focus on recent international trends in firearms suicides, discuss the significance of the issue of access to method, and review lessons from recent firearms massacres in Australia and elsewhere, in relation to the gun control debate and the future of the international gun control movement. Particular attention will be given to what social scientists and social activists can learn from each other in relation to the issue of firearms and suicide.

THE IASP–LUNDBECK PROJECT, FROM IDEA TO IMPLEMENTATION

O. Ekeberg,[1] J.P. Soubrier,[2] S. Mora, and R. Goldney[3] — [1]Denmark, [2]France, and [3]Australia

In 1995, following a successful incentive program for suicide prevention presented in France to 1200 psychiatrists, we started in collaboration with Lundbeck Foundation, a worldwide survey through the IASP network.

A draft of guidelines of educational program for physicians was sent for comments. With full approval from WHO, statistics were also asked to every IASP National Representative. At this date, 27 answers were received. Interesting results concerning statistics, epidemiology and variations of suicide rates with regional as well as polycultural differences were obtained. After open discussion of this presentation, a final guideline will be published.

A DUAL APPROACH TO SUICIDE AWARENESS & PREVENTION IN SCHOOLS

Leona L. Eggert, Elaine A. Thompson, Brooke P. Randell, and Liela J. Nicholas — Psychosocial and Community Health Dept., University of Washington, USA

The objective is to test and compare the efficacy of theory-based, indicated preventive interventions for reducing suicide potential among high-risk youth, potential high school dropouts, in 5 high schools.

Suicide-risk youth (n=105) participated in a 3-group, repeated-measures study, comparing: (1) the MAPS assessment interview plus a 1-semester experimental Personal Growth Class (PGC); (2) MAPS plus a 2-semester experimental PGC; and (3) MAPS-only control group. Data used were pre-intervention, 5-month, and 10-month follow-up assessments.

All 3 groups showed decreased suicide risk behaviors, depression, hopelessness, stress, and anger; and increased network social support and self-esteem, supporting the theoretic model undergirding the MAPS and PGC. However, increased personal control occurred only in the PGC groups, supporting its skills training theoretic model.

This study contributed to suicide prevention research efforts, demonstrating that suicide-risk youth:

1. were identified from within a school population and targeted for prevention research; and
2. responded positively on multiple indicators to both the MAPS interview and PGC.

Because the MAPS assessment interview demonstrated therapeutic effects, a 2nd study was funded and is currently being tested to compare 3 brief preventive interventions designed to reduce suicide risk. These findings will be ready for presentation at the time of the conference.

THE POWER OF RITUAL AND SUICIDE PREVENTION: A MULTIDISCIPLINARY EXPLORATION

Andrew Gardner[1] and Steve Price[2] — [1]Womens and Childrens Hospital and [2]Uniting Church in Australia

The objective is to explore the use of Ritual in Suicide Prevention.

A brief presentation of ideas and concepts of "Ritual" in Western culture, with an opportunity to explore the loss of transition rituals in Western culture and the use and abuse of replacement 'rituals'. Input will be invited by session participants regarding their own insights and experience. Examples of programmes which incorporate the use (consciously and unconsciously) of ritual will be examined, and participants will have the opportunity to work cross culturally and mulitdisciplinary in a process of ritual development.

What is ritual?, What makes for effective ritual?, Creation of therapeutic environments which support a search for meaning and connections beyond the individual.

Participants will have an appreciation of ritual as making a significant contribution to healthy psychological development, and to its application in therapy.

An approach, using Durkheim as a starting point, and the categories of Anomie and Egoistic suicide, that will allow exploration of the loss of ritual in Western culture and the effect that this has had on suicide rates, and suggested directions for further research and practice.

The encouragement of a rediscovery of the great myths and rituals that underpin human societies has an important part to play in issues of suicide prevention.

REDUCING SUICIDE BY CARBON MONOXIDE POISONING

Sandra Hacker and Stephen Roseman — Australia

Suicide by carbon monoxide (CO) poisoning is a serious and neglected problem, taking the lives of hundreds of Australians every year.

Deaths form CO poisoning currently account for about 20% of all suicides, with the highest rates recorded among men aged 20–50. Exhaust suicides have increased dramatically in both absolute numbers and as a proportion of methods of suicide.

The Australian Medical Association has been actively campaigning on this issue for over two years. In that time the AMA has collected a large quantity of data from a variety of sources on both the prevalence of the problem and strategies to prevent these deaths.

CO poisoning is highly lethal — unconsciousness will occur within about 5 minutes and death after about 12 minutes of exposure. If the poisoning is not fatal, victims can suffer severe brain injury which may not manifest itself until some weeks later.

As with most methods of suicide, issues such as access, availability and acceptability of CO poisoning are important factors in its popularity. It has been speculated that the male cultural association and familiarity with motor vehicles is the major reason for the disproportionate representation of men in exhaust suicides.

Several strategies have been suggested to reduce the number of deaths by CO poisoning.

Legislation enforcing catalytic converters has resulted in a reduction of CO output form newer cars (from 24.2g/km to 9.3g/km). New regulations will see a further reduction (to 2.1g/km). However, it is not yet clear if these reductions will decrease completed exhaust suicides. Another option is to reduce suicides by inserting baffles in the exhaust pipe. This method has the added benefit of being possible to fit to the existing fleet. The difficulties with modifying exhaust pipes relate to cost, car performance, ease of circumvention and appearance. CO detectors are another possibility. These sensors turn off the engine if the amount of CO in the cabin goes above a certain level. Problems with detectors include unintentional cut-off, cost, tampering or disabling and development of the sensor. Also it will only apply to new vehicles.

A final suggestion is to alter the chemistry of petrol to make the experience physically unpleasant for the victim while they are conscious. The evidence to support this method is based upon the small number of exhaust suicides from diesel vehicles, but more research is needed in this area.

Due to the international nature of the motor vehicle manufacturing industry, it seems difficult for a single country to enact these measures in isolation. The reason for discussing CO poisoning in this context is to encourage international support to reduce exhaust suicides in a global context.

SUICIDE MINIMISATION IN THE AUSTRALIAN CONTEXT: CAN WE ACHIEVE DEFINITIVE OUTCOMES?

T. Humphrey — Australian Mental Health Suicide Consumer-Alliance Inc. Club Speranza, Australia

What is suicide?: Suicide as a definition is not always an incontrovertible statement. And even if we know it to be it may not be recorded as such statistically. Are we all looking to prevent the same thing and should we? Do we include euthanasia? Euthanasia is actually much misunderstood. There are different kinds of aficionados to debate and love or hate eg; 'active', 'passive', 'assisted', 'involuntary', 'voluntary', 'non voluntary', 'advance directive'! Over 70% of the population want it. Religious groups oppose it.

Suicide prevention, a valid "blanket" statement? — Different dimensions: What do we prevent? What do you do when you know? What should be the focus? The individual. The program. The big scale. Small programs. Legislation. The levels of definitive outcome in prevention. Personal. Local. Global. What are the economics? What is practical and what is realism? What are the inhibitors? Money...time...availability/proximity, contrary mindsets. The aboriginal dimension. The Australasian dimension.

Research and its value: Suicidology versus treatment — consciousness raising — Awareness.

Consumerism, The Power of 1: Why not use the people who are experiencing the problem?

Suicide in the Big Picture, Valid Options, Some Opinions: What is already there? Where do we go from here? 'Here for Life', Australian Mental Health Suicide Consumer Alliance, Suicide Prevention Australia, Rose Education, State associations for mental health (NSW has a comprehensive suicide policy statement), Wesley Mission's 'Life Force' etc. National and state goals and targets and task forces. A national government and NGO approach.

EUTHANASIA AND ASSISTED SUICIDE: RESULTS OF IASP SURVEY AND WORKSHOP DISCUSSIONS

M.J. Kelleher, M.J.A. Kelleher, and P. Corcoran — Suicide Research Foundation, Ireland

Euthanasia and assisted suicide are matters of public debate. The drive for change often emanates more from the press, the judiciary, the lay man and the moral philosopher rather than from professional or voluntary carers. Holland in Europe, the Northern Territory in Australia and the state of Oregon in the US have sought change. Neighbouring areas have resisted this.

Clarification of these issues is being sought in three ways. Firstly a postal enquiry of all IASP members and national representatives was carried out using a specially constructed questionnaire. A half-day pre-conference workshop will consider euthanasia in Adelaide, the results of this survey as well as other related issues. A further half-day session on assisted suicide will be similarly organised in Adelaide.

The results of these three enquiries will be presented at the main conference.

Euthanasia — For and Against — Where do you stand?

The session will begin with a brief statement of the answers to the appropriate questions given in the IASP Task Force Postal Questionnaire Survey on Euthanasia. Following that the following issues (and any others raised from the audience) will be considered and discussed.

- Euthanasia — What does it mean?
- For whom is it meant?
- Is there a distinction between active and passive?
- Is there a distinction between voluntary, non-voluntary and involuntary valid?
- Must the person be terminally ill?
- Is it for physical illness only?
- What about mental illness?
- What about those who are not ill?
- Who should carry it out?

Euthanasia — Assisted Suicide — Morality and Practice

The session will begin with a brief statement reporting the responses to the appropriate questions taken from International Survey carried out by IASP into euthanasia and assisted suicide. Active audience participation will be invited. The issues to be considered are given below and will include appropriate issues put on the agenda from the floor.

- Should assisted suicide be allowed?
- What does it entail?
- Who should do it?
- Are professional responsibilities different from lay ones?
- Must the person be ill, either physically or mentally?
- Must the suffering be intolerable?
- Is advice different from prescribing the means?
- Should the professional remain neutral or has he an obligation to persuade?
- What are your criticisms?
- Should well enough be left alone?

STEPS FOR LIFE

Raymond King — Charles Sturt University , Australia

This workshop introduces a rationale for broad-based suicide awareness and prevention programs in schools. It then presents and demonstrates a specific example of a broad-based program "Steps for Life" which has been developed and is currently in use in Australian schools. The program involves the production of protocols for teaches and students.

Operational principles for practitioners advocating and initiating a climate of care in schools. The caring context of the school is featured as a vehicle for the "Steps for Life" program. Practical means for evaluating the caring context for schools, encompassing a school–community resources, and the efficacy of the "Steps for Life program, are discussed.

ADVOCATING THE "SUICIDE AWARE" SCHOOL

Raymond King, Margaret Appleby, and Gail Kilby — The Rose Foundation, Australia

The workshop introduces the concept of the "Suicide Aware" school and presents a rationale for suicide awareness programs in schools. It provides specific examples of Australian schools in which a climate of care has been developed which facilitates suicide awareness and prevention strategies and protocols for teachers and students.

The workshop then extracts some principles for practitioners creating the suicide aware school and suggests practical means for evaluating the development of a caring context for schools which encompasses the wider community.

Workshop topics:
1. Conceptualising the "Suicide Aware" school.
2. Theorising school-based suicide awareness and prevention programs.
3. Australian successes in creating a climate of care in schools that facilitates awareness of suicide prevention strategies.
4. Future directions in the evaluation of school-based programs towards the development of a caring context for schools.

PRINCIPALS OF POSTVENTION: APPLICATIONS TO TRAUMA AND SUICIDE IN SCHOOLS

Antoon A. Leenaars and Susanne Wenckstern

Postvention refers to "things done" to address and alleviate possible reactions to trauma, whether suicide, homicide or terrorist attack. This paper will outline the following principles, providing clinical associations, applications and cautions. The principles are:
1. In working with survivor victims of suicide, it is best to begin as soon as possible after the tragedy, within the first 24 hours if that can be managed,
2. Resistance may be met form the survivors; some — but not all — are either willing or eager to have the opportunity to talk to professionally oriented persons,

3. Negative emotions about the decadent (the deceased person) or about any trauma — irritation, anger, envy, shames, guilt, ane so on — need to be explored, but not the very beginning. Timing is so important,

4. The postventionist should pay the important role of reality tester. He/she is not so much the echo of conscience as the quiet voice of reason,

5. One should be constantly alert for possible decline in physical health and in overall mental well-being, even suicide risk,

6. Needless to say, pollyannish optimism, or banal platitudes should be avoided,

7. Trauma work is multifaceted and takes a while — from several months to the end of life, but certainly more than three weeks or six sessions,

8. A comprehensive program of health care on the part of a benign and enlightened community should include prevention, intervention and postvention.

Finally, the participants will be asked to dialogue about the issues and the direction of postvention in Australia.

COLLABORATIVE APPROACHES TO YOUNG PEOPLE AT RISK OF SUICIDE AND SELF-HARMING BEHAVIOUR

Tony McGuire — Australia

The workshop focuses on the collaborative development of best practice models addressing self-harm and suicidal behaviour amongst young people. The workshop programs optimise outcomes at tertiary, secondary and primary levels by mobilising either: (section 1) a network of health professionalism or (section 2) the wider community.

Section 1: Assisting Adolescents A.S.A.P — Service Provider Collaboration

A.Austin (clinical Psych), A. Bickerton (FRANZCP), C.O'Brien (Psych) St. George Youth Services

The Anti-Suicide-Adolescent Program (A.S.A.P) has been established to ensure a quicker response to suicidal youths and their families through collaboration between the youth service, hospital emergency department and psychiatric services. This section of the workshop will focus on the creation of this professional infrastructure in an environment of scarce resources. We will demonstrate how this process of collaboration provides the necessary pathway for better outcomes.

Section 2: Community Development Model and Peer Support Program

T.McGuire, E.Panaretos, K.Christmas: Wide Bay Young People At Risk Program

a. The establishment of a model that empowers the wider community with the skills and resources to implement early intervention and prevention strategies in addressing self-harm and suicidal behaviour that especially targets rural towns and provincial cities. This section details how a collaborative approach is maintained and resources/structures developed in rural communities.

b. The peer support training program has been developed through applied methods that highlights the benefits of intersectoral collaboration and young people's participation in community projects. This section of the workshop will focus on the development of this framework and young people's achievements in rural communities and provincial cities.

DRUG DEPENDENCE AND SUICIDE

Pam McKenna, Steve Alsop, and Hussain Habil

Alcohol and other drug problems and mental health are closely related. Many clients with alcohol and drug related problems also experience mental health problems, and patients with mental health problems are at high risk of hazardous and harmful drug use. Specifically, a number of studies have indicated a strong relationship between hazardous and harmful drug use and suicide risk. This session will explore this relationship in the context of structural barriers that impede effective responses. In particular, the experience of drug specialist and mental health services will be examined and resolutions to barriers explored. Specific reference will be made to common problems which arise in the management of heroin dependence, drawing on research from Malaysia, and this will include a focus on factors which contribute to depression and suicide risk. Finally, using current models of addiction behaviour, participants will be introduced to the clinical implications of different patterns of drug use. The process of giving up harmful drug use has substantial relevance for clinical endeavour and participants will be provided with a framework for treatment approaches.

DRUGS AND SUICIDE

Pam McKenna, Steve Alsop, and Habil Hussein — Befrienders International

The objective is to explore the link between alcohol and other drug use and suicidal self harming behaviours.

Through a workshop format, using group activity, delegates will be asked to:

- identify risk factors
- identify populations at risk
- identify resources available
- identify signs of suicidal ideation
- identify signs of heavy drug use

The generated information will be drawn together establishing links with current research findings.

OPPORTUNITIES AND CHALLENGES FOR BIOLOGICAL STUDIES OF SUICIDAL BEHAVIOUR

John Mann — New York State Psychiatric Institute, Columbia University

Measurement of suicidal behaviour that utilizes both a dimensional as well as the more traditional catorgorical approach may explain some of the variance in biological correlates such as CSF 5–HIAA, neuroendocrine studies and platelet indicies. For example, serotonergic indicies correlate with more lethal froms of suicide attempts. Most studies are retrospective and prospective studies are needed to test state and trait characteristics of correlates of suicidal behaviour. For example, most serotonergic correlates appear to be traits and may therefore predict future behaviour. New methods for assessing the serotonergic system include candidate gene studies and neuroimaging. The intial application of these techniques to suicide research will be discussed.

"KEEP YOUSELF ALIVE": A WORKSHOP ON GENERAL PRACTIONER AND GATEKEEPER TRAINING

Graham Martin, Sheila Clark, Paul Beckinsale, and Jeanne Lorraine — Southern CAMHS, Flinders Medical Centre

This workshop presents a rationale for the education and training of general practitioners in recognition of mental health problems and suicidal behaviours. The workshop will showcase a workshop package consisting of four videotapes:

- Youth Suicide: Recognising the Signs (21 minutes)
- Youth Suicide: What do I do now? (Crisis Intervention) (24 minutes)
- Youth Suicide: What do I do next? (Therapy) (30 minutes)
- Youth Suicide: Picking up the Pieces (Postvention) (30 minutes)

and 16×12 minute audio tapes about issues to do with Suicide, its aftermath and its prevention and a workshop manual.

The presenters will highlight key issues demonstrated by the videotapes and expect intense enthusiastic audience participation and discussion.

The workshop package is part of a national program "Keep Yourself Alive" funded under the Youth Suicide Prevention Initiative. The program will begin an extensive series of workshops in five states and territories of Australia (Queensland, New South Wales, ACT, Northern Territory and South Australia) following the official launch on April 11th 1997 at the Royal Australian College of General Practitioners in Adelaide.

AFTER SUICIDE: WHO COUNSELS THE CARE GIVER?

Konrad Michel, Graham Fleming, Carolyn Rosenbauer, Vanda Scott, and Yoshitomo Takahashi — Psychiatrische Poloklinik, Universitatsspital, Switzerland

A number of authors have looked in to the problems associated with the loss of a patient by suicide, and it is generally known how such an event should be dealt with in clinical practice. But what does reality look and feel like?

In this workshop panel members from different professional backgrounds will give short accounts of their personal experiences, and the participants will be invited to discuss what kind of help is needed and what we can do better in helping the care givers and collegues. Psychiatrists and psychotherapists working in in-and-out patients settings, GP's, nurses, social workers and volunteers, etc., are welcome in this workshop.

SURVIVAL ANALYSIS AND PSYCHOBIOLOGY OF SUICIDE RISK

Peter Nordstrom — Department of Clinical NeuroScience, Karolinska Institutet, Sweden

The serotonin hypothesis of suicide risk has received considerable empirical support during the last two decades and the suicide serotonin link has also stimulated a psychobiological approach to the study of tempremental vulnerability to suicide risk. Another major suicide risk predication hypothesis is that suicide occurs as the endpoint of a suicidal process with attempted suicide as the typical clinical presentation.

Survival analysis with median split subgrouping was thus applied in

1. Identification of mutual concerns regarding a fragmented approach to suicidal youth and their families;
2. Development of a model for combining scarce resources to maximise the impact of the interventions;
3. Formulating and conducting training sessions for professionals in hospital Emergency Department and Adult Mental Health Service;
4. Development and implementation of a collaborative clinical approach which provides a timely service.

This workshop will explore the development of the best practice model targeting suicidal adolescents and their families, and professionals who work with this group. The focus of the program is to optimise the use of limited resources through intersectorial collaboration between hospital and community health services.

The presenters will address the issues that are important in implementing a successful hospital and community health project to improve services for suicidal youth and their families. This includes a willingness to invest time in developing a shared context among the workers.

MANAGING YOUTH SUICIDAL BEHAVIOUR: THE 4RS WORKSHOP FOR GENERAL PRACTITIONERS

Jon Pfaff and Stephen Edwards — National General Practice Youth Suicide Prevention Project

The *aim* of the workshop is to present a simple and straight-forward model designed to train general practitioners to *recognise* young people at risk of suicide, to *raise* the issue of suicide with at risk patients, to *assess* current risk, and to *respond* to those at risk through appropriate management and prevention strategies. The *format* of the **4Rs** workshop is presented in five parts:

i. *issues* — setting the scene by exploring issues relating to youth suicide;

ii. *recognising the signs* — identifying the warning signs for youth suicide;

iii. *raising the issue* — encouraging disclosure of suicidal ideation;

iv. *risk assessment* — determining level of risk & urgency of clinical intervention;

v. *responding* — management and prevention strategies.

The workshop is *designed* for a small group of up to 16 General Practitioners, and is presented over a four-and-a-half hour time period (including coffee & lunch breaks). It provides an interactive experience for participants, who are challenged through various quizzes, role plays, and small group exercises.

The workshop is currently being used in a National demonstration project, funded by the Commonwealth of Australia, utilising the Divisions of General Practice in Tasmania, Victoria & Western Australia.

SUICIDALITY AND ADOLESCENT PEER RELATIONS

Ken Rigby — University of SA

Over the last decade or so there has been an increasing sensitivity among educators to the serious consequences of peer abuse or bullying in schools. In part, this has occurred as a result of media reports, published in many countries including Norway, England and Japan, of adolescent suicides allegedly following severe bullying in schools. Evidence derived from such reports of a relationship between peer victimisation and suicide is clearly open to many criticisms. It is known that diverse factors may contribute to suicide, and information collected retrospectively about a suicide victim's peer relations may have doubtful validity.An alternative or complementary approach to assessing the possible impact of adverse peer relations is through the use of surveys in which evidence is collected from children on the nature of their relations with other children and the extent to which they engage in suicidal ideation — or have actually taken steps to harm themselves. In this presentation I will present results from three studies undertaken in South Australia between 1994 and 1996 aimed at assessing the relative risk of suicide as a function of chidren's involvement in bully/victim problems at school.

SUICIDAL BEHAVIOUR AMONG TWINS

Alec Roy,[1] Nancy Segal,[2] Marco Sarchiapone,[3] and Gunnar Rylander[4] —
[1]UMDNJ-NJ Medical School, 2University of California, [3]Catholic University of Rome, and 4NJ & Karolinska Hospital

The objective is to examine for possible genetic contributions to suicidal behaviour.

We collected 176 twin pairs in which one or both twins had committed suicide. Seven of the 62 monozygotic (MZ) twin pairs were concordant for suicide compared with 2 of the 114 dizygotic pairs (11.3% vs 1.8%, P<0.01). However, no study has examined attempts at suicide among living cotwins of twin suicide victims.

We collected a new series of 35 twins whose cotwin had committed suicide. Eleven of the 27 living MZ cotwins had themselves attempted suicide compared with 0 of the 8 living DZ cotwins (40.7% vs 0%) Fisher's Exact Test, one tailed, P<0.04).

Studies show that MZ twin pairs have significantly greater concordance for both suicide and attempted suicide than DZ twin pairs.

These data suggest that genetic factors play a part in suicidal behaviour. We now personality, neurobiologic and molecular genetic studies in the living cotwins of the MZ suicide victims.

THE ESTABLISHMENT OF NANJING CRISIS INTERVENTION CENTRE

Zhai Shu Tao — Nanjing, China

The Nanjing Crisis Intervention Centre (NCIC) was established at July 1, 1991. NCIC is part of Nanjing Brain Hospital. Its function includes professional services and scientific researches.

Service activities. Since until Sep 30, 1996, we have had annually hot-line services for 4100 times, face-to-face assistance 6680 cases, letter counselling 423 times, women psychological counselling 1600 cases, family-social intervention 150 times.

NOMENCLATURE FOR SUICIDE RESEARCH

Morton M. Silverman — University of Chicago, Illinois USA

The clinical and research enterprise within the field of suicidology lack a standard nomenclature, as well as a standard classification for referring to suicide-related behaviours. This presentation will report on efforts held in the United States of America to develop a commonly defined set of terms. This set of clear and unambiguous term is based on a logical and minimum set of necessary component elements.

Such a nomenclature will improve the clarity and precision of communications within and among the clinical, research, and public health constituencies, advance suicidological research and knowledge, and improve the efficacy of clinical interventions. If this nomenclature is found to be acceptable, the next stage will be to develop standard, operational means for applying these definitions in clinical practice, research, and public health domains. Disseminating and encouraging the use of an operationalized nomenclature would constitute a third stage in this process.

ESTABLISHING A SUICIDE PREVENTION CENTRE

Alan Staines — Suicide Prevention Centre, Australia

Suicide prevention centre's have a rich history dating back to the first suicide prevention 'anti suicide' bureau established in the U.K. by the Salvation Army in 1907. The first suicide prevention centre in the U.S.A was founded in Los Angeles in 1958.

Since that time crisis centres/telephone hot lines have been established all over the world. Though services may differ from country to country many of the same dilemmas and challenges. Australia has a history of telephone counselling services but very little is being done in establishing suicide prevention crisis centres.

What does it take to establish a suicide prevention centre?

What is the future for suicide prevention centres in Australia?

PARTNERSHIP AT WORK IN MENTAL HEALTH — WORKING CREATIVELY WITH CONSUMERS, COLLEAGUES AND CASHIERS

Kathleen Stacey, Cindy Turner, CHAMPS Members, Trish Mundy, Barry Taylor, and Bruce Turley

This workshop will be presented by two teams, one from South Australia and the other from Victoria. Using case examples, a range of creative partnerships which have lead to sustainable programs on the ground will be explored.

An empowering consumer partnership will be discussed through the CHAMPS community development project which is based on principles of youth partnership and accountability. CHAMPS seeks to elevate young peoples' voices in dialogue about the issues which influence their mental health, how adults can provide respectful mental health services to young people and how young people can be empowered and enabled to take action for themselves and their peers. Young people and adult workers will co-present describing several health promotion projects including YARN, a youth to youth phone-based peer support network with young people trained as peer counsellors. Other projects include media liaison, a CHAMPS camp, conference presentations and CHAMPS by the River (the creation of a local youth-friendly recreational area). The adults will address what it means to live their intentions in working with young people.

Victorian examples of working in partnership with colleagues — one rural and the other metropolitan — explain the process and outcomes of establishing multi-agency youth suicide prevention teams in two localities. The localities self selected to be involved in the project because of locally identified needs. While there were some pre-existing partnerships, the forging of new links between the police, general practitioners, youth workers, teachers and recreational officers of local government around the issue of mental health promotion and youth suicide prevention took time and input. The lessons learned from facilitating local, active multi-agency groups will be presented.

The cashier's story is one of a successful partnership being facilitated by a funding agency — VicHealth, partnering two applicants — the Victorian Coroner's Office and Lifeline Victoria. Both agencies were interested in improving post-vention counselling and through a subsequent project carried out in partnership, several models of post-vention counselling are being trialed. The role of a funding agency in supporting project implementation through partnering agencies will be discussed in terms of the added value such relationships can bring.

This workshop is expected to be fun, stimulating, thought provoking, thoughtful, alternative and refreshing. The wisdom of the young partners add a challenge to all of us to extent our practices and partners beyond the traditional.

AUSTRALIAN ABORIGINAL SUICIDE

Polly Sumner, Nunkuwarrin Yunti, and Adelaide

I think it is fair to say that colonisation has found its way into the therapy room.

To treat the cause the therapist has to understand the history. The history is that anatomy of the social illnesses, that we see in our work.

Prevention: to decrease the incidents of suicide, education to service providers is paramount of a skills based nature; community based education and ongoing culturally appropriate supportive programs are essential.

IN THE FACE OF PAIN: A COMMUNITY BASED SUICIDE INTERVENTION TRAINING PROGRAM

Darien Thira and Sharon Thira — Vancouver Crisis Centre, Canada

The *In the Face of Pain* program is a three-day introduction to the knowledge and skills necessary for a community-based response to crisis and suicide. Through a highly interactive process that builds on the experience and skills within the participants the program offers a pragmatic understanding of crisis and suicide and explores the role that the whole community can play in crisis intervention and suicide prevention. Participants are trained to identify, assess and respond to a person in suicidal crisis, essential crisis counselling skills are practised, community resources are identified, and community postvention strategies are also explored. The program is designed to be modified (in content and length) to meet the needs of the specific community and has been very successfully used by aboriginal communities (urban and rural).

ENHANCING CAREGIVERS' GATEKEEPING COMPETENCE IN SUICIDE FIRST AID

Bryan Tanney and Bruce Turley — Lifeline, Australia

The objective is to improve caregivers' "gatekeeping" competence and confidence in performing a suicide first aid intervention with a person at risk and promote intersectoral co-operation in implementing these interventions in the community.

A Phase 4F Rothman field trial of a large-scale community-based intervention to enhance caregivers' ability and confidence to perform effective suicide first aid interventions with people at risk has been funded by the Australian Commonwealth Government. 72 presenters recruited from diverse community service organisations in three sites were trained to deliver two proven learning experiences to over 10 000 participants. These learning experiences comprised a 2-day workshop designed to promote informed, purposeful and effective interventions with people at risk and a modular 2–3 hour public awareness presentation. Process and outcome evaluations were conducted using standardised instruments administered to community focus groups, presenters, participants and controls. National dissemination is planned.

A progress report will highlight implementation issues for presenters and participating organisations in mounting community-scale suicide intervention strategies in diverse community settings. Trends emerging from preliminary data on both individual and organisational outcomes will be featured. Implications for future planning and action research in this field will be discussed.

SUICIDE RESEARCH AND THE GENERAL PRACTITIONER

Kees van Heeringen and Viviane van Casteren — Dept. of Psychiatry, University Hospital, Institute for Hygiene and Epidemiology, Brussels, Belgium.

General practitioners (GP's) play a crucial role in the prevention of suicidal behaviour. However, suicide research is mainly hospital-based, and a recent study in Belgium showed that general practitioners refer only approx. 50–60% of their attempted suicide patients to a hospital. This study aimed at investigating whether hospital-based data provide guidelines for the prevention of suicide that can be used by general practitioners.

Comparison of data from a hospital-based monitoring study (n=832) and data from the National Sentinel Network of General Practitioners (n=349) was made on suicide attempts in 1990–1991.

The presentation will focus, first, on comparing characteristics of patients and suicide attempts based on the two datasets. Secondly, comparisons will be made between patients seen by a GP but not referred to a hospital, and patients referred to a hospital but not seen by a GP.

The results will be discussed in the light of their contribution to suicide prevention in general practice.

ESTABLISHING A SUICIDE PREVENTION CENTRE

Lakshmi Vijayakumar,[1] Zhai Shu Tao,[2] and Pam Williams[3] — [1]India, [2]PR China, and [3]South Africa

The objective is to understand the complexities involved in establishing a suicide prevention centre.

The workshop is aimed at determing the type of suicide prevention centre and the various problems and pit-falls in starting one. The need to tailor the services to the cultural mileau of the region would be highlighted. The problems of selection of crisis intervention personnel, finding funds and the publicity for the suicide prevention centre would be discussed. The workshop would consist of lectures and discussion groups.

ESTABLISHING A SUICIDE PREVENTION CENTRE IN INDIA

Lakshmi Vijayakumar — India

Over 90,000 people commit suicide in a year in India. Despite the enormity of the problem there was hardly any initiative either by the Government or NGO's towards prevention of suicide. To fill this void Sneha, a voluntary befriending service which is affiliated to Befrienders International was started in Madras.

There are many difficulties in establishing a suicide prevention centre in a developing country like India. The priorities are sanitation, housing, education, immunisation etc., rather than mental health. It requires considerable effort to mobilise resources and interest for mental health and suicide prevention in particular.

The concept of volunteerism and external emotional support is rather new for India. Family responsibilities leave little time for voluntary work and seeking outside emotional support in a crisis is not the norm. But rapid urbanisation, industrialisation and changes in family structures result in the absence of traditional support systems and the need for external emotional support arises.

For a population of 940 million, there are only about 4000 psychiatrists. Hence suicide prevention centres like Sneh play a vital role in being the entry point for those who require the attention of mental health professionals.

Establishing a suicide prevention centre in India has its own challengers and opportunities, difficulties and constraints have only led to innovation.

COGNITIVE BEHAVIOUR THERAPY

J.M.G. Williams — School of Pyschology, University College of North Wales

Cognitive therapy is an active time-limited treatment for a range of psychological problems. It uses a collaborative approach in which therapist and client work together to examine how maladaptive patterns of thoughts, feelings and behaviour contribute to the onset and maintenance of emotional disorder. This workshop focuses on how the core techniques of cognitive therapy may be extended to address the special problems of clients who are hopeless and suicidal, drawing upon the latest research findings on the psychological processes underlying hopelessness.

ESTABLISHING A SUICIDE PREVENTION CENTRE IN SOUTH AFRICA

Pam Williams — Befrienders International, South Africa

From her experience in establishing suicide prevention centres among widely differing cultural groups in South Africa, the speaker will discuss some of the strengths and weaknesses, the benefits and the pitfalls, of setting up and maintaining a service which is initiated, staffed and monitored entirely by volunteers.

A PROPOSED PROCESS MODEL FOR SUICIDE INTERVENTION: 'BEING' DIFFERENTIATED FROM 'DOING'

Lin Young — Samaritan Befrienders Inc., Australia

This model essentially provides one of the first examples of a process orientation in suicide prevention. The model is limited and based on the experience of working with over 500 individuals who have attempted suicide or are expressing serious intent to commit suicide. It is not given as a step by step guide, rather as a reduction of what is useful. It addresses suicide intervention, not the preliminary steps in establishing rapport.

1. acknowledgment of suicide ideation
2. exploration of suicide plan
3. awareness of ambivalence
4. acknowledgment of their psychological struggle
5. understanding of the major issues that are impacting on a person
6. addressing their underlying loneliness
7. clarity in their responses to 'feeling' questions
8. awareness of how the person is repressing emotion
9. experience of repressed emotion
10. grounding
11. acknowledgment of their physical and psychological relief
12. some self acceptance and understanding
13. exploring options
14. no suicide' contract

POSTERS

TELEPHONE SUPPORT FOR THE SUICIDAL

Simon Armson and John Lawrie — The Samaritans, United Kingdom

This poster will trace the development of the introduction of a single telephone number by The Samaritans in the UK and Ireland. Though the Samaritan service is not uniquely offered by telephone, the majority of contact is by this medium. Until recently every Samaritan centre offered only its own local telephone number.

The poster will touch on the work done by The Samaritans which indicated that distance of a caller from a Samaritan centre inhibited the use of the service, yet such people tended to be in areas of high suicide risk.

The benefits and limitations of the single number will be examined in terms of the greater accessibility of the service and availability of Samaritan volunteers at times of crisis. The impact on the public perception of the promotion of the service will be evaluated and some tentative conclusions drawn from information now available about the use made of the service by those who call it.

THE SAMARITANS' RESPONSE TO A NATIONAL SUICIDE PREVENTION STRATEGY

Simon Armson, John Lawrie, and Sujata Ray — The Samaritans, United Kingdom

"The Health of the Nation" is a national strategy which identifies and sets targets for five key areas of public health within England and Wales. Mental illness is one of these areas and the performance measure is the suicide rate, of the nation as a whole and amongst those with severe mental illness. The targets are a 15% reduction in the national suicide rate and a 33% reduction in suicide by people with severe mental illness by the year 2000.

The Samaritans welcomes the focus on mental illness and particularly on suicide rates in England and Wales. The organisation has always believed that suicide is a major, preventable cause of death and has made a considerable contribution to suicide prevention nationwide.

The poster will focus on the broad principles for management action which underlie the Health of the Nation strategy and will demonstrate how The Samaritans has been and continues to work to such principles:

I. collaborative working between health, social services, voluntary agencies and local community groups;

II. the targeting of resources towards specific groups at high risk;

III. public education and awareness-raising to reduce the stigma associated with emotional problems.

"To reach out and listen is the first major step in reducing the level of suicidal despair." *(Dept of Health, 1994)*. The Samaritans has been reaching out and listening for 43 years.

PREPARING VOLUNTEERS TO PROVIDE EMOTIONAL SUPPORT

Simon Armson, John Lawrie, and Joan Guenault — The Samaritans, United Kingdom

There are valid questions to be asked about the suitability of deploying volunteers without medically oriented training in the support of people passing through emotional crisis maybe to the point of contemplating or actually attempting suicide.

The experience of The Samaritans UK is that, given proper selection and preparation of new volunteers for such work, and support by other more experienced volunteers while performing it, a volunteer-based service is a distinctive and valuable part of the wider picture of suicide prevention.

DATA SYSTEM FOR MONITORING "GOOD" PRACTICE IN THE HOSPITAL MANAGEMENT OF DELIBERATE SELF HARM

Diane Atkinson — Youth Self Harm Social Worker: Royal Perth Hospital, Australia

For the past two years Royal Perth Hospital, along with Sir Charles Gairdner Hospital and Fremantle Hospital, have been utilising a computer data entry system enables the collection of demographic information, the nature of presenting problem, precipitating factors, treatment received whilst in hospital, and follow up plans. Research has shown that clients are most likely to represent to hospital, in three months following a suicide/self-harm attempt, therefore it is vital that details of agencies referred to and percentage of clients attending their appointments are recorded, to determine annual report to Western Australia's Youth Suicide Advisory Committee. The Poster Presentation describes the role of the Youth Self Harm Social Worker and how this fits with other services provided by the Youth Suicide Advisory Committee.

YOU'RE WEIRD! EDUCATIONAL EXCEPTIONALITY AS A RISK FACTOR AT EARLY ADOLESCENCE

Nada Barraclough and Dona Matthews — Distress Centre Ontario, Canada

Early adolescence is a risk factor all by itself if, as well, you enter adolescence as a marked kid — officially categorised as different than others by virtue of some kind of labelling process — you're entering this very challenging period with more disabilities than just the one the label signifies.

We will consider educational exceptionality from a developmental psychopathology standpoint, looking at risks and resilience's associated with being Learning Disabled, Attention Deficit Disorder and /or Gifted at a critical period of early adolescence. The cumulative effects of additional risk factors such as divorce, ethnicity, sex and family conflict are examined.

The aim of this poster is twofold: to argue for an understanding of educational exceptionality as a risk factor in the early adolescent context, and to offer strategies for those working with young people through this development transition.

We will provide theoretical and/or empirical data from a variety of areas, including Development Psychopathology, Developmental Psychology, Cognitive/Neurological Psychology and Educational Psychology, to support our arguments and strategies, so that interested readers/participants can review the relevant literature as desired.

FACTORS MEDIATING ATTEMPTED SUICIDE REFERRAL FROM PRIMARY TO SECONDARY CARE

Agnes Batt,[1] P. Jarno,[1] Mo Frattini,[2] A. Tréhony,[2] and F. Eudier[3] — [1]Faculty of Medicine, Dept of Public Health, France; [2]ORSB, France; and [3]Dept of Psychiatry CHRU, France

This communication will review the factors mediating the referral of attempted suicides from primary to secondary care, as they were reported by general practitioners (GP's) asked to relate their experience in the course of semi-structured interviews. Guidelines for the interviews as well as basic data on the suicidal phenomenon in the catchment area were gathered in a booklet and sent to the practitioners by way of introduction to the interview.

Following analyses, elements collected were assembled into a questionnaire constructed from the GP's experience, in view of a prospective quantitative survey of attempted suicide first taken in charge by them. The first results of the prospective survey will be discussed.

This research is part of a wider program aiming at elaborating a postgraduate educational scheme in view of secondary prevention.

CANNABIS ABUSE AND SERIOUS SUICIDE ATTEMPTS

Annette Beutrais, Peter Joyce, and Roger Mulder — Canterbury Project, New Zealand

The relationship between cannabis abuse/dependence and risk of medically serious suicidal attempt was examined in subjects making suicidal attempts and in comparison subjects.

The association between cannabis abuse/dependence and suicidal attempt risk was examined in 302 individuals who made serious suicidal attempts and in 1028 randomly selected comparison subjects. Each subject completed a semi-structured personal interview; a significant other completed a parallel interview.

Of those who made serious suicide attempts, 16.2% met DSM-III-R criteria for cannabis abuse/dependence at the time of the attempt, compared with 1.9% of comparison subjects (OR = 10.3, 95% CI = 5095–17.8). Risks of serious suicidal attempt were significantly (p<.0001) related to a series of sociodemographic and childhood characteristics, and to mental disorders comorbid with cannabis abuse/dependence. When the association between cannabis abuse/dependence and suicidal attempt risk was controlled for sociodemographic factors, childhood factors, and concurrent psychiatric morbidity, there was no significant association between cannabis abuse/dependence and serious suicide attempt risk (OR = 2.0, 95% CI = 0.97–5.3, p>.05). These results suggest that the association between cannabis abuse/dependence and suicidal attempt risk arose because individuals who develop cannabis abuse/dependency tended to come from disadvantaged sociodemographic and childhood backgrounds which, independently of cannabis abuse, are associated with higher risk of suicidal attempt, or because cannabis abuse/dependence is comorbid with other mental disorders, which are independently associated with suicidal behaviour.

These results suggest that cannabis abuse/dependence, in the absence of psychosocial adversity and concurrent mental disorder, is not associated with risk of serious suicidal attempt.

#1 SUICIDE...THE ULTIMATE REJECTION
#2 SUICIDE...FURTHER DOWN THE TRACK
#3 AFTER SUICIDE...HELP FOR THE BEREAVED
(SET OF TWO VIDEOS WITH ACCOMPANYING BOOK)

Graeme Blakey, Marg Potter, Mat Potter, Sandi Hogben, Aaron Hogben, Liff Blakey, Kate Swaffer, Dianna Herd, Sarah Swain, John Mills, and Sheila Clark — Bereaved through Suicide Support Group Inc, Australia

The programs are divided into sections so that they can be shown as a whole or in individual segments appropriate to a seminar or counselling session.

These videos have been made to help people understand the tragedy of suicide and the great pain and disorganisation it has on family friends and colleagues. The people who bravely spoke on these programmes did so with the aim of helping others cope with the tragedy of suicide.

The first video relates experiences shortly after the suicides. The second follows some of the same people and others, some years down the track.

The outstanding assistive book arose from a desire to provide an easy-to-read,how-to-survive kit in one cover for those left behind after a suicide.It draws on the knowledge and feelings of several bereaved people involved in the postvention area as well as the specialized knowledge supplied by Dr Sheila Clark.

The three items complement each other but are able to be used effectively singularly or in any combination.

SOCIAL RISK FACTORS IN ACCOMPLISHED SUICIDE

Calin Scipcaru and Carmen Grigoriu — Institute of Legal Medicine, Romania

To establish the importance of existential ambiental factors in suicide determination, compared with pathological psychiatrical factors. We used morphological analyses, psychological and social enquiry on the relatives of the victims and also comparative methods concerning the risk of familial regressions determining, crimes. We studied 386 cases of familial violence in the same period (1992–1995).

Pathological risk factors represented 14.4% and from them, 22% in maniacal depressive psychosis, 12% in schisophrenia, 12% in pathological alcoholism, 10.5% in personality disharmonies and 5.2% in epilepsy. In the rest of 85.6% of the cases the cause was an existential psychological crisis determining reactive depressions. The analyses of suicide compared with familial homicide, revealed that a contention for an external aggression determined suicide and vice versa, a lack of contention determined homicide, on 15% of the cases, suicide followed a homicidal act.

The authors consider suicide like a behavioural perturbance at a fragile anomic personality, determining adaptive dysfunctions in connection with the environment. More than this, the authors revealed the value and the difficulties of a prophylactic management of suicidal risk.

KIDS HELP LINE

Julie Clarke — Kids Help Line, Australia

Kids Help Line is a national telephone counselling service for young people aged 5–18 years. It opened in 1991 and has operated nationally since 1993. Kids Help Line receives up to 25, 000 calls per week from young people and responds to 1 in 3 calls. Call code categories reflect the issues raised by young people. While the proportion of calls logged as suicide calls is relatively low, many of the other calls reflect significant issues that may contribute to suicidal thoughts or intention. It can be argued that KHL provides a significant preventative service that young people see as effective. The poster presentation would be descriptive of the Kids Help Line service and present data obtained over the 5 years that the service has been available.

NON-REGISTRATION OF DEATHS AS A SOURCE OF ERROR IN MORTALITY: DATA IN THE REPUBLIC OF IRELAND

John F. Connolly,[1] Anne Cullen,[2] and Deidre Smithwick[1] — [1]St. Mary's Hospital, Ireland and [2]Tyron and Fermanagh Hospital, Ireland

Deane & McLoughlin (1980) show that 6.1% of the samples of death in the West of Ireland were neither registered nor certified. Our own study, "Under reporting of suicide in an Irish county": (Connolly et al 1995), show that in a 15 year period in County Mayo 7.3% of deaths by suicide had not been registered. The present paper replicates the study of Deane & McLoughlin for County Mayo. Lists of people buried in the year 1992 were obtained from parish registers. These were compared with the official registry of deaths for County Mayo for that year. Additional information was obtained from the Central Statistics Office.

Results show that non registration of death continues to be a problem in a rural Irish county. The findings are discussed in depth and the international literature on under reporting of suicide and non registration of death is discussed. It is concluded that non registration of death, though a diminishing problem, continues to be a source of error in suicide mortality data particularly in rural areas.

DRAFT NATIONAL YOUTH SUICIDE PREVENTION STRATEGY FOR NEW ZEALAND

Maria Cotter — Ministry of Health, New Zealand

Like many countries New Zealand has seen the suicide rate of young people escalate dramatically over the past decade. New Zealand now boasts the unenviable position of having one of the highest youth suicide rates in the world.

Recently, the government agreed to formulation of a National Youth Suicide Prevention Strategy. This poster presentation will illustrate the major components of the Strategy, which is still under development, including the vision, aims, goals and objectives.

THE COMPARATIVE ANALYSIS OF SUICIDE IN LITHUANIA

Algirdas Dembinskas and Alvydas Navickas — Psychiatric Clinic, Vilnius University, Lithuania

We have compared the suicide rate during three periods with different political, economical and social setting:

- period 1 — 1930–1940 - Independent Lithuania;
- period 2 — 1980–1990 - End of Soviet Occupation;
- period 3 — 1991–1994 - New independent Republic.

We have studied the materials:

- of the Statistical Department of Lithuanian Government;
- of the Lithuanian State Archives;
- of the Lithuanian Centre of Forensic Medicine.

Period 1. During this period the suicide rate fluctuated insignificantly and was 8.5/100 000; for male — 10.7; for female — 5.5; in the urban area — 25.2; in the rural area — 5.7.

Period 2. During this period the suicide rate had significant changes and average was 31.7/100 000 (for instance in 1984:35.8; in 1986:25.1). The suicide rate for male was 52.8; for female — 10.9; in urban area was such as in the first period; though in rural area increased to 42.7.

Period 3. During this period the suicide rate increased very highly: 1991–30.4/100 000; 1994–45.8/100 000. The suicide rate increased in all groups: for male form 52.0 to

64.5; for female from 11.2 to 15.0; in the urban area form 22.0 to 37.0; in rural area form 48.9 to 64.5. The male suicide rate in rural area became very big — 105/100 000.

We can note that Lithuanian politics and economical situation has the great impact on the level of self-aggressiveness. We can see that this situation touches specially males in countryside.

We have investigated various social factors and influence of them on suicide.

YOUNG PEOPLE AT RISK: ACCESS, PREVENTION, AND ACTION

Steven Drew, Jo Ward, Tony McGuire, Eleesa Johnstone, and Andrew Nathan — Queensland Health, Australia

This presentation will outline the development and implementation of the Queensland Health 'Young People at Risk: Access, Prevention and Action'"' (YPAR) program which is aimed at the prevention of suicide and self harming behaviour amongst young people between 10–24 years of age.

YPAR is underpinned by the concepts of community development, intersectoral collaboration and health promotion. The program is being piloted on four different regions throughout Queensland. These are:

i. the rural /area of the South West incorporating Roma, Charleville, Cunnamulla and St George;
ii. the coastal/provincial area of Wide Bay covering Bunderberg, Monto, Mundubbera, Gayndah, Maryborough, Hervey Bay, Kingaroy, Murgon and Cherbourg;
iii. the metropolitan/rural area of West Moreton which includes Ipswich City and the rural Shires of Esk, Laidley and Boonah; and,
iv. the Brisbane South metropolitan area as represented by the City of Logan, to the south of Brisbane.

Each pilot is demographically diverse and the display will highlight these differences and will show the difficulties in developing a program which reflects the issues and meets the needs of particular communities, while endeavouring to identify similarities which may enable application across the State and still undertake a consistent and valid evaluation of the program at a statewide level as well as the local level.

FAMILY MOURNING, GRIEF, AND RECOVERY FOLLOWING A SUICIDE

Edward J. Dunne and Karen Dunne-Maxim — UMDNJ–UBHC, Office of Prevention, USA

The authors use examples of mourning rituals in different cultures to demonstrate how prescribed behaviors mediate grief. Gender and age specific methods of mourning impose cultural expectations which are then incorporated into the unstated expectations of family members about how they and others in the family should grieve. These expectations increase in importance when the death being grieved by the family is problematic as in suicide or murder. Differing expectations by family members lead to complications in the grieving process.

Clinical vignettes provide examples of grieving families to illustrate the points of the discussion. Suggestions for interventions which help the family negotiate this legacy of a suicide in the family are offered.

Economic and sociological factors once again proved very important as determinants of suicide; the concept of primary suicide prevention should take this into account.

REVIEW OF PARASUICIDALS BY POISONING IN VILNIUS 1994–1995

Julija Grebeliené — Vilnius University Emergency Hospital: Poison Centre, Lithuania

The objective is to evaluate the development of parasuicidal poisoning in Vilnius during 1994–1995.

Analysis of sociodemographical and clinical characteristics of 495 persons who tried to poison themselves. Compared sex, age, social status, circumstances of poisoning, materials used for suicide, frequency of parasuicides during a year. Evaluated psychopathology of suicides.

Number of parasuicides has increased; number of women increased significantly. Age of those who attempted suicide lowered, number of suicides in sober condition increased, more attempts to suicide by psychotropical medicines, while the number of affected with depressions and mental diseases has not changed.

Although overall suicidal level of 1994–1995 has not changed, there has been a further increase in the number of parasuicides. The data marks out the problem of women and youth and the increased use of psychotropical medicines.

It is expedient to use the data in planning prevention of parasuicides in Lithuania.

COMMUNITY LIFE PROMOTION — AN ABORIGINAL COMMUNITY APPROACH TO SUICIDE PREVENTION

Colleen K. Gray — Australia

Apunipima Cape York Health Council has implemented a Best Practice Pilot Project to establish a culturally appropriate Mental, Emotional and Social Health Service in the Aboriginal communities of Hopevale and Wujal Wujal. By using a community development approach to the planning and implementation of the Communities to plan and develop a program that has strong community ownership.

The Community Life Promotion Officers who were recruited from the Communities are experts in utilising Aboriginal networks and ways of working. Counselling and suicide prevention therapies involve the use of artwork to express the emotions and stories of our clients.

We appreciate the role mainstream services try to provide, and are working to develop collaborative approaches to bridge the cultural gaps between mainstream services and community workers and residents. One of our important roles has been to support and teach culturally appropriate ways of working to the mainstream mental health workers.

In this program we believe that suicide prevention begins at birth and along life's continuums. Our suicide support programs include counselling, referral, diversionary therapy, art therapy and linking up with appropriate community members. Our programs support the community at all stages. We are developing and running parenting workshops, youth groups and women groups. We provide debriefing and support for affected individuals and groups.

YOUTH LINK — REPORT ON A PROJECT TO IMPROVE ACCESS TO MENTAL HEALTH SERVICES FOR AT RISK ABORIGINAL YOUNG PEOPLE

Norman Grech — Youth Link, Australia

I wish to present a poster to the Congress, outlining a current project on improvement of access to mental health services for a risk and marginalised Aboriginal young people.

The poster will outline the components of the project, including outreach approaches, information seeking from the target group and agencies with whom they may have some contact, and will highlight information gained regarding the delivery of culturally appropriate mental health services for the target group.

The poster will also indicate any implications arising for future directions of Youth-Link, and other non-Aboriginal agencies seeking to address issues of accessibility and appropriateness for Aboriginal clients.

It is requested that this poster be allocated space alongside the other Youthlink poster, to be presented by Ms Jennifer Griffith's of YouthLink.

YOUTHLINK — AN INNOVATIVE MODEL OF MENTAL HEALTH SERVICE DELIVERY TO AT-RISK YOUTH

Jennifer Griffiths — Youth Link, Australia

The poster will outline an innovative community outreach model of mental health service delivery and highlight the contrast with the more traditional model of mental health service delivery to young people. The rationale for the model which is the improvement of access to services for the 'hard to reach' population will be indicated.

The poster will also indicate the model of the "pathways" followed by YouthLink in response to individual young people at risk of suicide.

MONITORING PARASUICIDE: CHANGES IN RATES AND SEX RATIO

Heidi Hjelmeland — Norwegian University of Science and Technology, Norway

The objective is to Monitor the incidence of Parasuicide over several years studying changes in rates and sex ratio.

All medically treated parasuicide patients were registered in the county of Sor-Trondelag, Norway, in the period 1989–1995.

The parasuicide rates had decreased in the monitoring period. For women the decrease was virtually continuous throughout the period. For men the rates remained rather stable though the period of 1989 to 1992, but seem to show a decreasing tendency from 1992 onwards.

If each year is considered separately, no clear decreasing tendency in sex difference in incidence was found in the 7 years of monitoring. However, if the monitoring period is divided into two parts, namely the period 1989–1992 (f/m ratio= 1.31) and 1993–1995 (f/m ratio= 1.22) and the female/male ratios are compared to those found in previous studies form the area in 1978 (f/m-ratio=1.50) and 1987 (f/m ratio= 1.34), a decline in the female/male ratio of parasuicide is identified.

EXCESSIVE MORTALITY AMONG CRIMINALS — MYTH OR REALITY?

Thomas Hjortsjo — Skaraborg College of Health Science, SWEDEN

A study has been conducted to throw light on the excessive mortality among young people with criminal records. This was achieved by linking and matching computer files on official statistics relating to criminal records, national registration and causes of death. The causes of death that have attracted the greatest attention are suicide, uncertain intent, traffic accidents and other causes of death. Two groups of young offenders, comprising 118,115 and 20,743 individuals respectfully, have been compared with two matched groups with clean records, comprising 15,771 and 17,579 individuals in the period 1970–1994.

The results unequivocally indicate that excessive mortality exists among young people with criminal records, measured in the form of relative risk and Chi-square. Suicide and uncertain intent predominate among the boys, while the girls show in addition to these two causes a large incidence of death from other causes. There are probably many factors that could account for this state of affairs, but one of the most fundamental is undoubtedly early social alienation. Intensification of the efforts made by schools to trace young people in the risk zone is urgent. Co-operation with local police and other institutions in the communities where these young people live may contribute to their being taken care of earlier and in a better way.

ADOPTION AND SUICIDE IN AUSTRALIA

Wendy Jacobs — Australia

As a mother who lost a child to adoption when he was born and then to suicide when he was 21, and having spoken to other mothers who have lost their children to adoption, I am interested in the question of whether adoption leads to a greater risk of suicide in these mothers and / or their adopted out children.

The only major peak in the rate of female suicide in Australia (1900–1985) coincides with the peak in adoption rates in late 1960's- early 1970's. Were any of these suicides related to the loss of a baby to adoption? Many women suffer life long grief and symptoms of post traumatic stress disorder as a result of relinquishing a baby to adoption.

The increase in youth suicide, dating from about 1960, coincides with the increase in the numbers of adopted people in the 15–29 age group. Adoption became popular from the mid 1940's as a solution to the problems of illegitimacy and infertility: newborn babies were taken from their unmarried mothers and given to childless married couples. High rates of psychiatric disturbances have been found in adopted children, but there are no statistics on the number of adoptees who commit suicide.

American scientists claim that depriving a baby of its mother soon after birth leads to alterations in brain chemistry. This may offer a biological explanation for the "primal wound" that American psychologist Nancy Verrier says is causes by separation from the mother.

Although very few babies are currently surrendered for adoption, there are moves in some quarters to bring back adoption as an alternative to abortion or single motherhood. More research is needed into the mental health consequences of adoption, for both mother and child, or we may run the risk of seriously damaging more lives in the future.

SUICIDE AND SEASONALITY — OR DO WE PAY ENOUGH ATTENTION TO THE WEATHER FACTOR?

Gert Jessens[1] and Peter Steffensen[2] — [1]Centre for Suicidological Research, Denmark and [2]Danish Meteorological Institute, Denmark

The objective is to carry out a series of systematic studies of various temporal variations in the relation between meteorologic factors and suicidal behaviour in Funen — a representative part of Denmark.

Suicides (2610, age +15) from the period 1970–1993. The meteorological data consists of daily information on precipitation, temperatures, wind velocities, hours of sunlight, etc.

This pilot study confirms findings of several previous studies, especially concerning the spring peak and significantly fewer suicides at week ends.

With regard to the covariations between climatological factors and the frequency of suicides, this pilot study only to some extent confirmed a direct relationship. One problem posed by the climatological variables is that they are intercorrelated. The pilot study shows that climatological factors, eg; changing weather, to some extent may have an impact on suicidal behaviour.

WHO IS HERE FOR LIFE

Amanda Johnson — Australia

Here For Life is a not-for-profit organisation that works directly with youth and the community to reduce the level of youth suicide through innovative educational and preventive projects.

Here For Lifes effectiveness in the prevention of youth suicide is based on its ability to harness the skills, experience, resources, commitment and vision of a diverse range of volunteers, professionals and organisations. Together we develop, facilitate and coordinate innovative projects, guided by professional advice aimed at addressing the needs of youth and the community as a whole. Our integrity stems form our genuine concern for

Australia's youth, our connection to the community and our adherence to appropriate professional methods.

The following projects and activities have been developed to support youth mental health and general well being;

> *Education and Awareness workshops* for school teachers, parents and other people working with youth.
> *Personal Development programs* for secondary school students.
> *Regional projects* driven by the community.
> *Community Resource Centre* specialising in youth suicide.
> *Research and Evaluation.*
> *Advocacy and Lobbying* to media and government.
> *National adolescent health campaigns.*
> *Referral and Contract* network.
> *Other projects* aimed at youth suicide prevention.

ACCESS TO FIREARMS AND RISK OF SUICIDE: A CASE-CONTROL STUDY

Peter Joyce, Annette Beautrais, and Roger Mulder — Canterbury Suicide Project, Christchurch School of Medicine, New Zealand

The objective of this study examined the association between access to a firearm and risk of suicide in a consecutive sample of individuals who made serious suicide attempts.

The study used a case-control design in which a sample of 197 individuals who died by suicide and 302 individuals who made medically serious suicide attempts was contrasted with 1028 randomly selected community control subjects.

Suicide attempts by gunshot accounted for 1.3% of all serious suicide attempts (with non-fatal outcome) and 13.3% of suicides. However, amongst those making serious suicide attempts, gunshot had a high rate of fatality (83.3%). Whilst access to a firearm was associated with increased risks that gunshot would be chosen as the method of suicide attempt (OR=107.9, 95% confidence interval= 24.8–469.5), this access was not associated with significant increases in the risk of suicide (OR=1.4, 95% confidence interval = 0.96–1.99).

For this sample, access to a firearm was not associated with a significant increase in the risk of suicide although such access was associated with an increased probability that gunshot would be chosen as the method of suicide attempt.

SUICIDE AND SCHIZOPHRENIA

M. Lonnqvist, H. Isometsa, E. Henriksson, M. Heikkinen, and M. Martunen — National Public Health Institute, Finland

The risk of suicide in schizophrenia is high. It is estimated that 10–13% of all sufferers commit suicide. Many studies of clinical characteristics of suicide victims with schizophrenia have been compromised by the relatively small numbers of subjects and thus inadequate representation of women for comparison between the sexes, the heterogenous diagnostic criteria used, and the frequent selection of the suicide population from hospital and data based only on patient records. Seven studies so far have investigated completed suicides using samples of 15 or more suicide victims with DSM-111 or DSM-111-R schizophrenia. In these studies, young adult age and male sex have characterised suicide victims with schizophrenia. Comorbid depressive symptoms, alcoholism and previous suicide attempts have also associated with suicide.

EMPLOYMENT STATUS INFLUENCES THE WEEKLY PATTERN OF SUICIDE AMONG ALCOHOL MISUSERS

S. Pirkoloa, E. Isometsa, M. Heikkinen, J. Lonnqvist — National Public Institute, Department of Mental Helath and Alcohol, Research, Department of Psychiatry, University of Helsinki, Finland

As part of the National Suicide Prevention Project in Finland, a nationwide psychological autopsy study of all suicide victims (N=1397) over a 12-month period were investigated concerning factors associated with any variation in suicide frequency between weekdays and weekends. In particular, employment status was expected to have influenced the weekly pattern of alcohol misuse, and thereby to have caused clustering of suicides at week-ends among the employed. Among suicide victims who had misused alcohol, those in employment were significantly more likely to have committed suicide at the week-end than those without work (52% vs 34%, p<0.001). The clustering of suicides at week-ends among employed alcohol misusers is probably explained by a similar pattern in the use of alcohol, which suggests that besides the established risk factors for suicide among alcohol misusers, the act of using alcohol per se also contributes to the suicidal act.

WHAT HAVE WE LEARNED FROM POSTMORTEM STUDIES OF SUICIDE VICTIMS?

John Mann — New York State Psychiatry Institute, USA

Studies of suicide victims have the important methodological advantage of examining the most severe form of suicidal behaviour. The disadvantages are that post mortem studies can involve a number of artifacts and limitations such as effects of the method of suicide, residual psychotropic drug effects and a lack of clinical information. Recent studies have overcome most of these methodological problems and have yielded valuable data about the biochemical abnormalities in the brain of suicide victims. Highlights of information that these studies have generated include: 1) the detection of serotonergic system abnormalities that are associated with suicide regardless of the underlying psychiatric disorder; 2) localisation of the serotonergic abnormalities to the ventral prefrontal cortex; 3) abnormalities in the noradrenergic system which may be related to stress or associated psychiatric syndromes; 4) pyschological autopsies have indicated that over 90% of suicide victims have a psychiatric disorder. Future directions of postmortem studies of suicide will be discussed.

THE SPECTRUM OF SUICIDE PREVENTION AT CAMHS, FLINDERS MEDICAL CENTRE

Martin, Allison, Roeger, Lorraine, Dadds, and K. Williams — Flinders Medical Centre, Adelaide

The Southern Child and Adolescent Mental Health Service (CAMHS), South Australia is a comprehensive multidisciplinary mental health service for children and adolescents (from birth to 18 years), their families and the community. It is a community outreach and in-patient service of Flinders Medical Centre with teams located in urban and rural community settings. The service assists individuals, their families and communities to reduce the limitations imposed by society through community education, mental health promotion, early identification of mental health problems and disorders, acute therapy, empathic support, and advocacy. A range of research and professional development projects have arisen from needs identified in the context of the delivery of our services.

The Outcomes Project is funded by the South Australian Health Commission to monitor and evaluate service satisfaction and the effectiveness of treatment for Southern CAMHS clients. In addition, Commonwealth funded projects at Southern CAMHS include:

- The Early Detection of Emotional Disorders Project is a prospective longitudinal community research study and intervention program for adolescents with emotional disorder and suicidal behaviours, conducted in government and independent secondary schools;
- *Keep Yourself Alive* is a comprehensive multimodal education and training program for general practitioners in the recognition, assessment, counselling and postvention related to young people who have suicidal behaviours;
- The Mood Disorders Unit for Young People will provide a multidisciplinary service to young people (15–24 years) with serious affective disorder;
- The National Early Psychosis Project, SA aims to assist mental health professionals and agencies to adopt 'best practice' early intervention service delivery in the identification, diagnosis and treatment of psychotic illness.

"SUICIDE PREVENTION PROGRAMS AT SOUTHERN CHILD AND ADOLESCENT MENTAL HEALTH SERVICES, FLINDERS MEDICAL CENTRE, SOUTH AUSTRALIA."

Graham Martin, Stephen Allison, Leigh Roeger, Vikki Dadds, Kerin Williams, Sharon Evans, Jeanne Lorraine, and Peter Parry — Southern CAMHS, Flinders Medical Centre, Bedford Park 5042, Australia

This poster presentation will show case four programs developed at Southern CAMHS which are designed to prevent suicidal behaviours in young people aged 15–24 years.

1. "Keep Yourself Alive" is a Commonwealth funded workshop package consisting of four videotapes, two audio tapes (16 x 12 minute segments) and a manual. Workshops will be presented nationally to general practitioners and other gatekeepers over six months from April 11th the date of the official launch.

2. "Early Detection of Emotional Disorders" in young people. This research program aimed at early detection and intervention has just completed the first two years of a prospective study into risk factors for youth suicide. The presentation will demonstrate the process, thecomplexities and key results to date.

3. "Out of the Blues". This recently funded Mood Disorders Unit for young people aged 15–24 years aims to adapt best internationalpractice in the management of first episode of major depression in young people. The Unit will act as a National Demonstration Program from which clinical practice, management practice, and research endeavour can be promoted.

4. "Outcomes in Child and Adolescent Mental". This program is funded by the South Australia Health Commission for a period of two years. The study will determine the degree to which treatment factors, such as the number of one to one contacts and treatment modalities used, predict improvements in problem ratings and satisfaction with treatment.

NETWORKS FOR THE FUTURE — YOUTH SUICIDE

Barry McGrath, Kate Swanton, Michael Greco, Elana Balak, Wayne Fossey, and Liz Hull — Here for Life Network, Australia

The Commonwealth's National Youth Suicide Prevention Program has funded three projects to upskill General Practitioners to more effectively identify, refer and treat youth at risk of suicide or self harm.

The *Here for Life Network* Project aims to mobilise the community in a coordinated and skilled response to the needs of young people at risk of self harm.

The project brings together an intersectoral consortium of stakeholders with expertise in youth suicide prevention - they operate and manage services within the local area, have established links to existing networks and live and work in the local community.

Based on close consultation with the local community and extensive needs assessment processes, the consortium members have developed and implemented strategies to raise community awareness about the problem, skill the community to identify, refer and treat youth at risk and link key individuals to ensure an ongoing response to young people. The project is being extensively evaluated within an action research framework, and if effective will be implemented Australian wide.

Inherent in the project is the issue of sustainability - the development of networks is the key to a coherent and continuing response to those in need. Unless links are established and networks sustained, the project will have failed in its goal of assisting vulnerable young people in our community.

EMOTION–ENVIRONMENT SYNDROMES OF SUICIDE/BIOCHEMICAL RESPONSES TO PERCEPTIONS

Joan McVay — USA

The objective is to present a visual clarification of the human and animal's biochemical reaction to perceptions of situations in the environment which are filtered by multi-factoral components: *Social*; self-image, self-esteem, family expectations, family history, societal mores, culture; *Environmental*; epidermal ultra-violet light reactions, toxins, diet; *Biochemical/Mind-BodySyndrome*; laughter, failure, sexual, apathy, and others. The poster presentation will demonstrate how negative syndromes can lead to suicide.

A summary of biochemical research is presented in a poster presentation to demonstrate the main theory in the author's book *Evolution of a Death: Suicide and its Pandemic Dimensions*. A number of studies are presented graphically to illustrate the self perception, social perception, environmental influence, brain-body biochemical response which leads to suicide. Other graphic representations will display the multifactorial variables which go together and results in the biochemistry of suicide. These include political, economic, religious, cultural, and family factors.

Graphic illustrations, charts, and graphs illustrate the multidimensional, multifactorial nature of the biochemical - emotional syndrome causes of suicide and demonstrate that a single treatment or narrow dimensional approach to suicide research will not change the world statistics nor help individuals who are at suicidal risk.

The social problems of the 21st Century will not be solved or prevented by methods of research or treatment used in the past. As other researchers have pointed out with multifactorial approaches to evolving viruses and bacteria; immune deficiency diseases; ocean pollution; and other issues, suicide must be approached with a multidisciplinary team in both research and treatment.

This poster presentation will not only illustrate the author's premise and theory, but also graphically illustrate the multidimensional approach to research, prevention, and treatment needed to approach the dimensions of suicide globally in the 21st Century.

SUICIDE REPORTING IN PRINT MEDIA:
AN EVALUATION OF THE EFFECT OF GUIDELINES
ISSUED TO EDITORS AND JOURNALISTS

Conrad Frey, Ladislav Valach, Kathrin Wyss, and Konrad Michel — Psychiatrische Poliklinik, Universitätsspital, Switzerland.

The objective is to assess the effect of issuing guidelines for suicide reporting on the actual practice of reporting in Swiss print media.

In 1991 we conducted an 8 months' survey of suicide reporting in all Swiss print media. In 1994 the results were presented in a widely published national press conference, and written guidelines for suicide reporting were sent to newspaper editors. In addition to this, a personal meeting with the chief editor of the main Swiss tabloid took place. Following this intervention, a second evaluation of suicide reporting covering all Swiss print media was carried out during 8 months. The main variables on frequency, form and content of the newspaper reports before and after the press conference were compared.

Altogether more articles on suicide reporting were found in the second study period. However, most of these articles were not rated as potentially suggestive to induce imitation. The quality of reporting had clearly improved, especially in the main Swiss tabloid, where articles were significantly shorter, less sensational, and contained fewer pictures.

It appears that the issuing of guidelines for suicide reporting had an effect on the actual practice of reporting. For the change of practice in the main tabloid paper the personal contact may have been most influential. It is possible, however, that the publicity given to the topic lead to an increase in the number of articles on suicide.

Michel K, Frey C, Schlaepfer B, Weil B, Valach V: Suicide reporting in the Swiss print media. I. Frequency, form and content of articles. European Journal of Public Health (1995) 5, 199–203.

THE PREVALENCE AND CHARACTERISTICS OF DELIBERATE SELF-HARM AMONG ADULTS IN THE COMMUNITY — A PILOT STUDY TO DEVELOP AND TEST A SUITABLE QUESTIONNAIRE

Shymala Nada-Raja, Keren Skegg, John Langley, Dianne Morrison, and Rob McGee — University of Otago Medical School: Injury Prevention Research Unit, Dept of Preventive and Social Medicine, New Zealand

Much deliberate self-harm (DSH) that is conventionally labelled "attempted suicide" (including many overdoses) does not in fact have suicide as its prime intent. In order to understand better the phenomenon of DSH and how it relates to attempted and completed suicide, a study was conducted to develop and pilot a suitable questionnaire on DSH, both suicidal and non-suicidal in intent.

Through discussion with individuals in the hospital setting and the community, appropriate research definitions for different types of non-fatal DSH were developed and an interview schedule was designed.

Preliminary findings from the study and the strengths and limitations of the methods used will be outlined.

It is intended that the questionnaire developed in this study will be suitable for clinic populations and the community to determine the prevalence and characteristics of a wide range of self harm behaviours among adults. In addition to investigating the frequency of DSH are associated with, or whether they occur largely in separate populations.

PREVENTION OR ASSISTED SUICIDE? A NEW TYPOLOGY

Sergio Perez Barrero — ISCM Dpto Psia Hosp "Carles M. Cespedes" Bayamo, Cuba

There exist more than ten typologies of suicide. A similar number may be in the minds of suicidologists ruling their work. Were reviewed the most popular: Mintz's Durkheim's, Menninger's, Baechler's and Shneifman's. At present, a new problem, which was not taken into account be previous typologies has emerged and it is assisted suicide.

One new typology, based on the kinds of doctor-patient relationships: active-passive, guided cooperation and mutual participation, was done. The application of the previous concepts to the field of suicidology suggest a new classification of suicides into not responsable, partly responsable and totally responsible.

The typology proposed harmonizes etiological, preventive and therapeutic aspects as well as the most dissonant aspect of modern suicidology; assisted suicide.

ADOPTION AS A RISK FACTOR IN YOUTH SUICIDE

Evelyn Robinson — Australia

Research from the United States has shown that adopted adolescents are over-represented in psychiatric care and in juvenile detention centres. Their loss and grief issues associated with their change of identify and seperation from their families of origin often result in anti-social behaviour. As the negative impact of adoption on young people is not widely understood, their specific needs often go unrecognised. Evidence form Australia points to the fact that adopted young people are greatly over-represented among youth suicides. The available statistics point to an urgent need for further research.

Adopted young women are more likely than non-adopted young women to relinquish their own children for adoption, thereby exposing themselves to the risk of emotional and psychological disability, which has been shown to accompany the loss of children to adoption. Unresolved grief associated with this type of loss can lead to depression and suicidal tendencies

Adopted people often experience a sense of alienation and of not belonging. This is intensified during the period of adolescence when the formation of identity is taking place. For this reason adolescent adopted people are at greater risk of psychological disturbance which could lead to suicide than non-adopted young people.

If the unique issues of adopted adolescents can be recognised and addressed by those who are working with them, this knowledge can be used as an important tool in the prevention of suicides among these vulnerable young people.

A RETROSPECTIVE STUDY OF SUICIDE ATTEMPTS IN ANKARA: TARGETS FOR PREVENTION

I. Sayil, O. Berksun, R. Palabiyikoglu, A. Oral, S. Guney, S. Binici, S. Haran, S. Gecim, T. Yücat, H. Yazar, D. Büyüksellik, and A. Beder — A.U.T.F Cebeci Kampusu

The purpose of this study is to detect the suicide attempts in the city of Ankara for the year 1995 and to compare with data of the study carried out by the authors in 1990.

Information about suicide attempters who were treated at 9 hospitals of Ankara was collected by the crisis staff from the emergency service records. A form concerning demographic features and characteristics of the suicidal behaviour (time, method etc,) was used to gather data.

Total of 2532 suicide attempts were detected in emergency records. 1600 cases were female (65%) and 830 were male (35%). In general females outnumbered males 2:1 in suicide attempters. The highest rate of suicide attempts were in 15–25 age group. Self poisoning was the most common method. The rate of suicide attempts in 1990 was 107 per 100,000 for Ankara, but for the year 1995 it was found to be 113 per 100,000. There was an increase in the rate of younger attempters in both sexes compared to the year 1990.

The records of the emergency room in each hospital was discussed and compared with the findings of 1990 study. Also incomplete registration of some hospitals were discussed.

Education of the emergency staff and preventative programs for the risk groups are suggested.

MUENCHAUSEN'S SYNDROME AND SUICIDAL BEHAVIOUR

A. Schmidtke, S. Schaller, and V. Hocke — Clinical Psychology, Psychiatric Clinic Wuerzburg

The symptoms of the Muenchausen's syndrome or factitious disorders often resemble suicidal behaviour. However, according to recent theories concerning the aetiology of Muechhausen syndrome, the differences between these behaviours can be seen in their functionality: While for suicidal behaviour the functionaltiy lies between the goal "Death" and appellative behaviour with manipulative consequences on the environment, the functionality of a Muenchausen syndrome mainly consists of contact with the medical system itself as well as medical professional and of the role of an ill person.

To test this hypothesis and to investigate the differences between both groups, we tested persons with diagnosis of or under suspicion of Muenchhausen syndrome and compared them with matched controls. The instruments administered were personality tests, checklists to evaluate biographical and social variables and the history of self-destructive and /or healthy behaviour. In general, persons with Muenchhausen syndrome were more often females, had more medical professions or professions with contact to the medical systems and their history of hospital admissions and discharges was different. They also had major treatments in hospitals more often, during which the different therapists or hospitals were not informed by the patients of former treatments or parallel treatments. The personality tests of persons with Muenchhausen showed high neuroticism scores, social isolation and inadequate coping strategies.

PHYSICAL ILLNESS AND PARASUICIDE: EVIDENCE FROM THE EUROPEAN PARASUICIDE STUDY INTERVIEW SCHEDULE

P. Scocco,[1] D. De Leo,[1] P. Marietta,[1] A. Schmidtke,[2] U. Bille-Brahe,[2] A.J.F.M. Kerkhof,[2] J. Lonnqvist,[2] P. Crepet,[2] E. Salander-Renberg,[2] D. Wasserman,[2] K. Michel, and T. Stile[2] — [1]University of Padua, Italy and [2]Steering Group WHO/DERO Multi Centre Study on Parasuicide

The importance of somatic pathology in the parasuicidal process was analysed under the umbrella of the European Multicentre Study on Parasuicide (Prediction/Repetition Study - EPSIS 1). 1269 parasuicidal subjects were assessed, following an attempted suicide, in 9 European centres, representing 7 countries, by means of a structured interview: the European Parasuicide Study Interview Schedule (EPSIS).

The rate of accomplished suicide was 12% with maximum frequency between 30 - 40 years old. The frequency at young ages was 19% of the whole number of cases, from which 27.6% had several hospitalised suicide attempts. We had 10 cases of accomplished suicide before 10 years old, from which one case at 5 years old. The motivation was opposition to parental abuse, lack of parental affection, fear of punishment for school conflicts, fear of abandonment of unwanted children. The breaking of psycho-affective connections with the family was very frequent at teenagers where it determined suicide or behavioural deviance.

We may introduce the term of "infantile existential syndrome" as a complex of causes potentially generating suicide.

ENHANCING CAREGIVERS' GATEKEEPING COMPETENCE IN SUICIDE FIRST AID

Bryan Tanney — Lifeline, Melbourne

The objective is to improve caregivers' "gatekeeping" competence and confidence in performing a suicide first aid intervention with a person at risk and promote intersectoral cooperation in implementing these interventions in the community.

Intervention to enhance caregivers' ability and confidence to perform effective suicide first aid interventions with people at risk has been funded by the Australia Commonwealth Government. 72 presenters recruited from diverse community service organisations in three sites were trained to deliver two proven learning experiences to over 10,000 participants. These learning experiences comprised of a 2-day workshop designed to promote informed, purposeful and effective interventions with people at risk and a modular 2–3 hour public awareness presentation. Process and outcome evaluations were conducted using standardised instruments administered to community focus groups, presenters, participants and controls. National disseminations is planned.

A progress report will highlight implementation issues for presenters and participating organisations in mounting community-scale suicide intervention strategies in diverse community settings. Trends emerging from preliminary data on both individual and organisational outcomes will be featured. Implications for future planning and action research in this field will be discussed.

PULLING THE THREAD TOGETHER:
INTERSECTORAL COLLABORATION IN PRACTICE

Barry Taylor — NEHCN, Victoria

The Statewide Youth Suicide Prevention is funded by the Victorian Health Promotion Foundation for two years to provide a focus to youth suicide prevention initiatives. The project has three components: statewide advisory and training service, statewide youth suicide prevention network and pilot projects in two communities focusing on intersectoral collaboration around youth suicide prevention.

The poster presentation will describe the activities of the project in each of the three areas and will include a discussion on the experience of developing and implementing a statewide project. The project was built around the principles of community development and health promotion and an analysis of the applicability of these models to youth suicide prevention will be given.

The major focus of the poster will be on the pilot projects in the two communities, one urban and one rural. The range of activities used in the project will be described as well as a reflection on what the project would do differently in hindsight. Activities of the project included an intersectoral forum, training on youth suicide, development of policies and guidelines and awareness raising about the mental health needs of young people in each community.

YOUTH SUICIDE PREVENTION PROGRAM

Raylee Taylor — With the support of GCIT, Suicide Prevention Working Party, Australia

The objective is to provide organisations working with youth, with a set of strategies which can be utilised to assist in decreasing the incidence of youth suicide within their community.

The Program is divided into four major modules.

1. Procedures — a model aimed at developing appropriate strategies to minimise the risk of suicide and related trauma and deal with critical incidents which relate to self harm. Suitable for educational establishments.
2. Awareness Training — Aimed at providing information to parents, teachers, community and youth workers, enabling them to identify young people at risk and respond in an appropriate manner.
3. Workshop — Provides a resource package for educational, youth or community organisations, enabling counsellors or similarly trained personnel to run a workshop, designed to provide Suicide prevention, intervention and postvention training.
4. Personal Management Program — this section aims to develop the participants' ability to adapt and manage daily issues and relationships. the knowledge and skills gained may assist in reducing the impact of crisis situations and/or self destructive behaviour.

The Program has launched on the Gold Coast Queensland (QLD), in May 1996. It is being utilised by TAFE institutes in QLD, Secondary schools in the South Coast Region of Qld. The program has also been purchased as a resource by the Queensland Health 'Young People at Risk' program. A wide range of educational establishments and community health organisations throughout Australia are also utilising the Program. As the program is in its infancy no evaluations have been conducted at this stage.

The Program provides a model for implementation, into educational, community or youth settings. It works on the basis of providing existing trained workers in the community, eg. Counsellors, Social Workers, Teachers and the Health profession, with a source enabling them to provide training in Suicide Prevention, Intervention and Postvention.

Judging from the response received, both from program participants and those who have accessed the program for their organisations, it appears that it is filling a gap in training material available and appropriate for use by organisations.

DEVELOPING EMOTIONAL SAFETY IN SUICIDE AWARENESS EDUCATION

Darien Thira — Vancouver Crisis Centre, Canada

The topic of suicide is an emotionally "risky" one for everyone, especially youth. A sense of emotional "safety" promotes participant's involvement, which is essential to the effective transfer and retention of information and, more importantly, attitude or behavioural change. Techniques for facilitators of suicide awareness seminars that will encourage the creation and maintenance of emotional "safety" in learners will be explored, along with the underlying philosophy that makes them work. Although simple to practice, these techniques have been found to have a profound effect on participation and group rapport and in the reduction of acting out by youth during seminars and workshops. Other tips for effective seminars with youth will be offered.

POST-SUICIDE BEREAVEMENT:
GUIDELINES FOR CAREGIVERS

Bruce Turley, Gil Matters, Lyn Bender, Michael Roberts, and Dave Mutton —
Lifeline

The objective is to develop good practice guidelines for caregivers responding to people bereaved by suicide.

Three strategies were employed to inform the development of guidelines for informal caregivers, counsellors, educators, health care providers and public officials. Interviews were conducted with 26 families from rural and urban Victoria who had experienced the suicide of a family member 14–25 months earlier. Themes relevant to caregivers were extracted from an extensive literature review on post suicide bereavement. A time-limited, professionally led, bereavement recovery group for eight recently bereaved survivors was conducted applying a pcychoeducational model.

Guidelines identified needs common to all bereavement along with recurring unique features associated with the legacy of suicide. Evaluations of the perceived helpfulness of typical responses by informal caregivers, professional workers and community institutions provided foundations for a more supportive community response to the bereaved. Strategies for addressing common barriers to help-seeking by the bereaved and to the provision of support by caregivers were offered. Safeguards, guidelines and process challenges in conducting groups for people bereaved by suicide were developed.

Learning from the experiences of survivors and addressing the challenges encountered by those who care for them provides a dynamic paradigm for ensuring that individuals and communities facilitate the healing and recovery of people bereaved by suicide.

SUICIDE ATTEMPTERS IN PRIMARY HEALTH CARE —
MODEL FOR GOOD PRACTICES

Hynninen Tuula, Upanne Maila, and Hakanen Jari — National Research and
Development Centre for Welfare and Health

In this project, which is part of the Suicide Prevention Project in Finland, a model for the care of suicide attempters was developed in order to make prevailing practices more systematic, effective, and easier to implement. After-care is demanding in many ways and practices vary. Yet good care of suicide attempters is one of the main challenges in suicide prevention.

In the model phases, prevailing problems and practices of care after a suicidal attempt are exemplified and principles and measures of good care defined. It is most essential to secure that the life situation of each attempter be assessed, at least short-term crisis-therapy provided, and open care and social support arranged. Main aims are to secure the continuity of care to prevent a possible second attempt.

The role of primary health care in the care of suicide attempters is growing. The model was prepared by collaborating with five health centres applying a cooperative process model developed earlier in the project. The model for good practices was published as a booklet and a free copy of it was delivered as an intervention to all (nearly 300) health centres in the country.

The project will be evaluated in two phases. In addition to the five collaborating health centres, all health centres in the country will be asked for feedback on the model.

THE ADELAIDE DECLARATION ON SUICIDE PREVENTION

Suicide is a significant health problem in every country in the world, being among the ten leading causes of death.

The world health organisation has six basic steps for the prevention of suicide. These are: 1. the treatment of mental disorders; 2. guns possession control; 3. detoxification of domestic gas; 4. detoxification of car emissions; 5. control of toxic substance availability; and 6. toning down reports in the media. These measures should result in a significant reduction in suicide in the world.

The International Association for Suicide Prevention calls on government health organisations, non-government health and welfare groups and volunteer organisations, to share with the general public the responsibility for the prevention of suicide and to work towards:

- the allocation of sufficient funds and human resources for research and suicide prevention strategies.
- the establishment of appropriate government agencies to provide leadership, co-ordination and resources to prevent suicide.
- the establishment of national and local networks of support and partnership for suicide prevention.
- the provision of resources to groups who may have special needs.

The International Association for Suicide Prevention accepts its responsibility to:

- place suicide prevention near the top of the agenda of the World Health Organisation.
- institute networks across the world to bring together professionals and non-professionals in the pursuit of suicide prevention.
- urge all countries to secure a budget allocation for suicide prevention.
- ensure that international, national and regional groups are co-ordinated and have access to the latest information about suicide prevention.
- encourage and promote research into the efficacy, effectiveness and feasability of suicide prevention programs.
- ensure the availability of reliable information about suicide prevention.
- ensure that adequare care is available to those affected by suicide.

Ratified by the Executive Board of the International Association for Suicide Prevention following the 19th congress of the International Association for Suicide Prevention held in Adelaide, Australia, 23rd–27th March, 1997.

AFTERWORD

Once again the International Association for Suicide Prevention has provided a unique opportunity for those concerned about suicide to share their experiences and familiarise themselves with the latest developments in suicide prevention. Almost 600 registrants including general medical practitioners, psychologists, psychiatrists, nurses, social workers, coroners, school counsellors, priests, legal practitioners and volunteers from national and international organisations, as well as carers and young people participated. This was very appropriate, as there is increasing recognition that it is only by a co-operative approach to suicide prevention that an impact upon the unacceptable suicide rates worldwide can be made.

With the diversity of cultures presented at the Congress it was evident that there would be no universal answers to suicide prevention across the world. Countries with widely differing methods of self destruction will require different legislation. Thus as indicated by the presenters firearm reform would be of little consequence in some developing countries, but other restrictions, such as the ready availability of organo-phosphate pesticides used for poisoning are clearly worth considering.

Significant advances in the treatment of emotional illnesses were documented, but unfortunately we still do not have strong evidence from controlled interventions to demonstrate that these treatments produce a reduction in suicide. However, the 'gold standard' of randomised controlled research trials may not be the most appropriate method to demonstrate the effectiveness of suicide prevention programs because of the low base rate of suicide.

Whilst it is important to be mindful of the need for evidence-based outcome research, the fact that the actual processes and techniques of intervention needs to be considered was also noted. This requires respecting a balance between the need to demonstrate the efficacy and effectiveness of our programs, and appreciating the interpersonal and humanitarian nature of our endeavours. This is particularly the case in the area of bereavement following suicide.

It is unfortunate that sometimes the outcome versus process investigations are seen to be mutually exclusive. To adopt such a stance can only alienate practitioners from researchers, and ultimately it is not those groups who are disadvantaged, but the very people who we are trying to assist.

The range of topics presented at the conference reflected a divergence of approaches, this represents the strength of the International Association for Suicide Prevention: it can provide a forum in which different viewpoints can be discussed and common ground can be reached.

The 19th conference of the International Association for Suicide Prevention set itself an ambitious task, that of addressing "Suicide Prevention — the Global Context." In the selected presentations in this volume, as well as in the abstracts which are included, it can be seen that to a large extent the aims have been realised. The body of knowledge presented here not only records what many researchers, clinicians and volunteers have achieved, but it also provides a catalyst for further work in suicide prevention.

At the conclusion of the conference a number of general points which could be brought to the attention of government health organisations and non-government health services, welfare and volunteer groups were documented. These have since been ratified by the Executive Board of the International Association for Suicide Prevention and are presented as "The Adelaide Declaration on Suicide Prevention."

Robert Goldney
President
International Association of Suicide Prevention
3 June 1997

INDEX